HARTY'S
# ENDODONTICS IN CLINICAL PRACTICE

*Commissioning Editor:* Michael Parkinson
*Project Development Manager:* Clive Hewat
*Project Manager:* Nancy Arnott
*Designer:* Erik Bigland

# HARTY'S
# ENDODONTICS IN CLINICAL PRACTICE

EDITED BY

## T. R. Pitt Ford BDS, PhD (University of London), FDS RCPS Glasgow, FDS RCS Edinburgh

Professor of Endodontology, Guy's, King's and St Thomas' Dental Institute,
King's College London, UK

## FIFTH EDITION

wright

EDINBURGH  LONDON  NEW YORK  OXFORD  PHILADELPHIA  ST LOUIS  SYDNEY  TORONTO
2004

WRIGHT
An imprint of Elsevier Limited

© 2004, Elsevier Limited. All rights reserved.

First published 1976
Second edition 1982
Third edition 1990
Fourth edition 1997
Fifth edition 2004
  Reprinted 2005, 2007

ISBN-13: 978 0 7236 1089 2
ISBN-10: 0 7236 1089 4

**British Library Cataloguing in Publication Data**
A catalogue record for this book is available from the British Library

**Library of Congress Cataloging in Publication Data**
A catalog record for this book is available from the Library of Congress

The Publisher's policy is to use paper manufactured from sustainable forests

Printed in Spain

# Preface

This book has been written for undergraduates and dental practitioners seeking to update their knowledge. It is primarily intended as the undergraduate text for dental students in the United Kingdom, and builds on the scientific basis of dentistry. It sets out to explain the why and the how of clinical endodontic treatment, which is the prevention and treatment of apical periodontitis. Students are becoming more analytical and ready to question clinical procedures that are not based on sound principles and evidence.

Recognized specialist practice in endodontics is now established in the United Kingdom, and is still in its infancy. It is of particular benefit to a growing number of patients, who can now be referred to specially trained practitioners for difficult or unusual endodontic procedures and can expect to receive a predictable outcome. As there is never likely to be a sufficient number of specialists to treat more than the most difficult cases, there is still a major place for undergraduates to be taught practical endodontics; indeed most endodontic treatment will be carried out in general dental practice. New graduates in the United Kingdom are required to undergo a formal period of training in dental practice, and this presents an opportunity to translate the teaching given in dental school into everyday clinical practice, and should result in more competent dental practitioners in the future. It is essential that general dental practitioners keep up to date,

and it is intended that this book should help them to do so, by supporting what they learn on short continuing education courses. The authorities in the United Kingdom now stress the importance of continuing education, and it is no longer acceptable for practitioners to rely on their teaching at dental school. Many treatment procedures taught even ten years ago have radically altered. When nickel-titanium alloys were first introduced into endodontics, few could have foreseen what a revolution would take place in root canal preparation, particularly by using files of greater taper rather than traditional files.

The book has been thoroughly revised and some new authors have been brought in to write up-to-date authoritative chapters and to maintain the international flavour. This is an easy-to-read handbook for busy practitioners, which is comprehensively referenced in a style that is unobtrusive.

I should like to express my thanks to all the contributors who have tirelessly given of their time and expertise to create this new edition, and in particular to Drs Walker and Frank who have contributed but not directly to this edition. I should also like to acknowledge the patience of my wife and family, together with the help of the publishers in bringing this book to fruition.

T. R. Pitt Ford
2004

# Contributors

**B. S. Chong** BDS MSc PhD MRD RCSEng
Honorary Research Fellow
Restorative Dentistry
Dental Institute
King's College London
London, England

**P. M. H. Dummer** BDS MScD PhD FDS RCSEd
Professor
Department of Adult Dental Health
Dental School
University of Wales College of Medicine
Cardiff, Wales

**M. P. Escudier** MBBS BDS FDS RCSEng
Senior Lecturer / Honorary Consultant
Oral Medicine
Dental Institute
King's College London
London, England

**A. L. Frank** DDS
Professor
Department of Endodontics
Loma Linda University
Loma Linda
California, USA

**J. L. Gutmann** DDS PhD
Professor
Department of Restorative Sciences
Baylor College of Dentistry
Texas A&M University System
Dallas
Texas, USA

**R. J. Ibbetson** BDS MSc FDS RDS
Professor
Edinburgh Postgraduate Dental Institute
University of Edinburgh
Edinburgh, Scotland

**C. Mason** BDS FDS RCSEng
Consultant
Great Ormond Street Hospital for Children
Great Ormond Street
London, England

**P. J. C. Mitchell** BDS MSc MRD RCSEd
Clinical Demonstrator
Restorative Dentistry
Dental Institute
King's College London
London, England

**D. Ørstavik** Cand Odont Dr Odont
Senior Scientist
Scandinavian Institute of Dental Materials
Haslum, Norway

**H. E. Pitt Ford** FDS RCSEng
Associate Specialist
Paediatric Dentistry
Guy's & St Thomas' Hospital NHS Trust
London, England

**T. R. Pitt Ford** BDS PhD FDS RCPS FDS RCSEd
Professor of Endodontology
Restorative Dentistry
Dental Institute
King's College London
London, England

**J. D. Regan** BDentSc MSc MS
Assistant Professor
Department of Restorative Sciences
Baylor College of Dentistry
Texas A&M University System
Dallas
Texas, USA

**J. H. Simon** DDS
Professor
Department of Endodontics
Loma Linda University
Loma Linda
California, USA

# Contents

Preface    v
List of contributors    vi

## 1 Introduction and overview
*T. R. Pitt Ford*

Introduction    1
Modern endodontics    2
Scope of endodontics    3
Role of microorgansisms    3
Tissue response to root canal infection    4
Quality assurance    4
Recent developments    5
References    6

## 2 General and systemic aspects of endodontics
*M. P. Escudier*

Introduction    9
Differential diagnosis of dental pain    9
Maxillary sinus    11
Systemic disease and endodontics    11
Use of antibiotics in endodontics    14
Control of pain and anxiety    14
Dental Practitioners' Formulary    15
References    15

## 3 Pulp space anatomy and access cavities
*T. R. Pitt Ford*

Introduction    17
Nomenclature    18
Accessory and lateral canals    19
Location of apical foramina    20
Variations in pulp space anatomy    21
Effects of irritation dentine on pulp space    21
Pulp space anatomy and access cavities    22
Pulp space anatomy of primary teeth    32
Apical closure    33
References    33

## 4 The dental pulp
*T. R. Pitt Ford*

Introduction    37
Pulp response to irritants    37
Diagnosis of pulp damage    38
Pulpal irritants    40
Management of deep caries    43
Pulp exposure    44
Traumatic injuries    45
Cracked cusps    45
Pulp response to periodontal disease and treatment    45
Pulp response to intra-alveolar surgery    46
References    46

## 5 Basic instrumentation in endodontics
*B. S. Chong*

Introduction 51
Basic instrument pack 51
Rubber dam 51
Instruments for access cavity preparation 56
Instruments for root canal preparation 57
Devices to determine working length 63
Irrigant delivery devices 65
Instruments for retrieving broken instruments and posts 66
Instruments for filling root canals 68
Storage and sterilization of endodontic instruments 71
Loupes, fibre-optic lights and operating microscopes 73
References 74

## 6 Preparation of the root canal system
*J. D. Regan and J. L. Gutmann*

Introduction 77
Preoperative assessment 78
Preparation of the clinical crown 80
Access cavity 81
Root canal orifices 83
Working length determination 84
Root canal irrigation 85
Instrumentation techniques 86
Nickel-titanium instruments 90
Controversies in root canal cleaning and shaping 90
References 91

## 7 Intracanal medication
*D. Ørstavik*

Introduction 95
History 96
Rationale and overview of applications 96
Microbes of the pulp 97
Antimicrobial agents 98
Resistance of oral microbes to medicaments 100
Concept of predictable disinfection in endodontics 101
Induction of hard tissue formation 103
Pain of endodontic origin 103
Exudation and bleeding 104
Root resorption 104
Tissue distribution of medicaments 105
Tissue toxicity and biological considerations 106
Suggested clinical procedures 106
References 108

## 8 Root canal filling
*P. M. H. Dummer*

Introduction 113
Canal anatomy 114
Access and canal preparation 114
Criteria for filling 114
Materials used to fill root canals 115
Sealers 115
Smear layer 117
Gutta-percha 118
Apical dentine plug 132
Other methods of root canal filling 132
Restoration of the root filled tooth 135
Follow-up 135
Criteria of success 135
References 136

## 9 Surgical endodontics
*J. L. Gutmann and J. D. Regan*

Introduction 143
Indications for periradicular surgery 143
Preoperative assessment 144
Surgical kit 145
Surgical technique 146
Periradicular surgery of particular teeth 168

Repair of perforation    170
Replantation/transplantation    171
Regenerative procedures    172
Success and failure – aetiology and
evaluation    173
Retreatment of surgical procedures    174
References    175


## 10  Endodontics in children
*C. Mason*

Introduction    183
Treatment of primary teeth    183
Treatment of immature permanent teeth    188
References    191


## 11  Endodontic aspects of traumatic injuries
*H. E. Pitt Ford and T. R. Pitt Ford*

Introduction    195
History, examination and immediate
management    195
Types of injury    197
Effects of trauma on the dental tissues    197
Management of primary teeth    197
Management of permanent teeth    198
Root canal treatment of immature teeth    206
Auto-transplantation of an immature premolar
into the incisor space    207
Complications    208
Orthodontic treatment    211
References    211


## 12  Marginal periodontitis and the dental pulp
*J. H. Simon and A. L. Frank*

Anatomy    215
Effect of necrotic pulp on the
periodontium    215

Effect of marginal periodontitis on the
pulp    216
Classification    217
Complications due to radicular anomalies    227
Anatomical redesigning    228
References    234


## 13  Problems in endodontic treatment
*T. R. Pitt Ford and P. J. C. Mitchell*

Emergency treatment    237
Failure of anaesthesia in acute
inflammation    239
Problems with preparation of the root canal
system    241
Problems with filling of the root canal
system    247
References    249


## 14  Restoration of endodontically treated teeth
*R. J. Ibbetson*

Introduction    253
Effects of endodontic treatment on the
tooth    253
Timing the restorative procedure    254
Anterior teeth    254
Posterior teeth    257
Posts    265
Metal posts with cast cores    268
Endodontically treated teeth as abutments    275
Elective devitalization    275
Conclusions    275
References    276


Index    279

# 1

# Introduction and overview

## T. R. Pitt Ford

Introduction 1

Modern endodontics 2

Scope of endodontics 3

Role of microorganisms 3

Tissue response to root canal infection 4

Quality assurance 4

Recent developments 5

References 6

## INTRODUCTION

Endodontic treatment can be defined as the prevention or treatment of apical periodontitis, that is the precautions taken to maintain the health of the vital pulp in a tooth, or the treatment of a damaged or necrotic pulp in a tooth to allow the tooth to remain functional in the dental arch. The concept of treating the pulp of the tooth to preserve the tooth itself is a relatively modern development in the history of dentistry and it may be useful to review, very briefly, the history of pulp treatment in order to appreciate better modern views on endodontic treatment. Toothache has been a scourge of mankind from the earliest times. Both the Chinese and the Egyptians left records describing caries and alveolar abscesses. The Chinese considered that these abscesses were caused by a white worm with a black head which lived within the tooth. The 'worm theory' was current until the middle of the 18th century when doubts were raised [21], but they could not be expressed forcibly because senior figures still believed in the worm theory [13]. The Chinese treatment for an abscessed tooth was aimed at killing the worm with a preparation that contained arsenic. The use of this drug was taught in most dental schools as recently as the 1950s in spite of the realization that it was self-limiting and that extensive tissue destruction occurred if minute amounts of the drug leaked into the soft tissues. Pulp treatment during Greek and Roman times was aimed at destroying the pulp by cauterization with a hot needle or boiling oil, or with a mixture of opium and hyoscyamus. At the end of the 1st century AD, it was realized that pain could be relieved by drilling into the pulp chamber to obtain drainage. In spite of modern antibiotics there is still no better method of relieving the pain of an abscessed tooth than drainage.

Endodontic knowledge remained static until the 16th century when pulpal anatomy was described. Before the latter part of the 19th century, root canal therapy consisted of alleviating pain from pulps and the main function of the opened root canal was to provide retention for a dowel crown [10,11]. At the same time, bridgework became popular and many dental schools taught that no tooth should be used as an abutment unless it was first devitalized [47]. Root canal therapy became commonplace partly for these reasons and also because the discovery of cocaine led to painless pulp extirpation. The injection of 4% cocaine as a mandibular nerve block was first reported in 1884 [11,50]; and 20 years later the first synthetic local anaesthetic, procaine, was produced. At this time reports of endodontic surgery appeared [23]. Shortly after the discovery of X-rays by Roentgen in 1895, the first radiograph of teeth was taken [10,20,22]. This

1

further popularized root canal therapy and gave the treatment respectability. About the same time dental manufacturers began to produce special instruments, which were used primarily to remove pulp tissue or clean debris from the canal. There was no concept of filling the root canals since the object of the procedure was to provide retention for a post crown.

By 1910 'root canal therapy' had reached its zenith and no self-respecting dentist would extract a tooth. Every root stump was retained and a crown constructed. Sinus tracts often appeared and were treated by various ineffective methods for many years. The connection between the sinus tract and the pulpless tooth was known but not acted upon. In 1911 William Hunter [12,27] attacked 'American dentistry' and blamed bridgework for several diseases of unknown aetiology. He reported recovery from these conditions in a few patients following extraction of their teeth. It is interesting to note that he did not condemn root canal therapy itself but rather the ill-fitting bridgework and the sepsis that surrounded it. About this time micro-biology became established and the findings of microbiologists added fuel to the fire of Hunter's condemnations. Radiography, which at first helped the dentist, now gave irrefutable evidence of apical periodontitis surrounding the roots of pulpless teeth.

Whilst the theory of focal infection was not enunciated by Billings [6] until 1918, Hunter's condemnations started a reaction to root canal therapy, and there began the wholesale removal of both non-vital and perfectly healthy teeth. The blame for obscure diseases was placed on the dentition, and, as dentists could not refute this theory, count-less mouths were mutilated. Naturally not all dentists accepted this wholesale dental destruction. Some, particularly in continental Europe, continued to save teeth in spite of the focal sepsis theory. It is difficult to know why dentists in continental Europe disregarded this theory and one expla-nation may be that their patients equated the loss of teeth with a loss of virility and therefore did not allow their dentists to mutilate their dentitions. Alternatively it could be that these practitioners were not so readily swayed by fashion as were their British colleagues.

## MODERN ENDODONTICS

The re-emergence of endodontics as a respectable branch of dental science began in the 1930s [19,40]. The occurrence and degree of bacteraemia during tooth extraction was shown to depend on the severity of periodontal disease and the amount of tissue damage at operation. The incongruity between microbiological findings in the treatment of chronic oral infection and the histological picture was demonstrated. When the gingival sulcus was disinfected by cauterization before extraction, microorganisms could not be demonstrated in the bloodstream immediately postoperatively.

Gradually, the concept that a 'dead' tooth was not necessarily infected began to be accepted. Further, it was realized that the function and usefulness of the tooth depended on the integrity of the periodontal tissues and not on the vitality of the pulp [34]. Another important advance was clarification of the 'hollow tube' theory [49] by research using sterile polyethylene tube implants in rats [61,62]. The tissue surrounding the lumina of clean, disinfected tubes, which were closed at one end, was relatively free of inflammation and displayed a normal capacity for repair. When such tubes were filled with muscle, the inflammatory reaction was only severe around the openings of the tubes containing muscle contaminated with Gram-negative cocci. These findings place stress on the microbial contents of the tube; if the tube contains microorganisms then the potential for repair is far less favourable than when the lumen of the tube is clean and sterile [64]. This infected situation is likely to be found in most root canals requiring treatment.

The concept that 'apical seal' was important led to the search for filling and sealing materials that were stable, non-irritant and provided a perfect seal at the apical foramen. With the more recent realization of the importance of coronal leakage [51,52] and the biodegradation of root canal fillings, total filling of the root canal space including lateral and accessory canals has assumed much greater importance.

Until recent decades dentists were preoccupied with a mechanistic approach to root canal treatment and to the perceived effects of various potent drugs on the microorganisms within the root canal rather than a total antimicrobial approach of effective cleaning, shaping and filling of the canal space. This preoccupation diverted attention from the effects of such drugs on the adjacent tissues. Antiseptics that kill bacteria may act for a short period and are toxic to living tissue [8]. The consequences of such materials passing out of the tooth into the surrounding vital tissues can be localized tissue necrosis. These avoidable problems cause distress to patients and can lead to litigation. Effective elimination of bacteria from root canals is achieved by instrumentation combined with irrigation.

## SCOPE OF ENDODONTICS

The extent of the subject has altered considerably in the last 50 years. Formerly, endodontic treatment confined itself to root canal filling techniques by conventional methods; even endodontic surgery, which is an extension of these methods, was considered to be in the field of oral surgery. Modern endodontics has a much wider field [2] and includes the following:

- diagnosis of oral pain;
- protection of the healthy pulp from disease or injury;
- pulp capping (both indirect and direct);
- pulpotomy (both conventional and partial);
- pulpectomy;
- root canal treatment of infected root canals;
- surgical endodontics, which includes apicectomy, hemisection, root amputation, and replantation.

## ROLE OF MICROORGANISMS

The Chinese believed that dental abscesses were caused by small organisms, worms, a view that persisted until the 18th century. At the end of the 19th century Miller [35] demonstrated the role of bacteria in root canal infection, and noted that different microorganisms were found in the root canal compared with the open pulp chamber. Shortly afterwards, systematic culturing of root canals was undertaken [42]. Unfortunately, these methods, which were potentially so valuable for improving root canal treatment, were used to condemn much of the dentistry done at the time [27]. During the 1930s microbiological techniques were used to re-establish the scientific basis of root canal treatment; techniques at that time, however, only readily identified aerobic bacteria, and led to confusing results in later clinical studies [3,53]. This resulted in clinicians being complacent about the role of microorganisms, and performing treatment simply as a technical exercise.

The development of anaerobic culturing allowed many unknown microorganisms present in root canals to be grown [36], which led rapidly to the demonstration that the majority of canal microorganisms were anaerobes [31,55], and the realization that canals previously considered sterile contained anaerobes alone. Furthermore, when traumatized teeth were examined, there was a close correlation between the presence of anaerobic bacteria in the root canal and a periapical radiolucency [55]. This was later demonstrated experimentally in teeth where the pulp tissue had been removed; only in those where the pulp was infected did periapical inflammation occur [37]. Although anaerobic culturing of root canals is not a technique for everyday clinical use, the research has given rational explanations for pulp disease and its treatment [56]. With the rapid increase in knowledge, anaerobic root canal bacteria are continually being reclassified. Only a few years ago Bacteroides were being reported as major pathogens of root canals [25], yet they have now been reclassified into two new genera, Prevotella and Porphyromonas, according to their ability to ferment carbohydrate [56]. Classification is now based on biochemical tests and is rapidly being dominated by molecular biologists. Bacteria, which previously could not be cultured and so were considered absent, are now being found with increasing frequency, and as knowledge expands it is likely that in a few years the flora of root canals will appear very different. The use of molecular biological techniques, such as Polymerase Chain Reaction (PCR), has enabled amplification of small amounts of nucleic acids from cell nuclei to allow identification of bacteria that would be undetectable by culturing techniques [15]. As in other aspects of science, PCR complements information from other methods rather than being a replacement, since it does not detect every organism detected by culturing.

Most root canal infections contain a mixture of bacteria [17,18,55], and it has been shown that the relative proportions of different bacteria are determined by environmental conditions [18]. If a mixture of bacteria are inoculated into root canals at a fixed proportion, their relative numbers change over time, with a decline in aerobes and an increase in anaerobes [18]. It has also been established that combinations of bacteria are more likely to survive than inocula of single species, eg, *Prevotella oralis* [17]. It is clear that one species can produce substances that others can metabolize in order to survive [56].

Bacteria are normally confined to the root canal system in pulpless teeth [38] and it is unusual for periapical lesions to contain bacteria unless there is an acute abscess. At the orifice of the root canal a large number of inflammatory cells that prevent bacteria from entering the tissues are normally found [44].

## TISSUE RESPONSE TO ROOT CANAL INFECTION

The role of infection in the demise of damaged pulps was demonstrated in a classic study by Kakehashi and coworkers in the 1960s [30], and eventually led to a biological approach to operative dentistry [4]. The presence of bacteria, their by-products or damaged tissue in the root canal can cause apical periodontitis, typically at the apical foramen but also around the foramina of any lateral or accessory canals or at a fracture. The periradicular inflammation prevents the spread of infection from the tooth into the alveolar bone, otherwise osteomyelitis would occur. The inflammatory lesion contains inflammatory mediators and numerous inflammatory cells, e.g. polymorphonuclear leucocytes, macrophages, B- and T-lymphocytes and plasma cells. The interaction between these cells and the antigenic substances from the root canal results in the release of a large number of inflammatory mediators. The inflammatory mediators include neuropeptides, the

complement system, lysozymes and metabolites of arachidonic acid [58]. Prostaglandins, leukotrienes and cytokines play an important role in the development of periradicular lesions [33,59,63].

As long as antigens emerge from canal foramina, there will be a continuing inflammatory response, mediated in a number of different ways. This is a very dynamic response to rapidly multiplying bacteria in the root canal, and may not be readily apparent to the clinician observing a radiograph or a histologist examining a slide of fixed cells. Effective elimination of the microorganisms allows inflammation to subside and healing to occur.

## QUALITY ASSURANCE

The general public across the world now expect professional people to deliver a high standard of service; dentistry, and endodontic treatment in particular, is no exception. The European Society of Endodontology has issued quality guidelines for endodontic treatment [16]. It is essential that dental practices have a quality control system to ensure that each step in history, diagnosis and treatment is carried out in a logical and consistent manner. This is to ensure a high standard of care and treatment, known as clinical governance. Patients are increasingly well informed and will not tolerate poor standards, e.g., in decontamination and sterilization procedures, or out-of-date views.

Those dentists who have undertaken further training to become specialists are expected to achieve consistently high standards in diagnosis and treatment. However, general practitioners cannot continue to practise in the way that they were taught at dental school many years ago; they must keep up to date and offer referral to an appropriate specialist when the treatment required is beyond their skill. This change has already occurred in the USA and is spreading to other countries. In the UK continuing professional development is now mandatory for recertification with the regulatory body.

Almost all endodontic procedures can be carried out with a predictable outcome. It has long been reported that root canal treatment has a success rate of over 90% [26,28,32], even though closer analysis reveals that retreatment of teeth with apical periodontitis is less successful than initial treatment in teeth without apical periodontitis [54]. It is essential that individual practitioners monitor their outcomes against published reports, and that their treatment protocols conform to published guidelines. Success of treatment can be measured in different ways and it is insufficient to rely on clinical evidence alone; the use of radiography for follow-up is essential [24].

## RECENT DEVELOPMENTS

Pulp damage in the main is caused by dental caries, infection consequent to trauma, or infection as a result of operative dentistry. With a reduced incidence of dental caries, greater emphasis on preventing sports injuries, and preparation of smaller cavities combined with better restorative materials in operative dentistry, the number of teeth with damaged pulps should decline. This will probably not result in lower demand for endodontic treatment as patient expectations will continue to increase. The degree to which adhesive restorative materials will be successful in preventing pulp damage in clinical practice is another unquantifiable variable.

Diagnosis of pulp disease is sometimes difficult, and hopes of new equipment to facilitate diagnosis of the state of the pulp have not yet been realized clinically, although research continues into laser Doppler flowmetry, which assesses blood flow, as opposed to established methods of stimulating neural activity [29,39,41]. The majority of research has involved young teeth with large pulps, and it may be challenging to develop equipment that produces good signals from a pulp that has receded in a heavily restored tooth.

Research into new radiographic imaging systems is still progressing [43]. Simultaneously, recent advances in film technology have achieved the maintenance of radiographic quality with a substantial reduction in radiation exposure [46]. The many problems with present radiographic methods can to a large extent be eliminated by accurate technique in film exposure and processing.

Preparation of root canals has altered substantially in recent years. File manufacturers have produced instruments with safe tips that will not readily create a ledge in preparations. This has allowed canal preparation techniques to incorporate some limited rotation of hand files, which was for a long time considered incorrect. Nickel-titanium alloys have been developed for root canal files [5,57]. These files are more flexible than stainless-steel files, so larger sizes can be taken round curved canals. This has led to files of greater taper being used to prepare root canals, achieving a superior shape with fewer instruments. Nickel-titanium rotary files have been developed and have been shown to be effective [48]. Research into canal filling has been concerned with developing new ways to introduce heated gutta-percha into the canal system. The controlling of the heat applied (e.g. System B) has made vertical condensation a much easier and more predictable method of filling canals prepared by files of greater taper [7].

There has been a quiet revolution in endodontic surgery. Apart from a reduction in indications, because root canal retreatment is more predictably successful than root-end surgery [1], root-end preparation and filling have altered. Gone is the indiscriminate use of a bur to cut the root-end cavity, and in its place is ultrasonic preparation with specially shaped tips that clean and shape the end of the root canal much more effectively and safely. The use of amalgam for root-end filling has ceased, with zinc oxide–eugenol materials being widely used [14,45]. The most exciting development has been the commercial production of a new root-end filling material, mineral trioxide aggregate (MTA) [60]. A high rate of success (92%) has been achieved with this biocompatible material in a recent clinical study [9].

The importance of good coronal restoration of root-filled teeth has been highlighted [52], and this is facilitated by the use of adhesive materials where appropriate, the placement of suitable bases, and well-fitting restorations.

Endodontic referral practice is undertaking more root canal retreatment because of technical deficiencies in the original treatment. In many cases this is difficult and challenging but success can be very rewarding particularly when in the past the alternative would have been extraction. It is encouraging that many more patients are refusing to allow a tooth with an exposed or infected pulp to be extracted, but instead ask for it to be saved by root canal treatment. It is essential that practitioners make a careful diagnosis and give a realistic prognosis of the proposed treatment based on the best available evidence. Good quality endodontic treatment makes a significant contribution to oral health.

## REFERENCES

1. Allen RK, Newton CW, Brown CE (1989) A statistical analysis of surgical and nonsurgical endodontic retreatment cases. *Journal of Endodontics* **15**, 261–266.
2. American Association of Endodontists (1994) Glossary – Contemporary Terminology for Endodontics. 5th edn. Chicago, IL, USA: American Association of Endodontists.
3. Bender IB, Seltzer S, Turkenkopf S (1964) To culture or not to culture? *Oral Surgery, Oral Medicine, Oral Pathology* **18**, 527–540.
4. Bergenholtz G, Cox CF, Loesche WJ, Syed SA (1982) Bacterial leakage around dental restorations: its effect on the pulp. *Journal of Oral Pathology* **11**, 439–450.
5. Bergmans L, Cleynenbreugel JV, Wevers M, Lambrechts P (2001) Mechanical root canal preparation with NiTi rotary instruments: rationale, performance and safety. Status report for the American Journal of Dentistry. *American Journal of Dentistry* **14**, 324–333.
6. Billings F (1918) *Focal Infection.* New York, NY, USA: Appleton.
7. Buchanan LS (1994) The Buchanan continuous wave of condensation technique. A convergence of conceptual and procedural advances in obturation. *Dentistry Today* **October**, 80–85.
8. Chong BS, Pitt Ford TR (1992) The role of intracanal medication in root canal treatment. *International Endodontic Journal* **25**, 97–106.
9. Chong BS, Pitt Ford TR, Hudson MB (2003) A prospective clinical study of Mineral Trioxide Aggregate and IRM when used as root-end filling materials in endodontic surgery. *International Endodontic Journal* **36**, 520–526.
10. Cruse WP, Bellizzi R (1980) A historic review of endodontics, 1689–1963, Part 1. *Journal of Endodontics* **6**, 495–499.
11. Cruse WP, Bellizzi R (1980) A historic review of endodontics, 1689–1963, Part 2. *Journal of Endodontics* **6**, 532–535.
12. Cruse WP, Bellizzi R (1980) A historic review of endodontics, 1689–1963, Part 3. *Journal of Endodontics* **6**, 576–580.
13. Curson I (1965) History and endodontics. *Dental Practitioner and Dental Record* **15**, 435–439.
14. Dorn SO, Gartner AH (1990) Retrograde filling materials: a retrospective success–failure study of amalgam, EBA, and IRM. *Journal of Endodontics* **16**, 391–393.
15. Dymock D, Weightman AJ, Scully C, Wade WG (1996) Molecular analysis of microflora associated with dentoalveolar abscesses. *Journal of Clinical Microbiology* **34**, 537–542.
16. European Society of Endodontology (1994) Consensus report of the European Society of Endodontology on quality guidelines for endodontic treatment. *International Endodontic Journal* **27**, 115–124.
17. Fabricius L, Dahlen G, Holm SE, Möller AJR (1982) Influence of combinations of oral bacteria on periapical tissues of monkeys. *Scandinavian Journal of Dental Research* **90**, 200–206.
18. Fabricius L, Dahlen G, Öhman AE, Möller AJR (1982) Predominant indigenous oral bacteria isolated from infected root canals after varied times of closure. *Scandinavian Journal of Dental Research* **90**, 134–144.
19. Fish EW, MacLean I (1936) The distribution of oral streptococci in the tissues. *British Dental Journal* **61**, 336–362.
20. Grossman LI (1976) Endodontics 1776–1976: a bicentennial history against the background of general dentistry. *Journal of the American Dental Association* **93**, 78–87.
21. Guerini V (1909) *History of Dentistry.* Philadelphia, PA, USA: Lea and Febiger.
22. Gutmann JL (1987) History. In: Cohen S, Burns RC (eds*)*, *Pathways of the Pulp*, 4th edn. St Louis, MO, USA; Mosby, pp. 756–782.
23. Gutmann JL, Harrison JW (1991) *Surgical Endodontics.* Boston, MA, USA: Blackwell Scientific Publications, pp. 3–41.
24. Gutmann JL, Pitt Ford TR (1992) Problems in the assessment of success and failure. In: Gutmann JL, Dumsha TC, Lovdahl PE, Hovland EJ (eds). *Problem solving in endodontics. Prevention, identification and management,* 2nd edn. St Louis, MO, USA; Mosby-Year Book, pp. 1–11.
25. Haapasalo M (1989) Bacteroides spp. in dental root canal infections. *Endodontics and Dental Traumatology* **5**, 1–10.
26. Harty FJ, Parkins BJ, Wengraf AM (1970) Success rate in root canal therapy – a retrospective study of conventional cases. *British Dental Journal* **128**, 65–70.
27. Hunter W (1911) The role of sepsis and antisepsis in medicine. *Lancet* **1**, 79–86.
28. Ingle JI, Bakland LK (1994) *Endodontics,* 4th edn. Malvern, PA, USA: Williams & Wilkins, pp 21–44.
29. Ingolfsson AER, Tronstad L, Riva CE (1994) Reliability of laser Doppler flowmetry in testing vitality of human teeth. *Endodontics and Dental Traumatology* **10**, 185–187.
30. Kakehashi S, Stanley HR, Fitzgerald RJ (1965) The effects of surgical exposures of dental pulps in germ-free and conventional laboratory rats. *Oral Surgery, Oral Medicine, Oral Pathology* **20**, 340–349.
31. Kantz WE, Henry CA (1974) Isolation and classification of anaerobic bacteria from intact chambers of non-vital teeth in man. *Archives of Oral Biology* **19**, 91–96.
32. Kerekes K, Tronstad L (1979) Long-term results of endodontic treatment performed with a standardized technique. *Journal of Endodontics* **5**, 83–90.

33. McNicholas S, Torabinejad M, Blankenship J, Bakland L (1991) The concentration of prostaglandin $E_2$ in human periradicular lesions. *Journal of Endodontics* **17**, 97–100.

34. Marshall JA (1928) The relation to pulp-canal therapy of certain anatomical characteristics of dentin and cementum. *Dental Cosmos* **70**, 253–263.

35. Miller WD (1894) An introduction to the study of the bacterio-pathology of the dental pulp. *Dental Cosmos* **36,** 505–528.

36. Möller AJR (1966) Microbiological examination of root canals and periapical tissues of human teeth. Thesis. Gothenberg, Sweden: Akademiforlaget, pp. 1–380.

37. Möller AJR, Fabricius L, Dahlen G, Öhman AE, Heyden G (1981) Influence on periapical tissues of indigenous oral bacteria and necrotic pulp tissue in monkeys. *Scandinavian Journal of Dental Research* **89**, 475–484.

38. Nair PNR (1987) Light and electron microscopic studies of root canal flora and periapical lesions. *Journal of Endodontics* **13**, 29–39.

39. Odor TM, Pitt Ford TR, McDonald F (1996) Effect of wavelength and bandwidth on the clinical reliability of laser Doppler recordings. *Endodontics and Dental Traumatology* **12**, 9–15.

40. Okell CC, Elliott SD (1935) Bacteriaemia and oral sepsis with special reference to the aetiology of subacute endocarditis. *Lancet* **2**, 869–872.

41. Olgart L, Gazelius B, Lindh-Stromberg U (1988) Laser Doppler flowmetry in assessing vitality in luxated permanent teeth. *International Endodontic Journal* **21**, 300–306.

42. Onderdonk TW (1901) Treatment of unfilled root canals. *International Dental Journal* **22**, 20–22.

43. Ong EY, Pitt Ford TR (1995) Comparison of Radiovisiography with radiographic film in root length determination. *International Endodontic Journal* **28**, 25–29.

44. Pitt Ford TR (1982) The effects on the periapical tissues of bacterial contamination of the filled root canal. *International Endodontic Journal* **15**, 16–22.

45. Pitt Ford TR, Andreasen JO, Dorn SO, Kariyawasam SP (1994) Effect of IRM root end fillings on healing after replantation. *Journal of Endodontics* **20**, 381–385.

46. Powell-Cullingford AW, Pitt Ford TR (1993) The use of E-speed film for root canal length determination. *International Endodontic Journal* **26**, 268–272.

47. Prinz H (1945) *Dental Chronology. A Record of the More Important Historic Events in the Evolution of Dentistry.* London, UK: Kimpton.

48. Rhodes JS, Pitt Ford TR, Lynch JA, Liepins PJ, Curtis RV (2000) A comparison of two nickel-titanium instrumentation techniques in teeth using microcomputed tomography. *International Endodontic Journal* **33**, 279–285.

49. Rickert UG, Dixon CM (1931) The controlling of root surgery. Paris, France: Eighth International Dental Congress. **IIIa**, pp. 15–22.

50. Roberts DH, Sowray JH (1987) *Local Analgesia in Dentistry,* 3rd edn. Oxford, UK: Wright, pp. 1–4.

51. Saunders WP, Saunders EM (1990) Assessment of leakage in the restored pulp chamber of endodontically treated multirooted teeth. *International Endodontic Journal* **23**, 28–33.

52. Saunders WP, Saunders EM (1994) Coronal leakage as a cause of failure in root-canal therapy: a review. *Endodontics and Dental Traumatology* **10**, 105–108.

53. Seltzer S, Turkenkopf S, Vito A, Green D, Bender IB (1964) A histologic evaluation of periapical repair following positive and negative root canal cultures. *Oral Surgery, Oral Medicine, Oral Pathology* **17**, 507–532.

54. Sjögren U, Hägglund B, Sundqvist G, Wing K (1990) Factors affecting the long-term results of endodontic treatment. *Journal of Endodontics* **16**, 498–504.

55. Sundqvist G (1976) Bacteriological studies of necrotic dental pulps. Thesis. Umea, Sweden: University of Umea, pp. 1–94.

56. Sundqvist G (1994) Taxonomy, ecology, and pathogenicity of the root canal flora. *Oral Surgery, Oral Medicine, Oral Pathology* **78**, 522–530.

57. Thompson SA (2000) An overview of nickel-titanium alloys used in dentistry. *International Endodontic Journal* **33**, 297–310.

58. Torabinejad M (1994) Mediators of acute and chronic periradicular lesions. *Oral Surgery, Oral Medicine, Oral Pathology* **78**, 511–521.

59. Torabinejad M, Cotti E, Jung T (1992) Concentration of leukotriene $B_4$ in symptomatic and asymptomatic periapical lesions. *Journal of Endodontics* **18**, 205–208.

60. Torabinejad M, Hong CU, Lee SJ, Monsef M, Pitt Ford TR (1995) Investigation of Mineral Trioxide Aggregate for root-end filling in dogs. *Journal of Endodontics* **21**, 603–608.

61. Torneck CD (1966) Reaction of rat connective tissue to polyethylene tube implants. Part I. *Oral Surgery, Oral Medicine, Oral Pathology* **21**, 379–387.

62. Torneck CD (1967) Reaction of rat connective tissue to polyethylene tube implants. Part II. *Oral Surgery, Oral Medicine, Oral Pathology* **24**, 674–683.

63. Trowbridge HO, Emling RC (1997) *Inflammation. A Review of the Process.* 5th edn. Carol Stream, IL, USA: Quintessence.

64. Wu MK, Moorer WR, Wesselink PR (1989) Capacity of anaerobic bacteria enclosed in a simulated root canal to induce inflammation. *International Endodontic Journal* **22**, 269–277.

# General and systemic aspects of endodontics

M. P. Escudier

Introduction  9

Differential diagnosis of dental pain  9
  Pain history  10
  Examination  10
  Idiopathic orofacial pain  10

Maxillary sinus  11

Systemic disease and endodontics  11
  Endodontics and infective endocarditis  12
  Endodontics in patients with prosthetic hip joints  13
  Endodontics in patients taking warfarin or steroids  13

Use of antibiotics in endodontics  14

Control of pain and anxiety  14
  Analgesics  15

Dental Practitioners' Formulary  15

References  15

## INTRODUCTION

The treatment of periapical infection by modern endodontic procedures is a safe and effective procedure provided it is appropriately applied and undertaken by competent clinicians.

In line with this a full assessment of both the medical history and the clinical situation should be undertaken prior to commencing treatment. Comprehensive and sensible treatment planning based on a careful analysis of the information gathered will help to protect the patient from harm and the dental surgeon from criticism, legal or otherwise.

The dental surgeon is largely dependent on the patient's medical history to identify systemic disease or therapy, that may affect the management.

It is therefore vital that this is comprehensive and regularly updated. In addition, any areas of uncertainty or concern should, if possible, be discussed with the patient's general medical practitioner prior to commencing treatment. Many patients have systemic disorders, which are well-controlled by therapy and therefore unlikely to influence the outcome of dental treatment. However, the treatment itself may influence the management, e.g. prednisolone, warfarin.

The assessment will initially consist of the history and a clinical examination, which will provide a differential diagnosis. It should be remembered that the history is the single most important factor in arriving at a diagnosis [14]. However, the clinical examination and subsequent investigations will increase the clinicians' confidence in the diagnosis, even though they contribute relatively few new facts [18].

The fear of transmission of HIV (human immunodeficiency virus) or hepatitis viruses as well as prions has highlighted the importance of the application of current guidelines for infection control in endodontics as in any other aspect of clinical dentistry [6].

## DIFFERENTIAL DIAGNOSIS OF DENTAL PAIN

The commonest cause of pain in the oro-facial region is dental disease leading to pulpal pain (see Chapter 4). As such, dental surgeons are experienced and competent in the diagnosis and management of this clinical problem. However, the differential diagnosis of pain in the teeth, jaws and face is far wider than is sometimes appreciated. Pain may be:

- referred from a distant origin, e.g. cardiac;
- of unusual local cause, e.g. osteomyelitis;
- psychogenic in origin, e.g. atypical facial pain;
- neurological, e.g. trigeminal neuralgia;
- modified by apparently unrelated factors, e.g. previous cerebrovascular accident.

This broader diagnostic sieve should be remembered, particularly if the pattern of presentation is unusual, the examination findings are sparse or conflicting, or if pain persists or develops in spite of apparently successful treatment.

The essence of good clinical practice is a methodical and disciplined approach (history, followed by examination, followed by special investigations – usually radiographic, followed by analysis and conclusion). In the case of oro-facial pain this is extremely well dealt with in other texts [26].

## Pain history

A thorough, structured pain history will indicate a diagnosis in the majority of cases and will identify those areas for further investigation. This should commence with the patient being asked to describe the pain in their own words, followed by direct questions. Certain core information should be elicited in all cases (Table 2.1) [26].

**Table 2.1** Pain history

| | |
|---|---|
| Duration | When did your pain start? Have you ever had a pain like this before? |
| Character | What type of pain is it? |
| Periodicity | When do you get the pain? Does it come and go? Is there any particular pattern to the pain? |
| Severity | How severe is your pain? |
| Site | Where is your pain? |
| Radiation | Does your pain spread to other areas? |
| Provoking factors | Does anything make your pain worse? |
| Relieving factors | Does anything make your pain better? |
| Associated factors | Have you noticed anything else about your pain? |

## Examination

The assessment of a patient starts with his or her entry to the clinical setting. This will enable observation of the general demeanour as well as any locomotor problems, walking aids or possible neurological deficits. It may enable identification of any facial swelling, and particular attention should be paid to symmetry, notably that of the cheeks, the mandibular angle region and the nasolabial folds. Observation of the patient's face during the history taking may reveal a subtle neurological feature requiring formal assessment of cranial nerve function. An assessment of the level of pain can be made using the facial expression [21], although it is important to remember that facial expression can be manipulated. Hence avoidance of, or flinching from, examination may be a more accurate indication of a trigger spot or tenderness than response to questioning during examination. The observation of mandibular movements is the essential preliminary to examination of temporomandibular joint function.

The features of a comprehensive examination of the teeth are described in Chapter 4. The soft tissues of the cheeks, palate, tongue and floor of the mouth may also yield vital information. The necessity for a detailed occlusal examination depends on the history and clinical setting. Similarly, the history will determine the necessity or desirability of formal assessment of the temporomandibular apparatus. The maxillary sinus as a cause of pain is considered below. Thermal or electrical stimulation of suspect teeth, differential local anaesthetic injections, and removal of restorations all have their place in diagnosis. In addition radiography is usually essential, but all these techniques must supplement the history and clinical examination, and never replace them.

## Idiopathic orofacial pain

The orofacial region (including the teeth) is a common site for the expression of pain or discomfort as a manifestation of underlying psychosocial disharmony. It may represent anything from a plea for help to a symptom of frank psychosis. The dental surgeon should avoid being manipulated by the patient, or patient's relatives, into undertaking treatment when the diagnosis is uncertain or the evidence conflicting. In such circumstances it is better to defer active treatment until a definitive diagnosis can be obtained. In many such cases the pain will either resolve spontaneously or provide further evidence to assist in the diagnosis, e.g. development of hemifacial rash of herpes zoster. A review appointment should be arranged with the caveat that the patient may return sooner should the need arise. The dental practitioner also has the opportunity to refer the patient for a second opinion at any time, particularly where the diagnosis continues to remain unclear.

Certain features in the history often help in the diagnosis of idiopathic facial pain. The pain is often unremitting and may have been present for months or even years. The stated severity may be out of proportion to the observed level of distress, disturbance of life or self-therapy. The pain may not follow anatomical boundaries and may be described as throbbing, nagging, aching, miserable or cruel in nature. It does not usually disturb sleep, although there may be a coincidental disturbance of sleep pattern. In addition, other chronic pain conditions such as headache, low back pain and abdominal or pelvic pain are often present. There may also be obvious secondary gain (family or social) for the sufferer. In such cases it is important to seek further information in relation to the patient's social history and family circumstances. There is often a history of long-term or recent distressing life events, e.g. bereavement, divorce or job loss [26].

Depression is common in chronic pain patients and may be effectively detected by two simple questions [23]: 'during the last month have you often been bothered by feeling down, depressed or hopeless?' and 'during the past month have you been bothered by having little interest or pleasure in doing things?' Psychiatric treatment or psychotherapy is often beneficial and may be curative. Such cases are often best referred to an oral physician as direct referral to a psychiatrist may meet with difficulties.

## MAXILLARY SINUS

The close proximity of the maxillary sinuses to the maxillary teeth can make the diagnosis of pain in these segments difficult. The distinction between pain of dental origin and sinusitis may be helped by the presence of obvious dental disease, or a typical acute or recurrent sinusitis with nasal discharge. Acute sinusitis rarely occurs without preceding symptoms of 'a cold', and tenderness to pressure of a whole quadrant of teeth is characteristic. In such cases the use of broad-spectrum antibiotics, e.g. amoxycillin 500 mg for 7–14 days, is of benefit [24]. Periapical infection of premolar or molar teeth may lead to purulent discharge into the sinus with associated pain. A further consideration is the risk of penetration of the sinus wall or even the sinus lining by endodontic instruments, or during periradicular surgery. This may result in acute sinusitis from bacterial contamination. The condition may resolve spontaneously but the prescription of a broad-spectrum antibiotic and nasal decongestant (see below) is usual practice but not shown to be necessary.

Small oroantral communications usually heal spontaneously, and in the case of periradicular surgery the replacement of the surgical flap is sufficient to seal the opening. The identity of microorganisms involved in sinus infection is often unclear and broad-spectrum antibiotics may be required, e.g. amoxycillin 500 mg tds. It is usual to continue therapy for 5 days although a one-off 3g dose of amoxycillin is equally effective [15]. If there is poor drainage of the sinus, e.g. a history of chronic sinusitis, nasal drops (0.5% ephedrine) should be prescribed. In addition, inhalations such as menthol and eucalyptus have a soothing effect and may be beneficial.

A connection between sinus disease and root canal treatment has been reported in a single study in Austria [5]. This related to aspergillosis of the maxillary antrum following root canal treatment with zinc-oxide based cements that are known to promote cultures of Aspergillus.

## SYSTEMIC DISEASE AND ENDODONTICS

Disabled or debilitated patients cannot be expected readily to tolerate complex and lengthy treatment procedures, but, even in severe ill-health, some patients have a strong desire to retain their natural teeth, and the dentist's duty is to try to respond. Even in terminal illness simple treatment can be a great aid to comfort, masticatory function and morale. Good decision-making is dependent on frank and thoughtful discussion with the patient and his or her medical advisers. In some conditions, e.g. cardiac abnormalities, endodontic treatment should only be carried out if a high standard of treatment can be achieved, which may involve referral.

Both the patient's general prognosis and the prognosis for the tooth being treated must be considered; this may lead to the decision to extract the tooth rather than undertake root canal treatment. In chronic diseases subject to cyclical remission, either spontaneously or with treatment, it is sensible to defer dental intervention until the optimum physical state is achieved. This is particularly true of haematological disorders, e.g. leukaemia, especially if the patient receives periodic transfusion or cycles of chemotherapy. Sufferers from haemorrhagic diatheses will not require factor replacement or anti-fibrinolytic therapy for root canal treatment alone, but may do if a local anaesthetic is to be given or endodontic surgery undertaken. In all such cases, the patient's haematologist should be consulted to discuss any necessary perioperative measures.

There is no evidence to show that the presence of systemic disease has a major influence on the healing of periapical lesions. Hence a positive approach should be taken to treatment even in immuno-compromised patients [13].

Progressive narrowing of pulp chambers and root canals (due to excessive dentine formation) in patients receiving substantial doses of corticosteroids following renal transplantation has been observed [17]. As infection of renal transplants is caused by different organisms from infective endocarditis, there would not appear to be a need for antibiotic prophylaxis. However, some renal transplant units still advise the need for antibiotic prophylaxis and in such cases it would be advisable to discuss the individual case with the unit concerned.

## Endodontics and infective endocarditis

Infective endocarditis is an uncommon but life-threatening condition with an overall mortality of 20%. However, during the last 50 years, the number of deaths due to streptococcal infective endocarditis has fallen by 90%.

The therapeutic management of patients at risk of infective endocarditis has been addressed by the Working Party of the British Society for Antimicrobial Chemotherapy [7–9,11]. The Working Party suggested that the only dental treatment procedures likely to produce significant bacteraemia were 'extractions, or scaling, or surgery involving the gingival tissues'. Endodontic procedures were excluded as it was felt that *significant* bacteraemia would not arise from manipulation of instruments within the root canal. This was based on experimental studies [3,4], indicating that only deliberate prolonged and exaggerated disturbance of the periapical tissues with an instrument passed through the apical foramen, or in the course of open periradicular surgery, could produce detectable bacteraemia.

However, this was intended as general advice, which could and should be modified in individual circumstances as appropriate. It would therefore, be prudent to use antibiotic prophylaxis for endodontic manipulation in the presence of acute periapical infection or suppurating marginal periodontitis. The antibiotic regime recommended, a single 3 g dose of amoxycillin taken orally under supervision 1 hour before treatment, produces a reliably high and prolonged blood level. This regime may be used twice in any 1 month and then not repeated in the following 3–4 months. In the case of hypersensitivity to penicillin or exposure more than once in the preceding month, clindamycin 600 mg is advised. This latter regime should not be repeated at an interval of less than 2 weeks.

Prophylaxis should be targeted on so called 'at-risk' patients who have an increased susceptibility to endocardial infection [11]. This includes all patients with known rheumatic or congenital heart disease, with murmurs associated with cardiac disease, who have undergone valve replacement, or who have previously suffered an attack of infective endocarditis. In the case of those who have suffered infective endocarditis, the risk is further increased and specific guidelines are provided. For all at-risk patients it is essential that endodontic treatment is carried out to the highest standard to minimize the risk of the root canal acting as a source of subsequent bacteraemia. Patients who have undergone coronary arterial bypass grafting are not at risk of endocarditis [11].

It is important to maintain optimum periodontal and dental health in patients at risk of endocarditis. In addition, the adjuvant use of a 0.2% chlorhexidine gluconate mouthwash, or 2% chlorhexidine gluconate gel preoperatively, further reduces the number of bacteria released into the circulation and hence the likely risk of infection.

Periradicular surgery falls within the definition of 'other surgery involving the gingival tissues', and antibiotic cover is indicated, but there are other considerations in at-risk patients. Surgery should only be undertaken where it is clearly indicated (see Chapter 9). Very occasionally root canal cleaning, shaping and filling, followed by periradicular surgery can be undertaken in a single visit instead of over a number of episodes each requiring antibiotic cover. Salvage procedures for teeth with poor prognosis (e.g. perforations) are inadvisable in at-risk patients. Replantation of avulsed teeth can be done in at-risk patients provided that the procedure is done under antibiotic cover and the endodontic follow-up is carried out by a specialist.

## Endodontics in patients with prosthetic hip joints

There is no special risk to patients with hip or knee prostheses from any form of dental treatment, and certainly not from endodontic procedures [10]. However, some orthopaedic patients are still advised of the need for antibiotic prophylaxis [1] and in such cases it would be advisable to discuss the individual situation with the surgeon concerned.

## Endodontics in patients taking warfarin or steroids

Increasing numbers of patients are taking regular medication for a variety of conditions. Amongst those of particular relevance to the management of dental patients are warfarin and steroids.

Warfarin is a commonly used oral anticoagulant used in the management of several medical conditions. Its action is monitored by means of the International Normalized Ratio (INR) and the desired therapeutic range (deep vein thrombosis INR ~ 2.5, prosthetic heart valve INR ~ 3.5–4.5) and the

duration of treatment depends on the medical condition. In such cases the first question is whether the warfarin therapy is to be discontinued at any time. If it is, then a decision can be made as to whether the proposed treatment can be deferred until this time. If treatment is required, however, or the warfarin therapy is ongoing, the INR will need to be considered. Warfarin therapy should not be stopped or altered prior to dental treatment without the agreement of the anticoagulant team. Endodontic treatment, with or without local anaesthesia, or periradicular surgery can safely be undertaken with an INR of 2.5 or less. The caveat is that the INR should be formally checked within 24 h of the procedure and ideally on the day of treatment. Whilst various treatments can be undertaken above this INR [22], consideration needs to be given to the site and extent of the therapeutic intervention. As such, periradicular surgery involving raising a mucoperiosteal flap and bone removal is contraindicated. Similarly, the use of inferior alveolar nerve blocks above an INR of 2.5 should be avoided. The use of low-dose aspirin as an antiplatelet drug is also unlikely to pose significant problems provided appropriate local measures are employed [2].

Steroids may be administered topically, via an inhaler or systemically. Systemic steroids taken above a dose of 7.5 mg (10 mg in some guidelines) daily for over one month, or in high doses (>40 mg per day) for periods as short as a week may cause adreno-cortical suppression. In the case of high doses for short periods ('pulsed') the effects are not clinically significant after one month off treatment and deferral of treatment until this time would be prudent. In the case of long-term steroid therapy prophylaxis is required and is best administered either orally or intravenously. Two regimes may be employed depending on the preference of the patient and clinician. The first requires that the patient doubles the normal daily dose the day before, day of and day after treatment. The second is a one-off dose of 100 mg hydrocortisone administered orally 1 h prior to treatment, or intravenously a few minutes before treatment.

It should also be noted that some inhaled steroids, e.g. fluticasone, may cause adrenal suppression. Similarly, potent topical steroids prescribed by dermatologists, e.g. eumovate, applied to large areas may also produce suppression and require steroid prophylaxis prior to dental treatment.

## USE OF ANTIBIOTICS IN ENDODONTICS

Antibiotics or other antimicrobial drugs are either bactericidal (kill susceptible bacteria) or bacteriostatic (arrest their multiplication), and so allow the natural defence processes to combat infection, and healing to progress (Table 2.2). They do not directly relieve pain nor reduce swelling and should not be used to treat pulpitis [16], but reserved to control a spreading cellulitis or a periapical abscess together with drainage. Overuse should be avoided to prevent further increase in resistant strains of organisms [25] and adherence to clinical guidelines is recommended [19].

Ideally, the choice of an antibiotic should be based on the results of identification and sensitivity testing of the micro-organisms responsible for the infection. This is seldom feasible in practice and requires culture techniques in a laboratory setting as simple Gram staining and microscopy is of little help. However, most of the bacteria associated with dentoalveolar infection are still sensitive to penicillins [15] and hence phenoxymethyl-penicillin 250 mg, or 500 mg, four times/day for five days, depending on the severity of the infection is appropriate. Amoxycillin 250 mg, three times a day, for five days

may be preferred because of its efficient absorption. Metronidazole 200 mg, or 400 mg, three times a day for five days will assist in the elimination of anaerobes and may be used alone or in combination with a penicillin. The newer penicillinase-resistant antibiotic Augmentin (amoyxcillin 250 mg and clavulanic acid 125 mg) may be preferred to this combination for ease of use and patient compliance. A potential unwanted side-effect of the use of broad-spectrum antibiotics is interference with absorption of the oestrogen component of combined oral contraceptives, with consequent loss of effect. Women taking such preparations concurrently should be advised not to rely on this method of contraception alone for one month after the end of the antibiotic course. In addition, antibiotics are known to potentiate the action of warfarin which may upset the therapeutic control. The patient should therefore be advised to contact their anticoagulant centre for appropriate follow-up.

## CONTROL OF PAIN AND ANXIETY

Pain and anxiety control are central to successful endodontic treatment. The drugs available for local analgesia and for sedation are both safe and effective, but, as with any potent therapeutic agent, need to be employed with skill and discretion,

---

**Table 2.2** Useful antibacterial drugs

**A. Treatment of infections**
*Phenoxymethyl-penicillin capsules, 250 mg*
One or two 6-hourly at least 30 minutes before food for 4–7 days
*Amoxycillin capsules, 250 mg*
One or two 8-hourly for 4–7 days
*Augmentin capsules, 375 mg*
One or two 8-hourly for 4–7 days
*Metronidazole tablets, 200 mg*
One or two 8-hourly for 5 days

**B. Infective endocarditis prophylaxis**
*Amoxycillin oral powder, 3 g sachet*
3g, administered 1 h preoperatively
*Clindamycin 150 mg capsules*
600 mg administered 1 h preoperatively

---

**Table 2.3** Useful analgesics

**Mild to moderate pain**
*Aspirin tablets, 300 mg (or aspirin tablets dispersible, 300 mg)*
One to three every 4–6 h as necessary, maximum 4 g/day
*Paracetamol tablets, 500 mg*
One to two every 6 h as necessary, maximum 4 g/day
*Ibuprofen tablets, 200 mg*
One to two every 4–6 h as necessary, preferably after food, maximum 2.4 g/day

**Moderate to severe pain**
*Dihydrocodeine tablets, 30 mg*
30 mg every 4–6 h as necessary after food, maximum 1.8 g/day

**Severe pain**
*Pethidine tablets, 25 mg*
Two to four every 4 h maximum 6 g/day

particularly in patients who are taking other medication regularly. A whole spectrum of techniques of control of pain and anxiety are applicable in endodontics as in other dental treatment (Table 2.3). These range from simple persuasion and a comforting and sympathetic manner, through to sedation. Local anaesthetic techniques are well established, and 2–4 ml lidocaine (lignocaine) 2% with 1:80 000 adrenaline (epinephrine) is a safe and effective preparation for all patients. An aspirating syringe system should be used to help to avoid inadvertent intravascular injection. Only in very rare cases where true allergy to lidocaine is proven, need an alternative solution, e.g. prilocaine with felypressin, be used.

Conscious sedation using either an inhaled mixture of nitrous oxide and oxygen, or intravenous administration of midazolam, is a safe and effective way of overcoming anxiety. Such techniques are only rarely required for root canal treatment, however, sedation may more often be required for periradicular surgery.

## Analgesics

Analgesics may be used to treat existing pain, or to reduce postoperative pain. Analgesics administered preoperatively are useful in reducing postoperative pain. Aspirin and paracetamol remain the most effective and widely used remedies for local pain of mild to moderate severity. Aspirin is contraindicated in patients with peptic ulceration, bleeding diatheses, or who are taking systemic steroids. It is also not advised in children because of the risk of causing Reye's syndrome. When paracetamol is used, it is essential to warn patients not to exceed the daily maximum dose of 4 g, because of the risk of severe and sometimes fatal liver damage. Other non-steroidal anti-inflammatory drugs (NSAIDs) such as ibuprofen may be used if preferred and may be used in combination with paracetamol if required.

Dihydrocodeine tartrate is used to relieve more severe pain, but frequently causes unpleasant side-effects, including dizziness and nausea, and may prove ineffective. On the rare occasions that severe pain persists, then pethidine 50 mg, one or two tablets four-hourly, can be given and the patient's condition reviewed the next day.

Local treatment, e.g. drainage and irrigation of a root canal, making a tooth free of occlusal contact, replacement of a failed temporary filling following root canal cleaning, or irrigation of a surgical wound, is a far more effective way of dealing with pain than the indiscriminate use of analgesics.

## DENTAL PRACTITIONERS' FORMULARY

This formulary [12], which is published together with the *British National Formulary* jointly by the British Dental Association, British Medical Association and the Royal Pharmaceutical Society of Great Britain, is a succinct and authoritative guide to prescribing for the dentist and is regularly updated. It is an invaluable source of advice and information and should be available in every dental surgery. The sections on antibiotics and analgesics as well as the tables of potential drug interactions, prescribing during pregnancy and the section on 'medical emergencies in dental practice' are particularly useful. Further information on medical aspects of dentistry, is available in *Medical Problems in Dentistry* [20].

## REFERENCES

1. American Dental Association/American Academy of Orthopaedic Surgeons (1997) Advisory statement: Antibiotic prophylaxis for dental patients with total joint replacements. *Journal of the American Dental Association* **128**, 1004–1008.
2. Ardekian L, Gaspar R, Peled M, Brener B, Layfer D (2000) Does low-dose aspirin therapy complicate oral surgical procedures? *Journal of the American Dental Association* **131**, 331–335.
3. Baumgartner JC, Heggers JP, Harrison JW (1976) The incidence of bacteremias related to endodontic procedures. I. Nonsurgical endodontics. *Journal of Endodontics* **2**, 135–140.
4. Baumgartner JC, Heggers JP, Harrison JW (1977) Incidence of bacteremias related to endodontic procedures. II. Surgical endodontics. *Journal of Endodontics* **3**, 399–402.
5. Beck-Mannagetta J, Necek D (1986) Radiologic findings in aspergillosis of the maxillary sinus. *Oral Surgery, Oral Medicine, Oral Pathology* **62**, 345–349.
6. British Dental Association (2003) *Infection Control in Dentistry*. London: British Dental Association.
7. British Society for Antimicrobial Chemotherapy (1982) The antibiotic prophylaxis of infective endocarditis. *Lancet* **2**, 1323–1326.

8. British Society for Antimicrobial Chemotherapy (1986) Prophylaxis of infective endocarditis. *Lancet* **1**, 1267.

9. British Society for Antimicrobial Chemotherapy (1990) Antibiotic prophylaxis of infective endocarditis. *Lancet* **335**, 88–89.

10. British Society for Antimicrobial Chemotherapy (1992) Case against antibiotic prophylaxis for dental treatment of patients with joint prostheses. *Lancet* **339**, 301.

11. British Society for Antimicrobial Chemotherapy (1992) Antibiotic prophylaxis and infective endocarditis. *Lancet* **339**, 1292–1293.

12. *Dental Practitioners' Formulary* (May 2002) London: British Medical Association.

13. DePaola LG, Peterson DE, Overholser CD, *et al.* (1986) Dental care for patients receiving chemotherapy. *Journal of the American Dental Association* **112**, 198–203.

14. Hampton JR, Harrison MJ, Mitchell JR, Pritchard JS, Seymour C (1975) Relative contributions of history-taking, physical examination and laboratory investigations to diagnosis and management of medical outpatients. *British Medical Journal* **2**, 486–489.

15. Lewis MAO, McGowan DA, MacFarlane TW (1986) Short-course high-dosage amoxycillin in the treatment of acute dento-alveolar abscess. *British Dental Journal* **161**, 299–302.

16. Nagle D, Reader A, Beck M, Weaver J (2000) Effect of systemic penicillin on pain in untreated irreversible pulpitis. *Oral Surgery, Oral Medicine, Oral Pathology, Oral Radiology and Endodontics* **90**, 636–640.

17. Nasstrom K, Forsberg B, Petersson A, Westesson PL (1985) Narrowing of the dental pulp chamber in patients with renal diseases. *Oral Surgery, Oral Medicine, Oral Pathology* **59**, 242–246.

18. Roshan M, Rao AP, (2000) A study on relative contributions of the history, physical examination and investigations in making medical diagnosis. *Journal of the Association of Physicians of India* **48**, 771–775.

19. *Adult Antimicrobial Prescribing in Primary Dental Care for General Dental Practitioners* (2000). Faculty of General Dental Practitioners, Royal College of Surgeons of England, London, UK.

20. Scully C, Cawson RA (1998) *Medical Problems in Dentistry.* 4th edn. Oxford: Butterworth-Heinemann.

21. Solomon PE, Prkachin KM, Farewell V (1997) Enhancing sensitivity to facial expression of pain. *Pain* **71**, 279–284.

22. Surgical management of the primary care dental patient on warfarin. www.ukmi.nhs.uk/med_info/documents/Dental_Patient_on_Warfarin.pdf.

23. Whooley MA, Avins AL, Miranda J, Browner WS (1997) Case-finding instruments for depression. Two questions are as good as many. *Journal of General Internal Medicine* **12**, 439–445.

24. Williams JW, Aguiler C, Makela M, Cornell J, Hollman DR, Chiquette E, Simel DL (2002) *Antibiotics for Acute Maxillary Sinusitis* (Cochrane Review). The Cochrane Library, Issue 3, Oxford.

25. World Health Organization (2001) *Antibiotic Resistance: Synthesis of Recommendations by Expert Policy Groups.* Online. Available: http://www.who.int/csr/drugresist/Antimicrobial_resistance_recommendations_of_expert_polic.pdf.

26. Zakrzewska J, Harrison SD (2002) In: Pain research and clinical management: Volume 14, Assessment and management of orofacial pain. Amsterdam: Elsevier.

# 3

# Pulp space anatomy and access cavities

T. R. Pitt Ford

Introduction  17

Nomenclature  18

Accessory and lateral canals  19

Location of apical foramina  20

Variations in pulp space anatomy  21

Effects of irritation dentine on pulp space  21

Pulp space anatomy and access cavities  22
  Maxillary central and lateral incisors  22
  Maxillary canine  23
  Maxillary first premolar  23
  Maxillary second premolar  25
  Maxillary first molar  25
  Maxillary second molar  27
  Maxillary third molar  27
  Mandibular central and lateral incisors  27
  Mandibular canine  28
  Mandibular premolars  29
  Mandibular first molar  30
  Mandibular second molar  31
  Mandibular third molar  31

Pulp space anatomy of primary teeth  32
  Primary incisors and canines  32
  Primary molars  33

Apical closure  33

References  33

## INTRODUCTION

The major factors involved in the development of apical periodontitis are loss of integrity of coronal tooth substance and the entry of microorganisms into the dentine and pulp space. The chemo-mechanical removal of microorganisms, their substrate and products from the dentine and pulp space is the primary aim of root canal treatment, with the second being the three dimensional obliteration and sealing of the pulp space to prevent bacterial recontamination.

A clear understanding of the anatomy of human teeth becomes an essential prerequisite to achieving the objectives of access, thorough cleaning, disinfection, and obturation of the pulp space. Many of the problems encountered during endodontic treatment occur because of an inadequate understanding of the pulp space anatomy of teeth or the pulp response to irritation. Both students and clinicians alike need to familiarize themselves with the irregularities, complexities and aberrations that are likely to occur within the pulp space. The importance of developing a visual picture of the expected locations and numbers of canals in a particular tooth cannot be overstressed.

Clinical radiographs show the forms of roots and pulp canals in two planes only. A third plane exists in a buccolingual direction. The pulp space volume is always much greater than the normal clinical radiograph would suggest. The internal anatomy of human teeth has been studied by many investigators, who have provided a valuable insight into the size, shape and form of the pulp space. Methods of study have included replication techniques [10,20,30,65], ground sections [3,24,62], clearing techniques [36,45,53,58,82,84] and radiography [5,35,41,42,48, 49,57,59,68,98]. Present-day knowledge of pulp space anatomy is based on research findings and individual case reports.

## NOMENCLATURE

Anatomically, the dental pulp space is surrounded by dentine to form the pulp-dentine complex. Dentine forms the bulk of the mineralized tissue of the tooth. The dentinal tubules, which are interconnected, make up 20–30% of the total volume of dentine [21,31]. The number of tubules per square millimetre more than doubles and the area occupied by tubules increases three-fold from the dentine near the amelodentinal junction, to that near the pulp [16]. These differences have a significant clinical effect on the permeability of dentine. It is now realized that the dentinal tubules are an important reservoir of microorganisms when pulpal necrosis occurs [52]. Exposure of infected tubules during root-end resection may serve as a direct route of contamination from unclean root canals into the periradicular tissues [26,73].

The *pulp space* is divided into two parts: the *pulp chamber*, which is usually described as that portion within the crown; and the *pulp canal* or *root canal*, which lies within the confines of the root. The pulp chamber is a single cavity, the dimensions of which vary according to the outline of the crown and the structure of the roots. Thus if the crown has well-developed cusps the pulp chamber projects into well-developed *pulp horns*. In multirooted teeth the depth of the pulp chamber depends upon the position of the root furcation and may extend beyond the anatomical crown. In young teeth the outline of the pulp chamber resembles the shape of the exterior of the dentine. With age the dentinal tubules and the pulp chamber become reduced in size by the laying down of *intratubular dentine, secondary dentine* and *irritation dentine* particularly in areas where there has been caries, tooth wear and exposure to operative treatment (Fig. 3.1). The pulp chamber may then become irregular in outline. There is also a gradual decrease with age in pulp space volume, the number of nerves, blood vessels and cells within, but an increase in the fibrous and mineral components. The rate at which pulps age, varies from one tooth to another, and from one

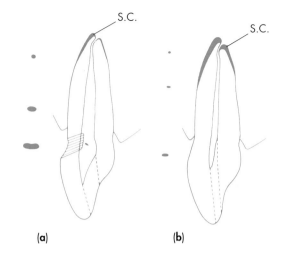

**Figure 3.1** Alteration of pulp size with age. (**a**) Tooth of young adult; large pulp chamber with irritation dentine under tubules affected by cervical abrasion; small amount of secondary cementum (SC) at apex. (**b**) Tooth of older patient showing smaller pulp space and greater amounts of secondary cementum that have altered the relationship of the apical constriction to the foramen. Access cavities are indicated by dotted lines. To the left: cross-sections of the root canals are shown at selected levels.

patient to another. Calcific changes can lead to the pulp space appearing entirely obliterated radiologically. A residual canal, although radiologically unidentified, may remain within the root and be the route for bacteria to reach the apex and cause a periradicular radiolucency.

The pulp of root canals is continuous with the pulp chamber and normally the greatest diameter is at the pulp chamber level. Because roots tend to taper towards their apex, the canals also have a tapering form which is constricted at the end, *apical constriction*, before emerging at the *apical foramina*, near the root end; rarely do foramina open at the exact anatomical apex of the tooth. During root development the pulp and periodontal tissues become separated, maintaining neural and vascular connections through the apical foramina.

The pulp space is complex and canals may divide and rejoin, and possess forms that are considerably more involved than many textbooks of anatomy have implied. Many roots have additional canals and a variety of canal configurations. Eight separate pulp space configurations have been identified [84] (Fig. 3.2). Generally, roots have a single canal and

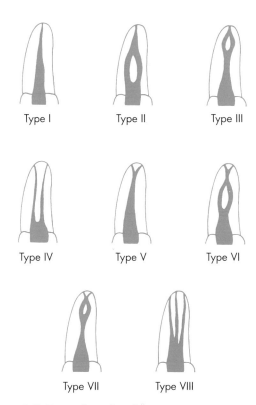

Type I  Type II  Type III

Type IV  Type V  Type VI

Type VII  Type VIII

**Figure 3.2** Types of canal configuration.

single apical foramen (Type I); it is not uncommon, however, for other canal complexities to be present and exit the root as one, two or three apical canals (Types II–VIII).

Since roots tend to be broader buccolingually than they are mesiodistally, the pulp space is similar and oval in cross-section. The diameter of the root canal decreases towards the apical foramen and reaches its narrowest point 1.0–1.5 mm from the foramen. This point, the apical constriction lies within dentine just prior to the first layers of cementum and is the narrowest point to which the canal tapers.

During root development the apical part of the pulp is described as being 'open'. As the tooth matures, the funnel-shaped foramen closes and constricts to a normal root shape with a small apical foramen. The position of the apical foramen may also alter its position relative to the root apex with the deposition of secondary cementum.

## ACCESSORY AND LATERAL CANALS

The pulpal and periodontal tissues not only maintain connection through the apical foramina but also through *accessory* and *lateral* canals. A lateral canal can be found anywhere along the length of a root and tends to be at right angles to the main root

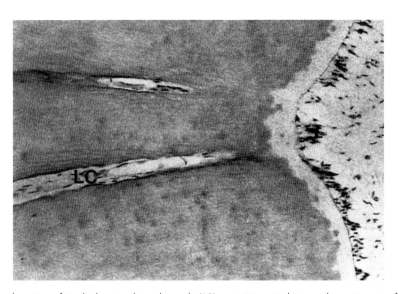

**Figure 3.3** Histological section of tooth showing lateral canals (LC) containing vital tissue; the main part of the pulp is to the right.

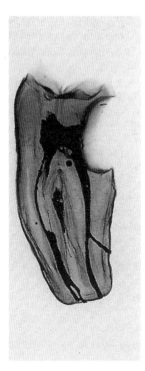

**Figure 3.4** Cleared mandibular molar with a lateral canal in the distal root.

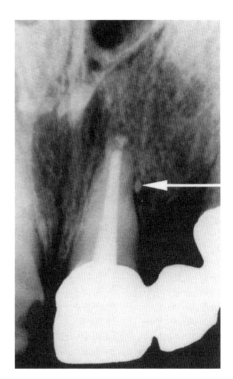

**Figure 3.5** Radiograph of root-filled incisor showing sealer in a lateral canal and excess in the periradicular tissues (arrowed).

canal. Accessory canals usually branch off the main root canal somewhere in the apical region. The presence of lateral canals in the furcation areas of molar teeth is well documented and their incidence is relatively high. Patent lateral canals are present in the coronal or middle third of 59% of molars [44]; 76% of molars are reported to have openings in the furcation [9]. It has been shown using a vascular injection technique that these accessory canals often had a greater diameter than the apical foramina, and the blood vessels passing through them often had a greater diameter than those in the apical foramina [38]. The accessory and lateral canals may be demonstrated by histological examination (Fig. 3.3), clearing techniques (Fig. 3.4), or clinical radiographs (Fig. 3.5). The presence of these canals in teeth with necrotic pulps allows bacterial toxins to stimulate inflammatory responses in the periradicular tissues.

## LOCATION OF APICAL FORAMINA

The majority of endodontists consider that the apical extent of canal preparation should be determined by the position of the apical constriction in the region of the dentine–cementum junction (Fig. 3.6). Provided that this constriction is not destroyed, the periradicular tissues are not damaged during root canal preparation and obturation.

Studies indicate that the apical foramen rarely coincides in position with the anatomical apex. According to various radiological and morphological studies of different teeth [2,8,13,17,22,23,37,40, 43,80], the mean distance between the apical foramen and the most apical end of the root is between 0.2 and 2.0 mm. Furthermore, the apical constriction tends to occur about 0.5–1 mm from the apical foramen [13]. Ideally the apical constriction should be used as a natural 'stop' in root canal treatment, and the integrity of the constriction should be maintained during treatment if complications are to be avoided. This position can usually be located accurately with an apex locator [34,64].

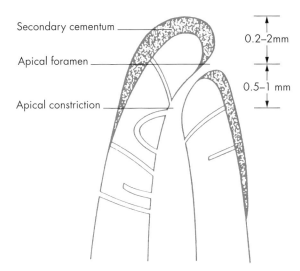

Secondary cementum

0.2–2mm

Apical foramen

0.5–1 mm

Apical constriction

**Figure 3.6** Diagrammatic section through apical third of root. The position of the apical foramen varies with age and may be 0.2–2.0 mm from the anatomical apex. The apical constriction may be 0.5–1.0 mm from the foramen.

## VARIATIONS IN PULP SPACE ANATOMY

Variations in tooth form have interested scientists and anthropologists as well as dentists. These studies of variation have primarily been concentrated on the systematic description of dental crown morphology rather than root form. Variations in root form and number are likely to have a direct influence upon the configuration of the root canals in affected teeth. One variation, which has received some attention, is the three-rooted mandibular first molar; surveys of mongoloid populations indicate a high prevalence [54,75,77,78]. The prevalence of other mongoloid root traits has been less well studied. In clinical practice it is not always possible to observe these variations from radiographs.

In the condition *dens invaginatus*, the surface of the tooth was formed into a deep pit into the pulp space during tooth development, and it is subsequently a route for infection into the pulp. Depending on the severity of the condition, endododontic treatment will be difficult or very challenging. The most commonly affected tooth is the maxillary lateral incisor [15,32].

In the opposite condition *dens evaginatus*, the surface of the tooth was formed into a very

protuberant cusp during tooth development. There is a high risk of this cusp being fractured off during function. This creates a route for infection to enter the pulp space. The mandibular premolar is most frequently affected and is more often found in mongoloid people [79]. It is best managed by prophylactic treatment [39].

The descriptions of the frequently occurring root and canal forms of permanent teeth are based largely on studies conducted in Europe and North America, and relate to teeth of predominantly caucasoid origin. The descriptions may not be wholly applicable to teeth of non-caucasoid origin. For example, the average lengths of teeth, around which there is wide variation, apply to caucasoid populations. Practitioners who regularly treat mongoloid populations are aware that roots are usually shorter.

## EFFECTS OF IRRITATION DENTINE ON PULP SPACE

Irritation dentine is formed by odontoblasts in response to irritation from caries, restorative dentistry or tooth wear. The amount formed is dependent on the degree and duration of irritation. The function of this dentine is to wall off the pulp from the irritants; it is generally of great benefit to operative dentists. However, when root canal treatment becomes indicated, the coronal pulp is then exceedingly small and therefore difficult to locate. In addition, canal orifices become narrowed by deposition of irritation dentine making their identification difficult.

There is no substitute for a good knowledge of pulpal anatomy, however the clinician is aided by a good quality preoperative radiograph, from which the depth and direction of the root canals can be gauged. The correct application of a rubber dam clamp can indicate the central position of the pulp. When inside the centre of the tooth and attempting to locate the pulp space, illumination and magnification are a major asset. Whilst this can be provided by a headlamp and loupes, it is best achieved by a surgical microscope. The increased illumination reveals the different colours of circumpulpal and irritation dentine, so that the access to the root canals can be correctly orientated.

## PULP SPACE ANATOMY AND ACCESS CAVITIES

Each line drawing (Figs 3.7–3.28) accompanying the description of pulp space anatomy represents, from left to right:

- longitudinal mesiodistal section, viewed from the lingual in anterior teeth and from the buccal in posterior teeth;
- longitudinal buccolingual section viewed from the mesial, and also the axial angulation of the tooth relative to the horizontal occlusal plane;
- horizontal sections through the root(s): (above) 3 mm from apex; (below) at the cervical level;
- incisal or occlusal view.

The outline of the access cavity is shown as a dotted line. The size of the pulp cavity shortly after completion of root formation is shown as a shaded area, and in old age by a black area. Line drawings are accompanied by photographs of cleared specimens to give an insight into the variations of canal form that exist in the adult dentition.

### Maxillary central and lateral incisors

The outlines and pulp cavities of these teeth are similar (Figs 3.7 and 3.8). Central incisors are larger with a mean length of 23 mm. Lateral incisors are shorter with a mean length of 21–22 mm. The canal form is usually Type I, and it is extremely rare for these teeth to have more than one root or more than

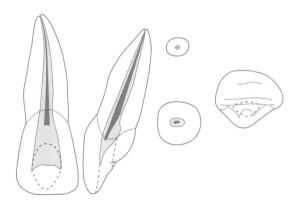

**Figure 3.7** Maxillary central incisor with a type I configuration.

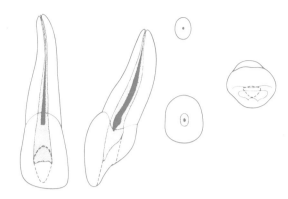

**Figure 3.8** Maxillary lateral incisor with a type I configuration.

one root canal. Where abnormalities do occur they seem to affect the maxillary lateral incisor, which may present with an extra root, second root canal, dens invaginatus, gemination or fusion [7,29,60,72,].

The pulp chamber, when viewed labiopalatally, is seen to be pointed towards the incisal and widest at the cervical level. Mesiodistally both pulp chambers follow the general outline of their crowns and are thus widest at their incisal levels. The central incisors of young patients normally have three pulp horns. Lateral incisors usually have two pulp horns, and the incisal outline of the pulp chamber tends to be more rounded than that of central incisors.

The root canal differs greatly in outline when viewed mesiodistally and labiopalatally. The former view generally shows a fine straight canal that is seen on a radiograph. Labiopalatally the canal is very much wider and often shows a constriction just apical to the cervix; this view is rarely seen on radiographs and it is important to remember that all canals have this third dimension when they are being treated. The canal is tapered with an oval or irregular cross-section cervically that becomes round only very near the apex. There is generally very little apical curvature in central incisors. However, the apex of lateral incisors is often curved, generally in a distal/palatal direction.

As the teeth age the anatomy of the pulp space alters with the deposition of secondary dentine. The roof of the pulp chamber recedes, in some cases to the cervical level, and the canal appears very narrow mesiodistally on a radiograph. It is often possible to negotiate a canal that appears very fine or non-existent on a preoperative radiograph. When some incisors are traumatized, their pulps may mineralize, that is, pulp canal obliteration; and subsequent root canal treatment is extremely difficult as mineralization frequently occurs throughout the length of the pulp space.

### Access cavities to maxillary incisors

Access cavities in anterior teeth will vary in size and shape according to the dimension of the pulp. They should be designed so that instruments can reach the apical third of the root without bending, or binding against the walls of the access cavity or root canal. An access cavity that is too small and close to the cingulum leads to severe stresses in the instrument with binding against the access cavity walls and possible ledge formation apically (Fig. 3.9).

The access cavity should extend far enough incisally to allow the instrument to reach the apical part of the canal. Sometimes the incisal edge must be involved if access is to be adequate.

As the pulp is broader incisally than it is cervically the outline should be triangular and must extend far enough mesially and distally to include the pulp horns. Once adequate access has been made into the pulp chamber, the cervical constriction should

be removed by files or Gates-Glidden burs to facilitate instrumentation of the apical part.

Correct access cavity design is particularly important in the older patient because the pulp space is more difficult to find. It is wise to design the access cavity close to the incisal edge so that the pulp space can be approached in a straight line.

### Maxillary canine

This is the longest tooth (mean length 26.5 mm), and therefore longer root canal files are often required. It seldom has more than one root canal; the pulp chamber is quite narrow, and as there is only one pulp horn the pulp is pointed incisally. The general shape of the pulp space is similar to the incisors (Fig. 3.10).

The Type I root canal is oval and does not begin to become circular in cross-section until the apical third. The canal is usually straight but may show a distal apical curvature; the curvature depends on the movement of the tooth during eruption.

### Maxillary first premolar

This tooth generally has two roots with two canals. The frequency of single-rooted maxillary first premolars ranges 31–39% in caucasians [6,10,49,85]. In people of mongoloid origin the frequency of maxillary first premolars with one root is in excess of 60% [50,55,89,90]. Three roots have been reported in 6% [10]. A typical caucasoid specimen has two well-developed fully formed roots that normally begin in the middle third of the root (Fig. 3.11). The

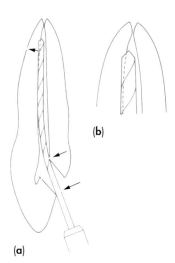

(b)

(a)

**Figure 3.9** (a) The access cavity is too small and close to the cingulum, therefore instruments do not lie passively in the canal and may create a ledge apically. The incorrect access also hinders cleaning of the pulp chamber and near the apex. (b) Enlargement of the apex showing labial ledge and uninstrumented palatal side.

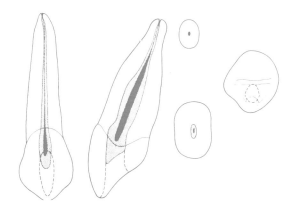

**Figure 3.10** Maxillary canine with a type I configuration.

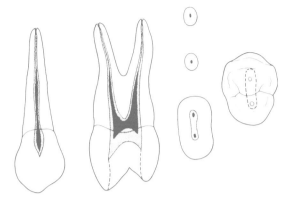

**Figure 3.11** Maxillary first premolar with two roots.

single-rooted condition prevalent in mongoloid people represents a fusion of two separate roots.

Irrespective of origin, this tooth normally has two canals, and in the case of single-rooted specimens these canals may open through a common apical foramen. Many types of canal configuration are to be found in this tooth (Fig. 3.12) and the presence of

lateral canals, particularly in the apical region can be as high as 49% [85]. The three-rooted form tends to have three canals, two located buccally and one palatally. Careful study of a preoperative radiograph should reveal the root morphology.

The mean length of first premolars is 21 mm. The pulp chamber is wide buccopalatally with two distinct pulp horns, but it is much narrower mesiodistally. The floor is rounded with the highest point in the centre and generally just apical to the level of the cervix. The orifices into the root canals are funnel-shaped and lie buccally and palatally. As the tooth ages the dimensions of the pulp chamber do not alter appreciably except in a cervico-occlusal direction. Secondary dentine is deposited on the roof of the pulp chamber and this has the effect of bringing the roof very much closer to the floor. The floor level remains apical to the cervix and the thickened roof may reach apical to the cervix. The root canals are normally separate, and very rarely blend into the ribbon-like type of canal frequently seen in the second premolar. They are usually straight with a round cross-section.

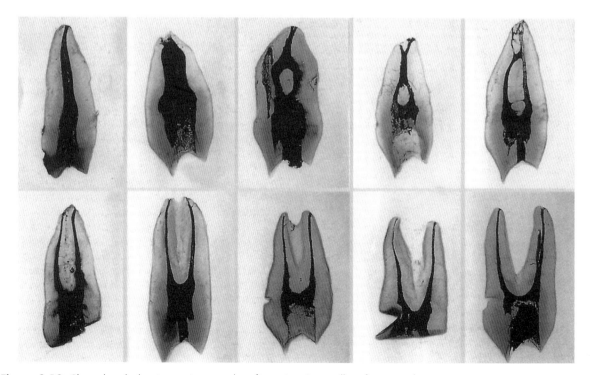

**Figure 3.12** Cleared teeth showing various canal configurations in maxillary first premolars.

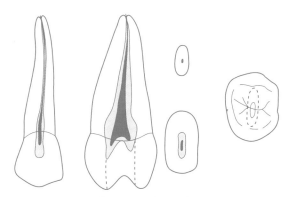

**Figure 3.13** Maxillary second premolar with a type I canal configuration.

## Maxillary second premolar

The maxillary second premolar tends to be single-rooted. The Type I canal form is prevalent; however, over 25% of these teeth may present as Types II and III, and a further 25% may have Types IV–VII forms with two canals at the apex [86,89]. Thus the typical maxillary second premolar may be envisaged as having one root with a single canal (Fig. 3.13). Less frequently two roots may be present, and while the outward appearance may be similar to the first premolar the floor of the pulp chamber is well apical to the cervix. The mean length of the second premolar is slightly longer than the first at 21.5 mm.

The pulp chamber is wide buccopalatally and has two well-defined pulp horns. The root canal is also wide buccopalatally but narrow mesiodistally. It tapers apically but rarely develops a circular cross-section except in the apical 2–3 mm. Often the root of this single-rooted tooth branches into two sections in the middle third of the root. These branches almost invariably join to form a common canal, which has a relatively large foramen. The canal is usually straight but the apex may curve to the distal. As the tooth matures the roof of the pulp chamber recedes away from the crown.

### Access cavities to maxillary premolars

Access must always be through the occlusal surface, to allow files to negotiate the canals. The shape of the access cavity is ovoid in a buccolingual direction. In the case of the first premolar the orifices of the root canal are readily visible as they lie just apical to the cervix. The second premolar root canal is ribbon-shaped and, because it lies well apical to the cervix, may not be readily visible. In preparing an access cavity, an inexperienced operator may incorrectly assume that the pulp horns are the canal orifices.

## Maxillary first molar

Maxillary first molars are generally three-rooted with four root canals (Fig. 3.14). The additional canal is located in the mesiobuccal root. The canal form of the mesiobuccal root has been thoroughly investigated. Studies *in vitro* indicate that a second canal is present in up to 74% of teeth [33,41,56,57,58,62, 71,81]. Canal configuration is usually Type II (Fig. 3.15), however the presence of a Type IV form with two separate apical foramina has been reported to be as high as 48% [57]. Studies in vivo have produced much lower figures for the prevalence of the second mesiobuccal canal, and show the difficulty in locating the extra canal when a surgical microscope is not available. In clinical studies mesiobuccal

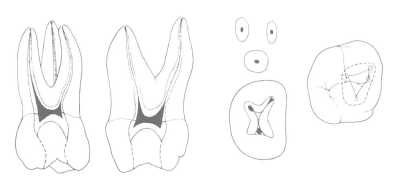

**Figure 3.14** Maxillary first molar.

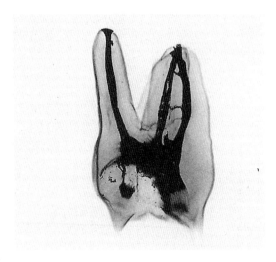

**Figure 3.15** Cleared maxillary first molar with a type II canal configuration in the mesiobuccal root.

roots with two canals could only be demonstrated in up to 50% [1,28,58,62,66,94]. The palatal and distobuccal roots usually present a Type I configuration.

In caucasians, the length of this tooth is 22 mm, the palatal root being slightly longer than the buccal roots. In mongoloid teeth there is a tendency for the roots to be closer together and the average length slightly shorter. The pulp chamber is quadrilateral in shape and wider buccopalatally than mesiodistally. It has four pulp horns, of which the mesiobuccal is the longest and sharpest in outline. The distobuccal pulp horn is smaller than the mesiobuccal but larger than the two palatal pulp horns. The floor of the pulp chamber is normally just apical to the cervix, and is rounded and convex towards the occlusal. The orifices of the main pulp canals are funnel-shaped and lie in the middle of the appropriate root. The second mesiobuccal canal, if present, lies on a line joining the main mesiobuccal and palatal canal orifices. If this line is divided into thirds, the second mesiobuccal canal is normally found near the first division adjacent to the main mesiobuccal canal under a lip of dentine (Fig. 3.14). Further, the transverse cross-sectional shape of the pulp chamber 1 mm above the pulpal floor is trapezoidal in most teeth [71]. For this reason the mesiobuccal canal opening is closer to the buccal wall than is the distobuccal orifice. The distobuccal root (and hence the opening into the root canal) is closer to the middle of the tooth than to the distal wall. The palatal

root canal orifice lies in the middle of the palatal root and is normally easy to identify.

The cross-section of the root canals varies considerably. The mesiobuccal canals are usually the most difficult to instrument because they leave the pulp chamber in a mesial direction. The second mesiobuccal canal is generally very fine and tortuous and usually joins the main canal. The orifice of this canal may be concealed by a dentine lip, which needs to be removed to detect the orifice [74]. As both mesiobuccal canals lie in a buccopalatal plane they are often superimposed on the preoperative radiograph. A further complication occurs because the mesiobuccal root often curves distopalatally in the apical third of the root.

The distobuccal canal is the shortest and finest of the three canals and leaves the pulp chamber in a distal direction. It is ovoid in shape and again narrower mesiodistally. It tapers towards the apex and becomes circular in cross-section. The canal normally curves mesially in the apical half of the root.

The palatal canal is the largest and longest of the three canals and leaves the pulp chamber as a round canal, which gradually tapers apically. In 50% of roots it is not straight but curves buccally in the apical 4–5 mm. This curvature is not apparent on a clinical radiograph.

As the tooth ages the canals become much finer, and the canal orifices become more difficult to find. Secondary dentine is deposited chiefly on the roof of the pulp chamber; thus the pulp chamber becomes very narrow between roof and floor. The presence of irritation dentine further complicates canal location. It is relatively easy for the inexperienced operator (particularly with high-speed handpieces) to perforate the floor of the pulp chamber. To prevent this accident it is important to measure on a preoperative radiograph, taken by the paralleling technique, the distance from cusp tips to roof of the pulp chamber. This distance may then be marked on the bur as a depth gauge. It is wise to restrict the use of high-speed handpieces to removal of superficial tooth substance or restorative materials, and to complete the access cavity with a round bur in a low-speed handpiece.

The variable nature of the pulp space anatomy of the maxillary first molar has received emphasis in recent clinical case reports. The occurrence of teeth

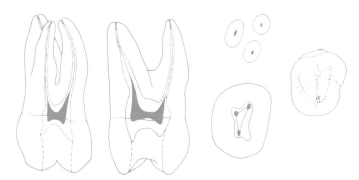

**Figure 3.16** Maxillary second molar.

with two palatal roots and multiple palatal canals has been reported [4,11,27,67,70,96].

## Maxillary second molar

The maxillary second molar is usually a smaller replica of the first molar (Fig. 3.16). The roots are less divergent, and fusion between two roots is much more frequent than in the maxillary first molar. Teeth with three canals and three apical foramina are prevalent, but a recent study has shown a high incidence of second mesiobuccal canals [51]; the mean length is 21 mm.

Root fusion has been demonstrated in up to 55% of caucasoid maxillary second molars [18,88], while in mongoloid groups this figure may be up to 85% [54,77,89]. Where root fusion does occur, canals and their orifices are much closer together (Fig. 3.17).

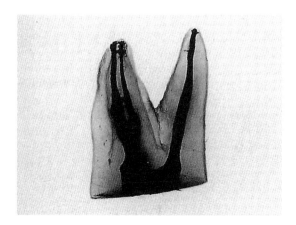

**Figure 3.17** Cleared maxillary second molar with fused buccal roots.

## Maxillary third molar

The maxillary third molar displays a great deal of variability. It may possess three separate roots, but more often partial or complete fusion occurs [51]. The pulp space anatomy is less predictable and these teeth may have a reduced number of canals. Root canal treatment is not frequently undertaken because of a lack of clinical indications and restricted access.

### Access cavities to maxillary molars

The traditional access cavity outline for maxillary teeth is normally in the mesial two-thirds of the occlusal surface leaving the oblique ridge intact, and is triangular with the base of the triangle towards the buccal, and the apex palatally. It has been suggested that this traditional shape should be modified in the case of the first molar to a trapezoid shape [94]. Because the distobuccal canal is not as close to the buccal surface as the mesiobuccal canal, less tooth need be removed from this area. The walls of the occlusal half of the access cavity should flare occlusally to prevent the accidental forcing of the temporary filling into the pulp chamber during mastication, and thus prevent bacterial contamination occurring between visits.

## Mandibular central and lateral incisors

Both teeth have a mean length of 21 mm, although the central incisor may be a little shorter than the lateral incisor. The root canal morphology may be placed into one of three configurations [5]:

27

- *Type I* – a single main canal extending from the pulp chamber to the apical foramen (Fig. 3.18).
- *Type II/III* – two main root canals that merge in the middle or apical third of the root into a single canal with one apical foramen (Fig. 3.19).
- *Type IV* – two main canals that remain distinct throughout the length of the tooth and exit through two major apical foramina (Fig. 3.20).

Studies indicate that the Type I canal form is most prevalent, Types II and III less prevalent, and Type IV least prevalent. The presence of two canals has been recorded to be as high as 41% [5]; however, the highest recorded figure for two separate apical foramina (Type IV) is 5% [59]. There is some evidence to suggest that there is a lower frequency of

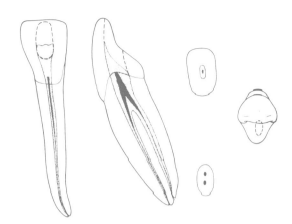

**Figure 3.20** Mandibular lateral incisor with a type IV canal configuration.

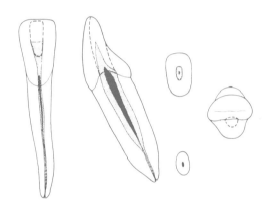

**Figure 3.18** Mandibular central incisor with a type I canal configuration.

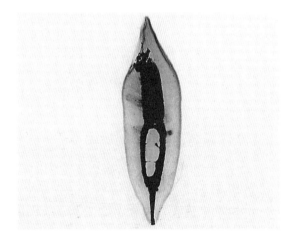

**Figure 3.19** Cleared mandibular central incisor with a type II canal configuration.

two canals in mandibular central and lateral incisors in mongoloid people [91].

The pulp chamber is a smaller replica of that in the maxillary incisors. It is pointed incisally with three pulp horns that are not well developed, is oval in cross-section, and wider labiolingually than it is mesiodistally. When the tooth has a single root canal it is normally straight but may curve to the distal and less often to the labial. The tooth ages in a similar way to the maxillary incisors, and the incisal part of the pulp chamber may recede to a level apical to the cervix. The pulps of these teeth may mineralize in response to traumatic injury.

### Mandibular canine

This tooth resembles the maxillary canine, although its dimensions are smaller. It rarely has two roots and the mean length is 22.5 mm. The Type I canal form is most prevalent (Fig. 3.21); the frequency of two canals is 14% [35]. However, less than 6% of mandibular canines display the Type IV canal form with two separate apical foramina [57,82].

### Access cavities to mandibular incisors and canines

Essentially these cavities are similar to those in maxillary incisors. However, because of the more pronounced labial curvature of the crown and because the canals (particularly in older patients) are so fine, it is sometimes necessary to involve the incisal edge of the tooth.

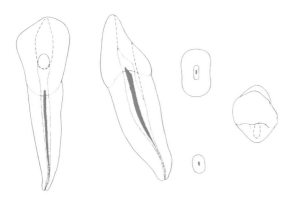

**Figure 3.21** Mandibular canine with a type I canal configuration.

## Mandibular premolars

These teeth are usually single-rooted; however, the mandibular first premolar may occasionally present with a division of roots in the apical half. The Type I canal configuration is the most prevalent (Fig. 3.22). Where two canals are present they are more prevalent in the first premolar and may involve up to one-third of teeth [57,76,83,89]. Additional canals may be suspected if the root canal that is visible in the coronal part of the root appears to stop abruptly as it is traced apically. Where division of canals occurs, the tendency is for them to remain separate to produce a Type IV/V form (Fig. 3.23). The Type II/III forms are seen in less than 5% of these teeth (Fig. 3.24). The highest reported frequency of a second canal in second premolars is 11% [98]. Less than 2% of first premolars have three canals

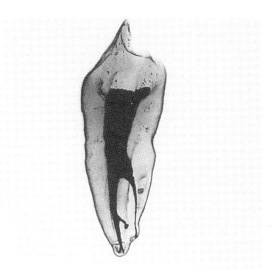

**Figure 3.23** Cleared mandibular first premolar with a type IV canal configuration and a lateral canal.

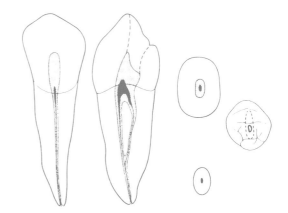

**Figure 3.24** Mandibular first premolar with a type II canal configuration.

[57,83,89,98]. The presence of multiple canals has been reported [12,61,63,95].

In one report, African Americans had nearly three times as many mandibular first premolars with more than one canal than caucasian patients [76]. A study of mandibular first premolars in the southern Chinese population of Hong Kong would also seem to indicate a high prevalence of teeth with more than one canal [89].

The pulp chamber is wide buccolingually, and while there are two pulp horns, only the buccal is well developed. The lingual pulp horn is very slight in the first premolar but better developed in the

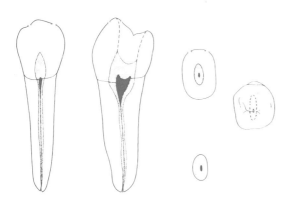

**Figure 3.22** Mandibular second premolar with a type I canal configuration.

second premolar. The canals of these two teeth are similar, although smaller than the canines, and are thus wide buccolingually until they reach the middle third of the root, where they constrict.

### Access cavities to mandibular premolars

These must be through the occlusal surface. In the first premolar with two canals it may be necessary to extend the cavity onto the buccal surface.

## Mandibular first molar

The mandibular first molar usually has two roots, a mesial and a distal. The latter is smaller and usually rounder than the mesial. There is a mongoloid variation in which there exists a supernumerary distolingual root; the frequency of this trait ranges from 6 to 44% [25,92]. The two-rooted molar usually has a canal configuration of three canals (Fig. 3.25), and the mean length is 21 mm. Two canals are usually located in the mesial root with one in the distal. The mesial root in 40–45% of cases has only one apical foramen [57,65,87]. The single distal canal is usually larger, centrally placed buccolingually and more oval in cross-section than the mesial canals, and in 60% of cases emerges on the distal side of the root surface short of the anatomical apex [69].

The incidence of two distal canals in mandibular first molars has been reported as 38% [65]. The orifices are sited buccal and lingual, and are small. The tendency for the mandibular first molar in mongoloid people to have three roots appears to be associated with the frequency of the second distal canal, which approaches half of these teeth [92].

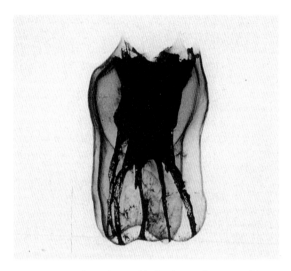

**Figure 3.26** Cleared mandibular first molar viewed from the mesial showing five canals.

Specimens with three canals in the mesial root [19] and a total of five canals have also been observed (Fig. 3.26).

The pulp chamber is wider mesially than it is distally and may have five pulp horns, the lingual pulp horns being longer and more pointed. The floor is rounded and convex toward the occlusal and lies just apical to the cervix. The root canals leave the pulp chamber through funnel-shaped openings of which the mesial tend to be much finer than the distal. Of the two mesial canals, the mesiobuccal is the more difficult canal to negotiate because of its tortuous path. It leaves the pulp chamber in a mesial direction, which alters to a distal direction in the middle third of the root. The

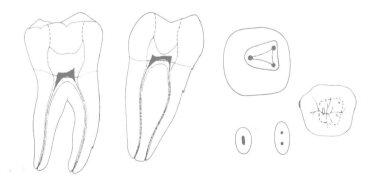

**Figure 3.25** Mandibular first molar, with a type IV canal configuration in the mesial root (second from left).

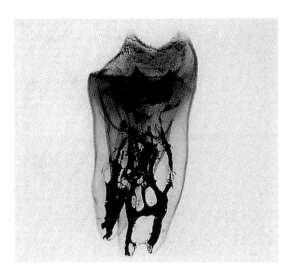

**Figure 3.27** Cleared mandibular first molar viewed from the mesiobuccal showing connections between the mesial canals.

mesiolingual canal is slightly larger in cross-section and generally follows a much straighter course, although it may curve mesially towards the apical part. These canals may have a latticework arrangement of connections along their length (Fig. 3.27). When a second distal canal is present on the distolingual aspect it tends to curve towards the buccal. With age the pulp chamber recedes from the occlusal surface and the canals become constricted.

## Mandibular second molar

In caucasoid populations the mandibular second molar presents as a smaller version of the mandibular

first molar with a mean length of 20 mm. The mesial root has two canals and, unlike the first molar, there is usually only one distal canal. The mesial canals tend to fuse in the apical third to give rise to one main apical foramen (Fig. 3.28).

Studies [14,46,47,93,97] have highlighted the tendency for mandibular second molars to have fused roots in up to 52% of the Chinese. The fusion gives rise to a horseshoe shape when the roots are viewed in cross-section. Where there is incomplete separation of roots there may also be incomplete division of canals giving rise to the C-shaped canal, which increases the likelihood of canal interconnections and unpredictably placed canal orifices. One such orifice has now been termed the median buccal canal orifice [97], which leads to the median buccal canal (Fig. 3.29).

## Mandibular third molar

The form of this tooth is often very varied. It generally has as many root canals as there are cusps. The roots and thus the pulp canals are normally shorter than other molars. It is generally relatively straightforward to carry out root canal treatment on mandibular third molars because access is facilitated by the mesial inclination of these teeth, however aberrant forms of the pulp do exist. Careful preoperative assessment is essential.

### Access cavities to mandibular molars

The prevalence of the second distal canal in mandibular first molars necessitates a rectangular outline. The access cavity should be placed in the

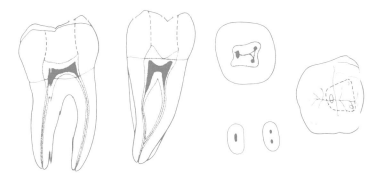

**Figure 3.28** Mandibular second molar, with a type II canal configuration in the mesial root (second from left).

31

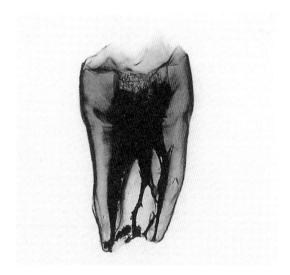

**Figure 3.29** Cleared mandibular second molar with fused roots viewed from the buccal showing the median buccal canal.

mesial three-quarters of the occlusal surface. Care should always to taken to remove the roof of the pulp chamber completely without causing damage to the floor of the pulp chamber. Where improved visual identification of canal orifices is required, e.g. in the case of anomalies, the access cavity may be extended. The walls of the access cavity should diverge towards the occlusal to resist masticatory forces and prevent dislodgement of the temporary restoration.

## PULP SPACE ANATOMY OF PRIMARY TEETH

The object of endodontic treatment in primary teeth is to preserve the tooth in function. The techniques used to achieve this have been different from those in permanent teeth.

The pulp cavities in primary teeth have certain common characteristics:

- Proportionally, they are much larger than in permanent teeth.
- The enamel and dentine surrounding the pulp cavities are much thinner than in permanent teeth.
- There is no clear demarcation between the pulp chamber and the root canals.

- The pulp canals are more slender and tapering, and are longer in proportion to the crown, than the corresponding permanent teeth.
- Multirooted primary teeth show a greater degree of interconnecting branches between pulp canals.
- The pulp horns of primary molars are more pointed than suggested by cusp anatomy.

### Primary incisors and canines

The pulp chambers of both maxillary and mandibular incisors and canines follow closely their crown outlines. However, the pulp tissue is much closer to the surface of the tooth, and the pulp horns are not as sharp and pronounced as in permanent teeth (Fig. 3.30). The pulp canals are wide coronally and taper apically, and there is no clear demarcation between pulp chamber and root canal. Occasionally the canals of mandibular incisors may be divided into two branches by a mesiodistal wall of dentine.

Maxillary primary incisors are 16 mm long, while the laterals are slightly shorter. Mandibular central incisors are 14 mm, and mandibular lateral incisors are 15 mm. The canines are the longest primary teeth, the maxillary canines being 19 mm and the mandibular 17 mm. As the root apices undergo resorption because of the developing permanent tooth, the roots are frequently shorter in older children.

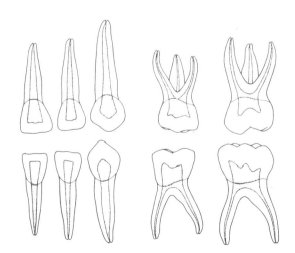

**Figure 3.30** Pulpal anatomy of the primary teeth.

## Primary molars

As in the permanent dentition the maxillary molars are three-rooted (two buccal and one palatal) whilst the mandibular molars only have two roots (mesial and distal) (Fig. 3.30). The pulp chambers are large in relation to tooth size, and the pulp horns are well developed, particularly in the second molars. From a restorative point of view it is important to remember that the tip of the pulp horns may be as close as 2 mm from the enamel surface, and thus great care must be taken in preparing cavities in these teeth if pulpal exposure is to be avoided. Because of the relatively large size of the pulp chamber there is relatively less hard tissue protecting the pulp.

The furcation of the roots is also very much closer to the cervical area of the crown and thus damage to the floor of the pulp chamber may lead to perforation. Mandibular molars normally have two root canals in each root, and the mesiobuccal root canal of the maxillary molars may divide into two. Thus both maxillary and mandibular primary molars frequently have four canals.

## APICAL CLOSURE

While calcification and cementum deposition at the apex continue throughout life, apices can be considered as fully formed several years after eruption, and approximate ages are shown in Table 3.1.

**Table 3.1** Ages when root apices are considered fully formed

| Tooth type | Age (years) |
| --- | --- |
| Primary incisor | 2 |
| Primary canine and molar | 3 |
| Permanent first molar | 9 |
| Permanent central incisor | 10 |
| Permanent lateral incisor | 11 |
| Permanent premolar | 15 |
| Permanent second molar | 17 |
| Permanent third molar | 21 |

## REFERENCES

1. Adachi Y (1978) The incidence and the location of secondary mesio-buccal canals in maxillary molars. *Japanese Journal of Conservative Dentistry* **21**, 65–72.
2. Altman M, Guttuso J, Seidberg BH, Langeland K (1970) Apical root canal anatomy of human maxillary central incisors. *Oral Surgery, Oral Medicine, Oral Pathology* **30**, 694–699.
3. Barrett MT (1925) The internal anatomy of the teeth with special reference to the pulp with its branches. *Dental Cosmos* **67**, 581–592.
4. Beatty RG (1984) A five-canal maxillary first molar. *Journal of Endodontics* **10**, 156–157.
5. Benjamin KA, Dowson J (1974) Incidence of two root canals in human mandibular incisor teeth. *Oral Surgery, Oral Medicine, Oral Pathology* **38**, 122–126.
6. Bernaba JM, Madeira MC, Hetem S (1965) Contribuicao para o estudo morfologico de raizes e canais do primeiro premolar superior humano. *Arquivos do Centro de Estudos da Faculdade Odontologia da UFMG* **2**, 81–92.
7. Brook AH (1975) Variables and criteria in prevalence studies of dental anomalies of number, form and size. *Community Dentistry and Oral Epidemiology* **3**, 288–293.
8. Burch JG, Hulen S (1972) The relationship of the apical foramen to the anatomic apex of the tooth root. *Oral Surgery, Oral Medicine, Oral Pathology* **34**, 262–268.
9. Burch JG, Hulen S (1974) A study of the presence of accessory foramina and topography of molar furcations. *Oral Surgery, Oral Medicine, Oral Pathology* **38**, 451–455.
10. Carns EJ, Skidmore AE (1973) Configurations and deviations of root canals of maxillary first premolars. *Oral Surgery, Oral Medicine, Oral Pathology* **36,** 880–886.
11. Cecic P, Hartwell G, Bellizzi R (1982) The multiple root canal system in the maxillary first molar: a case report. *Journal of Endodontics* **8,** 113–115.
12. Chan K, Yew SC, Chao SY (1992) Mandibular premolar with three root canals – two case reports. *International Endodontic Journal* **25**, 261–264.
13. Chapman CE (1969) A microscopic study of the apical region of human anterior teeth. *Journal of the British Endodontic Society* **3**, 52–58.
14. Cooke HG, Cox FL (1979) C-shaped canal configurations in mandibular molars. *Journal of the American Dental Association* **99**, 836–839.
15. De Sousa SM, Bramante CM (1998) Dens invaginatus: treatment choices. *Endodontics and Dental Traumatology* **14**, 152–158.
16. Dourda AO, Moule AJ, Young WG (1994) A morphometric analysis of the cross-sectional area of dentine occupied by dentinal tubules in human third molar teeth. *International Endodontic Journal* **27**, 184–189.
17. Dummer PMH, McGinn JH, Rees DG (1984) The position and topography of the apical canal constriction and apical foramen. *International Endodontic Journal* **17,** 192–198.

18. Fabian H (1928) *Spezielle Anatomie des Gebisses*. Leipzig, Germany: Werner Klinkhardt.

19. Fabra-Campos H (1989) Three canals in the mesial root of mandibular first permanent molars: a clinical study. *International Endodontic Journal* **22**, 39–43.

20. Fischer G (1907) Ueber die feinere Anatomie der Wurzelkanäle menschlicher Zähne. *Zahne Deutsche Monatsschrift für Zahnheilkunde* **25**, 544–552.

21. Garberoglio R, Brännström M (1976) Scanning electron microscopic investigation of human dentinal tubules. *Archives of Oral Biology* **21**, 355–362.

22. Green D (1956) A stereomicroscopic study of the root apices of 400 maxillary and mandibular anterior teeth. *Oral Surgery, Oral Medicine, Oral Pathology* **9**, 1224–1232.

23. Green D (1960) Stereomicroscopic study of 700 root apices of maxillary and mandibular posterior teeth. *Oral Surgery, Oral Medicine, Oral Pathology* **13**, 728–733.

24. Green D (1973) Double canals in single roots. *Oral Surgery, Oral Medicine, Oral Pathology* **35**, 689–696.

25. Gulabivala K, Aung TH, Alavi A, Ng YL (2001) Root and canal morphology of Burmese mandibular molars. *International Endodontic Journal* **34**, 359–370.

26. Gutmann JL, Pitt Ford TR (1993) Management of the resected root end: a clinical review. *International Endodontic Journal* **26**, 273–283.

27. Harris WE (1980) Unusual root canal anatomy in a maxillary molar. *Journal of Endodontics* **6**, 573–575.

28. Hartwell G, Bellizzi R (1982) Clinical investigation of in vivo endodontically treated mandibular and maxillary molars. *Journal of Endodontics* **8**, 555–557.

29. Henry PJ (1970) Two rooted central incisor. *Oral Surgery, Oral Medicine, Oral Pathology* **30**, 380.

30. Hess WL (1917) Zur Anatomie der Wurzelkanale des menschlicher Gebisses mit Beruechsichtigung der feineren Verzweigungen am Foramen apicale. *Schweizer Vierteljahrschrift für Zahnheilkunde* **27**, 1–52.

31. Hoppe WF, Stuben J (1965) Uber die messung des volumen der dentinkanälchen und über das Verhältnis des kanalvolumens zum gesamtdentinvolumen. *Stoma* **18**, 38–45.

32. Hulsmann M (1997) Dens invaginatus: aetiology, classification, prevalence, diagnosis, and treatment considerations. *International Endodontic Journal* **30**, 79–90.

33. Imura N, Hata GI, Toda T Otani SM, Fagundes MI (1998) Two canals in mesiobuccal roots of maxillary molars. *International Endodontic Journal* **31**, 410–414.

34. Jenkins JA, Walker WA, Schindler WG, Flores CM (2001) An in vitro evaluation of the accuracy of the Root ZX in the presence of various irrigants. *Journal of Endodontics* **27**, 209–211.

35. Kaffe I, Kaufman A, Littner M, Lazarson A (1985) Radiographic study of the root canal system of mandibular anterior teeth. *International Endodontic Journal* **18**, 253–259.

36. Keller O (1928) Untersuchurgen zur Anatomie der wurzelkanale des menschlichen Gebisses nach dem Aufhellungsverfahren. *Schweizer Monatsschrift für Zahnheilkunde* **38**, 635–657.

37. Kerekes K, Tronstad L (1977) Morphometric observations on root canals of human anterior teeth. *Journal of Endodontics* **3**, 24–29.

38. Kramer IRH (1960) The vascular architecture of the human dental pulp. *Archives of Oral Biology* **2**, 177–189.

39. Koh ET, Pitt Ford TR, Kariyawasam SP, Chen NN, Torabinejad M (2001) Prophylactic treatment of dens evaginatus using mineral trioxide aggregate. *Journal of Endodontics* **27**, 540–542.

40. Kuttler Y (1955) Microscopic investigation of root apices. *Journal of the American Dental Association* **50**, 544–552.

41. Lane AJ (1974) The course and incidence of multiple canals in the mesio-buccal root of the maxillary first molar. *Journal of the British Endodontic Society* **7**, 9–11.

42. Laws AJ (1971) Prevalence of canal irregularities in mandibular incisors: a radiographic study. *New Zealand Dental Journal* **67**, 181–186.

43. Levy AB Glatt L (1970) Deviation of the apical foramen from the radiographic apex. *Journal of the New Jersey State Dental Society* **41**, 12–13.

44. Lowman JV, Burke RS, Pelleu GB (1973) Patent accessory canals: incidence in molar furcation region. *Oral Surgery, Oral Medicine, Oral Pathology* **36**, 580–584.

45. Madeira MC, Hetem S (1973) Incidence of bifurcations in mandibular incisors. *Oral Surgery, Oral Medicine, Oral Pathology* **36**, 589–591.

46. Manning SA (1990) Root canal anatomy of mandibular second molars. Part I. *International Endodontic Journal* **23**, 34–39.

47. Manning SA (1990) Root canal anatomy of mandibular second molars. Part II C-shaped canals. *International Endodontic Journal* **23**, 40–45.

48. Miyoshi S, Fujiwara J, Tsuji Y, Nakata T, Yamamoto K (1977) Bifurcated root canals and crown diameter. *Journal of Dental Research* **56**, 1425.

49. Mueller AH (1933) Anatomy of the root canals of the incisors, cuspids, and bicuspids of the permanent teeth. *Journal of the American Dental Association* **20**, 1361–1386.

50. Nelson CT (1938) The teeth of the Indians of Pecos Pueblo. *American Journal of Physical Anthropology* **23**, 261–293.

51. Ng YL, Aung TH, Alavi A, Gulabivala K (2001) Root and canal morphology of Burmese maxillary molars. *International Endodontic Journal* **34**, 620–630.

52. Oguntebi BR (1994) Dentine tubule infection and endodontic therapy implications. *International Endodontic Journal* **27**, 218–222.

53. Okumura T (1927) Anatomy of the root canals. *Journal of the American Dental Association* **14**, 632–639.

54. Pederson PO (1949) The East Greenland Eskimo dentition. Numerical variations and anatomy. *Meddelelser om Gronland* BD 142, No. 3.

55. Pineda F (1959) Investigacion de la forma, numero y direccion radiculares sobre 4252 dientes. *Revista de la Asociacion Dental Mexicana* **16**, 241–253.

56. Pineda F (1973) Roentgenographic investigation of the mesiobuccal root of the maxillary first molar. *Oral Surgery, Oral Medicine, Oral Pathology* **36**, 253–260.

57. Pineda F, Kuttler Y (1972) Mesiodistal and buccolingual roentgenographic investigation of 7,275 root canals. *Oral Surgery, Oral Medicine, Oral Pathology* **33**, 101–110.

58. Pomeranz HH, Fishelberg G (1974) The secondary mesiobuccal canal of maxillary molars. *Journal of the American Dental Association* **88**, 119–124.

59. Rankine-Wilson RW, Henry P (1965) The bifurcated root canal in lower anterior teeth. *Journal of the American Dental Association* **70**, 1162–1165.

60. Reid JS, Saunders WP, MacDonald DG (1993) Maxillary permanent incisors with two root canals: a report of two cases. *International Endodontic Journal* **26**, 246–250.

61. Rhodes JS (2001) A case of unusual anatomy: a mandibular second premolar with four canals. *International Endodontic Journal* **34**, 645–648.

62. Seidberg BH, Altman M, Guttuso J, Suson M (1973) Frequency of two mesiobuccal root canals in maxillary permanent first molars. *Journal of the American Dental Association* **87**, 852–856.

63. Serman NJ, Hasselgren G (1992) The radiographic incidence of multiple roots and canals in human mandibular premolars. *International Endodontic Journal* **25**, 234–237.

64. Shabahang S, Goon WW, Gluskin AH (1996) An in vivo evaluation of Root ZX electronic apex locator. *Journal of Endodontics* **22**, 616–618.

65. Skidmore AE, Bjorndal AM (1971) Root canal morphology of the human mandibular first molar. *Oral Surgery, Oral Medicine, Oral Pathology* **32**, 778–784.

66. Slowey RR (1974) Radiographic aids in the detection of extra root canals. *Oral Surgery, Oral Medicine, Oral Pathology* **37**, 762–772.

67. Stone LH, Stroner WF (1981) Maxillary molars demonstrating more than one palatal root canal. *Oral Surgery, Oral Medicine, Oral Pathology* **51**, 649–652.

68. Sykaras S, Economou P (1970) Root canal morphology of the mesiobuccal root of the maxillary first molar. *Odontostomatologica Procodos* **24**, 99–107.

69. Tamse A, Littner MM, Kaffe I, Moskona D, Gavish A (1988) Morphological and radiographic study of the apical foramen in distal roots of mandibular molars. Part 1. The location of the apical foramen on various root aspects. *International Endodontic Journal* **21**, 205–210.

70. Thews ME, Kemp WB, Jones CR (1979) Aberrations in palatal root and root canal morphology of two maxillary first molars. *Journal of Endodontics* **5**, 94–96.

71. Thomas RP, Moule AJ, Bryant R (1993) Root canal morphology of maxillary permanent first molar teeth at various ages. *International Endodontic Journal* **26**, 257–267.

72. Thompson BH, Portell FR, Hartwell GR (1985) Two root canals in a maxillary lateral incisor. *Journal of Endodontics* **11**, 353–355.

73. Tidmarsh BG, Arrowsmith MG (1989) Dentinal tubules at the root ends of apicected teeth: a scanning electron microscopic study. *International Endodontic Journal* **22**, 184–189.

74. Ting PCS, Nga L (1992) Clinical detection of minor mesiobuccal canal of maxillary first molars. *International Endodontic Journal* **25**, 304–306.

75. Tratman EK (1938) Three rooted lower molars in man and their racial distribution. *British Dental Journal* **64**, 264–274.

76. Trope M, Elfenbein L, Tronstad L (1986) Mandibular premolars with more than one root canal in different race groups. *Journal of Endodontics* **12**, 343–345.

77. Turner CG (1967) The dentition of the Arctic peoples. PhD thesis. Madison, WI, USA: University of Wisconsin.

78. Turner CG (1971) Three rooted mandibular first permanent molars and the question of American Indian origins. *American Journal of Physical Anthropology* **34**, 229–241.

79. Uyeno DS, Lugo A (1996) Dens evaginatus: a review. *ASDC Journal of Dentistry for Children* **63**, 328–332.

80. Vande Voorde HE, Bjorndahl AM (1969) Estimating endodontic 'working length' with paralleling radiographs. *Oral Surgery, Oral Medicine, Oral Pathology* **27**, 106–110.

81. Vertucci FJ (1974) The endodontic significance of the mesiobuccal root of the maxillary first molar. *US Navy Medicine* **63**, 29–31.

82. Vertucci FJ (1974) Root canal anatomy of the mandibular anterior teeth. *Journal of the American Dental Association* **89**, 369–371.

83. Vertucci FJ (1978) Root canal morphology of mandibular premolars. *Journal of the American Dental Association* **97**, 47–50.

84. Vertucci FJ (1984) Root canal anatomy of the human permanent teeth. *Oral Surgery, Oral Medicine, Oral Pathology* **58**, 589–599.

85. Vertucci FJ, Gegauff A (1979) Root canal morphology of the maxillary first premolar. *Journal of the American Dental Association* **99**, 194–198.

86. Vertucci F, Seelig A, Gillis R (1974) Root canal morphology of the human maxillary second premolar. *Oral Surgery, Oral Medicine, Oral Pathology* **38**, 456–464.

87. Vertucci FJ, Williams RG (1974) Root canal anatomy of the mandibular first molar. *Journal of the New Jersey Dental Association* **45**, 27–28.

88. Visser JB (1943) Uber Wurzelverschmelzungen an den oberen Molaren des menschlichen Gebisses. *Acta Neerlandica Morphologica* **5**, 1–10.

89. Walker RT (1987) A comparative investigation of the root number and canal anatomy of permanent teeth in a southern Chinese population. PhD thesis. Hong Kong. University of Hong Kong.

90. Walker RT (1987) Root form and canal anatomy of maxillary first premolars in a southern Chinese population. *Endodontics and Dental Traumatology* **3**, 130–134.

91. Walker RT (1988) The root canal anatomy of mandibular incisors in a southern Chinese population. *International Endodontic Journal* **21**, 218–223.

92. Walker RT (1988) The root form and canal anatomy of mandibular first molars in a southern Chinese population. *Endodontics and Dental Traumatology* **4**, 19–22.

93. Walker RT (1988) Root form and canal anatomy of mandibular second molars in a southern Chinese population. *Journal of Endodontics* **14**, 325–329.

94. Weller RN, Hartwell GR (1989) The impact of improved access and searching techniques on detection of the mesio-lingual canal in maxillary molars. *Journal of Endodontics* **15**, 82–83.

95. Wong M (1991) Four root canals in a mandibular second premolar. *Journal of Endodontics* **17**, 125–126.

96. Wong M (1991) Maxillary first molar with three palatal canals. *Journal of Endodontics* **17**, 298–299.

97. Yang ZP, Yang SF, Lin YC, Shay JC, Chi CY (1988) C-shaped root canals in mandibular second molars in a Chinese population. *Endodontics and Dental Traumatology* **4**, 160–163.

98. Zillich R, Dowson J (1973) Root canal morphology of the mandibular first and second premolars. *Oral Surgery, Oral Medicine, Oral Pathology* **36**, 738–744.

# 4

# The dental pulp

T. R. Pitt Ford

Introduction  37

Pulp response to irritants  37

Diagnosis of pulp damage  38
  Clinical tests  39

Pulpal irritants  40
  Dental caries  40
  Cavity preparation  41
  Dental materials  42
  Bacterial leakage  42
  Exposure of dentine  43

Management of deep caries  43

Pulp exposure  44
  Pulp capping  44
  Pulpotomy  44

Traumatic injuries  45

Cracked cusps  45

Pulp response to periodontal disease and treatment  45

Pulp response to intra-alveolar surgery  46

References  46

## INTRODUCTION

All clinicians should be aware that the best root canal filling is healthy pulp tissue, and how to prevent damage. It should not be assumed that every damaged pulp must be extirpated and that pulp conservation is an unsatisfactory procedure.

The dental pulp is in the centre of the tooth and is the tissue from which the dentine was formed during tooth development. It remains throughout life and provides nourishment for the odontoblasts that line its surface. These odontoblasts have long processes that extend approximately one third as far as the amelodentinal junction [14]. The tubules beyond the odontoblast processes are normally patent and filled with tissue fluid. When irritants are applied to the distal ends of the dentinal tubules, the odontoblasts will form more dentine, within tubules as intratubular dentine, or within the pulp as irritation dentine as well as lead to the occlusion of tubules by mineralized deposits known as tubular sclerosis.

The pulp and dentine can thus be regarded as one interconnected tissue, the dentinopulpal complex. This is normally protected from irritation by an intact layer of enamel. When enamel is destroyed by caries, erosion or operative procedures, the pulp is at risk. In a young patient the tubules are wider and the pulp closer to the surface, so a similarly sized breach of enamel will have a greater effect on the pulp than one in an older patient. The more the area of exposed dentine, the greater is the effect on the pulp, therefore the potential damage of crown preparations and large cavities is greater than that of small cavities.

## PULP RESPONSE TO IRRITANTS

The pulp response to irritation is inflammation and formation of hard tissues, irritation dentine and tubular sclerosis; these hard tissues attempt to wall off the irritants from the pulp, which will then cease to be inflamed.

It has been shown that if buccal cavities are prepared in otherwise sound teeth and the cavities left open to salivary contamination, the pulp underneath the exposed tubules becomes inflamed [62]. Furthermore when severe irritants, namely micro-organisms in carious dentine, are placed on the cavity floor under a restoration, the pulp reaction is always severe. If the irritant is removed and a restoration with a lining (base) placed, the pulpal inflammation subsides and irritation dentine is formed [63]. Thus it has been demonstrated experimentally that damaged pulps have the capacity to recover.

## DIAGNOSIS OF PULP DAMAGE

The dentist who intends to restore a broken-down or decayed tooth needs to determine whether the pulp of the tooth is dead, dying or alive, for treatment to be successful. There is as yet no routine test that directly indicates the vitality of the pulp. Currently available tests assess the function of nerves in the pulp, by the application of electric current or a rapid change in temperature. Several studies have reported on the experimental use of laser Doppler flowmetry to measure blood flow in teeth [40,65, 66,68], but the technique has not been developed commercially for routine clinical use.

In symptomless teeth with damaged pulps, the response to thermal or electric testing may come from the significant amount of remaining normal pulp, because pulpal inflammation is often localized; this response indicates a healthier state than exists. Conversely, when the pulp does not respond to testing, it cannot always be assumed to be dead, for the pulp may have formed large amounts of irritation dentine and retreated sufficiently far from the stimulus not to respond. The correlation between histological findings and the results of pulp tests is satisfactory at a crude level but is poor when exacerbating or relieving factors, or the nature of the pain have been correlated [31,56,79]. In view of this poor correlation, clinicians have rejected previous complex histopathological classifications and developed a simple clinical classification of the state of the pulp:

- normal pulp;
- reversible pulpitis;
- irreversible pulpitis;
- pulp necrosis.

Inflammation in the pulp can be very localized; for example, a pulp horn may display a micro-abscess while the opposite pulp horn is normal and uninflamed [86]. These marked variations within a single pulp obviously hinder diagnosis. The concept that increased pulpal pressure causes strangulation of the vessels in the apical part of the root, because the tooth provides a rigid closed system, is an oversimplification, as there are physiological mechanisms to prevent this [44,51,94].

*Pulpitis* which causes symptoms is regarded as *acute*, whereas if it is symptomless it is classified as *chronic*; these clinical descriptions refer to the incidence of pain not to the type of inflammatory cells found on histological examination. Pain may range from short sharp bouts, through a continuous dull ache, to a severe throbbing pain. The pain may arise by stimulation such as drinking a cold liquid, or be spontaneous. Its character and occurrence usually change with time as the disease progresses. A patient may give a history of initial short bouts of pain stimulated by drinking cold liquids, which developed into a continuous dull ache; when the appointment was made, the tooth was throbbing, but by the time that the patient is examined the pain has gone. It is very likely that the pulp initially exhibited reversible inflammation, which progressed through irreversible inflammation to become necrotic.

Often the dentist will be restoring symptomless teeth but some will be causing pain. In either case it is necessary to determine the state of the pulp before commencing restorative treatment. If in doubt a period of observation may be appropriate, but if advanced restorative treatment is planned and the state of the pulp is suspect, root canal treatment may be indicated rather than risk the embarrassment of needing to perform this later, when careful diagnosis would have revealed the state of the pulp initially. This subject has been reviewed [78].

A number of clinical tests are available to assess the state of the pulp; none is totally reliable because they may be ineffective, or may elicit only a response from a normal part of the damaged pulp. After all the tests, the practitioner must use his or her judgement to decide the probable state of the pulp and the most appropriate treatment.

## Clinical tests

The following clinical tests are used:

- application of electric current;
- application of cold;
- application of heat;
- examination of radiograph;
- assessment of blood flow;
- cavity preparation without anaesthesia.

### Application of electric current

Electric current is usually applied from a battery-operated 'electric pulp tester'. The pulp tester is usually monopolar with an electrode being placed on the tooth under investigation; the circuit is completed by the patient contacting a ground electrode or the handle of the pulp tester. The teeth being investigated should be isolated and dried before the electrode, coated with a conducting medium, e.g. fluoride gel, is applied to the tooth. The current is variable, either under the operator's control or increased automatically over a period of time. Pulp testers produce negative pulses of electricity of the order of several hundred volts with a maximum current of a few milliamps, but the waveform of each type is different [33]. When the patient feels a sensation, he or she lets go of the handle of the pulp tester, thus breaking the circuit; the reading of the lowest current to elicit a response is recorded. Sound teeth respond over a range of values, with posterior teeth requiring higher settings than anterior teeth [32]. Teeth with acutely inflamed pulps tend to respond at lower levels than sound control teeth, while teeth with partially necrotic pulps tend to respond at higher levels. The position of the electrode on the tooth affects the readings obtained, with the lowest readings at the incisal edge [3].

A response at a high setting may occur with a damaged pulp, by leakage through the periodontal tissues, or through a receded normal pulp. A lack of response may occur because a tooth is root-filled, a pulp is necrotic, a vital pulp has receded, the pulp is in a state of shock (e.g. in traumatized teeth), or if the circuit is incomplete.

### Application of cold

Cold is usually applied to a dried tooth by touching it intermittently with a pledget of cotton wool covered in ice crystals as a result of evaporation of ethyl chloride. It may also be applied by a stick of ice; this may be conveniently made by filling a sterilized discarded needle cover with water and placing it in a freezer. The application of cold usually elicits a painful response in a healthy anterior tooth as the small amount of tooth substance is cooled very rapidly; the test may work less well on posterior teeth because of their greater mass. A response indicates that the nerve fibres in the pulp are alive; an exaggerated response may indicate an inflamed pulp, while no response may occur when the coronal pulp is necrotic, the pulp has receded, insufficient cooling occurred, or the pulp is in a state of shock in traumatized teeth. A prolonged and lingering response to the application of a cold stimulus, usually indicates an irreversibly damaged pulp [31].

### Application of heat

Heat is usually applied by a heated stick of gutta-percha temporary filling material being placed intermittently on the dried tooth surface, with a small amount of vaseline being used as a lubricant. A response indicates that the nerve fibres in the pulp are active. A lack of response may occur if the pulp is necrotic, the pulp has receded or insufficient heating occurred. Heat is generally considered particularly effective in diagnosing a pulp with irreversible pulpitis, for pain that lingers after the application of heat is often as a result of C-fibre stimulation; however in one clinical study, heat was not found to be more effective than cold for diagnosis [31].

### Examination of radiographs

Three radiographic views may be examined: the bitewing film, the periapical film, and the dental pantomogram. The bitewing film provides information about the crown of the tooth and the superficial part of the root. It gives a two-dimensional view of the extent of restorations, the extent of caries, the presence of recurrent caries, the amount of irritation dentine, the size of the pulp chamber and evidence of internal resorption. The periapical film additionally provides evidence of periradicular radiolucencies. The dental pantomogram has typically had a less clear image than an intraoral film, and it has been poor at displaying radiolucencies around the apices of maxillary teeth. More recent apparatus has improved image quality, which is focused on a narrow slice within the tooth. Where teeth have large restorations, the distance between the base of the cavity and the pulp is small; and irritants could therefore affect the pulp more readily than in a tooth with a small restoration. The closer the caries is to the pulp and the larger the lesion, the greater is the threat to the pulp. The formation of irritation dentine in response to caries indicates that the pulp has most probably responded success-fully to the irritant, as does a diminutive-sized pulp chamber. On the other hand, the lack of irritation dentine formation to caries and an abnormally large-sized pulp chamber compared with the other teeth in the mouth could indicate that the coronal pulp became necrotic at an earlier age. Internal resorption, which should not be confused with external resorption, indicates that there has been irreversible pulpitis. Periradicular radiolucencies, which may not always be at the apex, indicate pulp necrosis, which may be partial or total.

### Assessment of blood flow

Laser Doppler flowmeters may be used to assess blood flow in teeth, but as yet no flowmeter has been developed specifically for dental use. The technique involves directing a low-energy laser beam along a fibre-optic cable to the tooth surface, where the light passes along the direction of enamel prisms and dentinal tubules to the pulp [67]. Some light is reflected off moving red blood cells in the peripheral capillaries of the pulp. The reflected light is passed back to the flowmeter where the frequency-shifted light is detected for strength of signal and pulsatility. The clinician must interpret whether the pulp is alive and healthy, or dead; diagnosis may be improved by frequency analysis of the signal [65]. Laser Doppler flowmetry has been used to detect pulp vitality in traumatized teeth at a stage when other tests are inconclusive [66,68].

### Cavity preparation without anaesthesia

This procedure is only performed when all other tests have failed to give a diagnosis, and inter-vention is indicated. If the dentine is sensitive to drilling, it indicates that the pulp is alive but not necessarily healthy, for the pulp could be inflamed. A lack of sensitivity occurs if the pulp is necrotic. In a tooth with healthy pulp that has receded a long way, there may be no sensitivity because the tubules being drilled do not connect with odonto-blast processes as a result of tubular sclerosis or formation of irritation dentine.

### Diagnosis

After performing as many tests as the clinician deems appropriate, it may be possible to arrive at a diagnosis. If the diagnosis is uncertain in a symp-tomless tooth, it is usual to assume that the pulp is normal in the absence of definite contrary evidence. However, if the tooth has caused symptoms but is now quiet, the pulp must be regarded as suspect. While a policy of observation may be appropriate in some cases, root canal treatment should be carried out if advanced restorative procedures are planned on a tooth with a questionable pulp.

## PULPAL IRRITANTS

The dental pulp may be irritated by dental caries, cavity preparation, dental materials, bacterial leak-age around restorations, traumatic injuries or expo-sure of dentine. These will now be considered in detail.

### Dental caries

This has been regarded as the main cause of pulpal injury. When dental caries first affects dentine, the odontoblasts respond by tubular sclerosis and irritation dentine formation [81,93]. Tubular sclerosis is an accelerated form of intratubular dentine but the process continues further than normal with complete occlusion of the affected tubules by apatite crystals. It is a protective mechanism and occurs at the distal extremities of the odontoblast processes. This sclerotic dentine is more highly mineralized than the original dentine, and if examined in a ground section by transmitted light would appear trans-parent [84]. Irritation dentine can be considered an accelerated form of regular secondary dentine;

because it has been formed more quickly its tubular pattern is less regular, and the degree of irregularity indicates its rate of formation. It is confined to the tubules affected by the carious lesion. Where odontoblasts are destroyed by the irritant, new dentine may be formed from progenitor cells in the pulp [81].

If the carious lesion progresses, the enamel surface breaks down and bacteria enter the dentine; the rate of decay usually accelerates. The lesion may be divided into zones: an outer zone of destruction, a middle zone of bacterial penetration and an inner zone of demineralization. The pulp responds by continued irritation dentine formation. The zone of destruction contains dentine partially destroyed by proteolytic enzymes from the mixed flora of microorganisms. The tubules are filled with microorganisms and they can be found particularly in shrinkage clefts in the rotten dentine. This dentine can be readily removed by hand excavators in active lesions and often has a light colour. In slowly progressing or arrested lesions this dentine is darker and has a harder consistency.

The next zone, the zone of penetration, contains microorganisms within the dentinal tubules. The structure of the dentine when examined in a demineralized histological section is otherwise normal; some tubules are deeply infected while others contain no microorganisms. A variety of microorganisms have been recovered from this zone; many *lactobacilli* have been found but fewer *streptococci* [34]. More recently deep carious dentine has been shown to contain predominantly anaerobic bacteria (*propionibacteria, eubacteria, arachnia* and *lactobacilli*) [46]. Ahead of the zone of microorganism penetration is a zone of demineralization, frequently considered to be devoid of bacteria because the conditions for bacterial survival are too unfavourable; however, small numbers of anaerobic bacteria have been demonstrated in this zone [47].

When dental caries affects the superficial dentine, the pulp is normally protected by the zone of tubular sclerosis and by irritation dentine, and is likely to be of normal histological appearance. No foci of inflammatory cells can be observed in the pulp until caries has penetrated to within 0.5 mm [77]. As the early dentine carious lesion progresses, the sclerotic zone of dentine becomes demineralized and the lesion subsequently advances into the irri-

tation dentine. When bacteria invade this dentine, severe pulp changes such as abscess formation often occur. Therefore until the caries is very deep, the pulp is likely to be no more than reversibly damaged. Treatment should normally consist of removal of carious dentine and insertion of an effective restoration. This has been shown to result in recovery of the pulp [63].

The pulp is not infected until late in the carious process, typically when the irritation dentine is invaded. Infection of the inflamed pulp is localized to necrotic tissue in a pulp abscess [59]. Wider infection of the pulp only occurs after necrosis.

## Cavity preparation

The preparation of dentine with rotary instruments can have a damaging effect on the pulp unless measures are taken to minimize injury. Cavity preparation without waterspray causes significantly more pulp damage than when waterspray is used [64,87]. The waterspray must be continuously directed at the revolving bur; if the spray is obstructed by tooth structure or the bur allowed to stall or to cut when the operator has ceased to press the activating switch, pulp damage may occur. Various studies into the pulpal effects of high-speed instrumentation have been reviewed [82], and it was found to be acceptable provided adequate water coolant spray was used; the use of air coolant alone was considered unsatisfactory.

The area of dentine prepared can have a profound effect on the pulp response. The more tubules that are exposed, the more routes there are for irritants to reach the pulp. Small cavities are likely to be less damaging to the pulp than large ones; in addition, in a small cavity prepared to treat a carious lesion most of the exposed dentinal tubules will be blocked by tubular sclerosis as a result of the carious lesion. The deeper the cavity, the greater is the potential for damage: the pulp is closer, odontoblast processes may have been cut, more tubules will have been exposed, and the deeper tubules have a larger diameter. However no correlation between thickness of remaining dentine and pulp damage has been shown [64,74]. Only when cavities are very deep, with the remaining dentine less than 0.3 mm thick, does some pulp damage occur [87]. Prolonged drying of cavities causes odontoblast aspiration, i.e.

their cell bodies move into the dentinal tubules, but there is no permanent damage to the pulp [8].

Veneer crown preparations are potentially the most damaging to the pulp, and on occasions irreversible pulp damage has been caused by preparation with insufficient waterspray [4]. When local anaesthetics containing adrenaline (epinephrine) are used for crown preparation, the pulp is at particular risk of damage because of its reduced blood flow [52].

The pulp response to the use of lasers for cavity preparation has been reported to have no long-term adverse effects [61,88,89,96]. However, one study has found pulp damage when a laser was used to treat exposed pulp [49].

## Dental materials

There is a considerable volume of literature on the irritant effects of dental filling materials [38,75,76]. However, during the last 20 years, much of the earlier work on the irritancy of various materials has been brought into question [4,5,10,17,21,27,95].

Silicate cement was long regarded as the most irritating restorative material due to its acidity [85,99], however the cement *per se* has been shown to be bland, as it is the manner in which it is used that causes the pulp reaction [18]. The cement contracts on setting causing a gap to occur between it and the tooth, into which gap bacteria grow [16]; inflamed pulps have been found in teeth containing bacteria in the gap [5]. When bacteria were deliberately excluded, there was an excellent pulp response to the material itself [18,27]. Elimination of bacteria has been achieved experimentally by surface-sealing the restoration with zinc oxide–eugenol cement. The clinical significance is that such a restoration must be lined by a base material which effectively prevents bacterial leakage.

Composite resin has also been regarded as irritant to the pulp, but the blandness of this class of material has now been demonstrated together with the important contribution of bacterial contamination to pulp reaction [15,91]. It is important to treat the cavity margins to allow the composite resin to seal the margins of the restoration and thereby eliminate bacteria from the cavity [15]. From a clinical standpoint, both etching enamel margins and the use of a cavity liner have been considered necessary not only to prevent a pulpal inflammatory reaction, but also to reduce the reaction should the seal be imperfect.

The use of dentine bonding agents to prevent marginal leakage around composite resin restorations has been investigated for many years, but initially their long-term stability was a matter of concern. In recent years considerable development of these agents has been undertaken, and a favourable pulp response has been reported to some [28,36,97], but not where a total etch technique was performed [69].

Pulp damage may occur from temporary crown materials, not so much because of their inherent toxicity but more as a result of marginal leakage and bacterial invasion of dentinal tubules. It is recommended that temporary crowns should not be used for long periods and they must always be adequately cemented [12,13].

Although there is now considerable evidence to show the blandness of dental filling materials placed in teeth, many materials, particularly when freshly mixed, have been shown to be toxic to cell cultures [19]; however, dentine has a moderating effect [60].

## Bacterial leakage

Bacterial leakage around restorations is not solely confined to composite resin and silicate cement materials, as a similar pattern occurs with amalgam restorations [5]. The bacteria from the oral cavity colonize the space around the restoration after its placement, rather than surviving from the time it was placed. The lack of importance of bacterial contamination at the time of cavity preparation has been shown in a study of pulpal exposures [25]. There is a good correlation between bacterial leakage around restorations and pulpal inflammation [20,21].

Pulps respond to irritation from bacterial leakage by inflammation, tubular sclerosis and formation of irritation dentine so that after some months the bacteria cease to irritate [90]. However, measures should be taken to prevent pulp damage during the period before the pulp has walled itself off; these consist of cavity lining, use of cavity varnish in appropriate instances, use of a dentine-bonding agent and etching of enamel for resin-based materials, or use of an adhesive cement.

In operative dentistry the main reason for placing a cavity lining (in some parts of the world referred to as a base) is to prevent damage to the pulp from bacterial leakage around restorations. Former reasons such as material irritancy or thermal protection have been severely criticized [12,18].

The choice of lining material in cavities without pulpal exposures would appear to be a matter of operator preference in many instances. Cements based on calcium hydroxide, glass ionomer, zinc phosphate, zinc polycarboxylate or zinc oxide eugenol would all appear to be satisfactory under amalgam, and have been widely used. Zinc oxide–eugenol cement has the benefit of prolonged anti-bacterial activity. Under resin-based restorative materials zinc oxide–eugenol cement is inappropriate, unless separated by a covering layer of alternative cement (e.g. glass ionomer), as otherwise the eugenol may plasticize the resin. The durability of some calcium hydroxide cements has been questioned particularly if the overlying restoration has an imperfect seal [12,28].

### Exposure of dentine

This may occur by fracture of part of the tooth, by a restoration failing to cover the entire area of prepared dentine, or by abrasion and erosion of the overlying cementum or enamel. In the early period after exposure of dentine by trauma or cavity preparation, the pulp is sensitive to stimuli and may become inflamed, particularly if bacteria colonize the surface of exposed dentine and enter the tubules. The pulp responds to the low-grade irritation by tubular sclerosis and formation of irritation dentine, thereby protecting itself and making it less sensitive to stimuli [70].

Some patients complain of dentine sensitivity in undamaged or non-restored teeth, usually at their necks where there is exposed dentine. The affected tubules are open and communicate with the pulp. Sensitivity may be reduced by application of potassium oxalate, which not only occludes the tubules but also reduces nerve activity [70]. The good work of repair can be undone by assault with acidic solutions, particularly in patients who continue to erode their teeth either with acidic drinks and foods, or by regurgitation [12].

## MANAGEMENT OF DEEP CARIES

With the treatment of any carious cavity in dentine, it is accepted that the margins, and the amelo-dentinal junction in particular, must be caries-free as detected by an absence of softening with a probe. However, there has been less agreement over whether all carious dentine overlying the pulp should be removed [37]. In a tooth that is considered to have a healthy pulp, the prognosis for the pulp is better if exposure during caries removal is avoided [24].

A view prevails that if carious dentine remains, it will allow the carious process to continue. There is an opposite view that clinical evidence supports leaving a small amount of caries under a well-executed restoration; in the circumstance the caries becomes arrested [35]. Since very few restorations form an hermetic seal [5,16], a high incidence of recurrent caries would be expected if the former view were entirely correct. The latter view is full of clinical imprecision; how much is a little caries, and when does a little become an unacceptably large amount? A two-stage approach of step-wise excavation in which most of the carious dentine is removed at the first visit and the tooth dressed, before re-entering the tooth at a second visit, has been shown to be successful [7,58]. What is meant by carious dentine? Clinical opinions conflict with scientific evidence in deciding if a cavity is caries-free. In one study only 64% of clinically hard dentine floors were bacteria-free [80]; therefore, in a third of teeth where the clinician thought there was a clean floor, the diagnosis was wrong. The problem has been addressed by use of an indicator dye placed in the prepared cavity; the dye stains the superficial infected dentine but not the deeper demineralized non-infected dentine [39]. This deeper non-staining layer has been shown to remineralize thereby justifying its retention. The use of dye may lead to excessive removal of carious dentine, in that it may not conserve all remineralizable dentine [50].

Many operators erroneously rely on the colour of affected dentine for deciding when a cavity is caries free; a lighter colour is usually indicative of more active caries. A deep lesion may extend into dentine modified by tubular sclerosis or dead tracts, or into irritation dentine; these are darker than normal dentine, but must not be regarded as carious simply because of their colour. Hardness of carious dentine is a better indicator of disease activity than colour.

If carious dentine is left in a cavity, the clinician is unaware whether it has extended to involve the pulp. If the pulp is already inflamed, it becomes an expensive error to crown such a tooth when the crown later needs to be modified or destroyed to carry out root canal treatment. If removal of all the cariously infected dentine leads to the pulp, then root canal treatment is appropriate and should be carried out, except in the case of an immature tooth where pulpotomy may be indicated (see Chapter 10). Some operators when treating symptomless teeth with deep carious lesions, prefer to perform step-wise excavation. The remaining carious dentine is removed several months later; this has been referred to as indirect pulp capping. The procedure allows the pulp to lay down defences prior to complete caries removal.

Following removal of the carious dentine, a protective lining should be placed in a very deep cavity; a calcium hydroxide material, which stimulates pulp repair, is commonly used. Over this an antibacterial base should be placed; zinc oxide–eugenol cement is very effective because it slowly leaches eugenol, which will kill any remaining microorganisms [48], and is a more effective bactericide than calcium hydroxide materials [53]. The durability of calcium hydroxide cement as the sole base under amalgam has been questioned by the finding of softened material on removal of the overlying restoration 1–2 years later [12,26,28].

## PULP EXPOSURE

Exposure of the pulp may arise as a result of traumatic injury to the tooth, or accidentally by instruments during cavity preparation. In both instances the pulp can be regarded as being normal prior to the injury. Treatment is usually by pulp capping or pulpotomy; provided that treatment is not unnecessarily delayed, a good outcome can be achieved.

### Pulp capping

The pulp wound should be cleaned of debris and the haemorrhage arrested by careful swabbing with sterile cotton buds or paper points laid across the wound. When the wound is dry, the pulp capping material should be placed over the exposure. This should be followed by a zinc oxide–eugenol base and a permanent restoration [42].

The most widely used materials for pulp capping have contained calcium hydroxide [72,83,98]. Under favourable circumstances, the pulp responds by stimulating progenitor cells within the pulp to lay down irritation dentine under the exposure site to form a dentine bridge. With most proprietary materials this bridge forms close to the capping material, but with calcium hydroxide itself the barrier is formed further away from the material [92]. The dentine bridge is not formed by calcium from the pulp capping material [2].

The importance of preventing bacterial contamination at the time of exposure has previously been stressed [71], however it is now known that contamination for periods up to 24 h does not adversely affect pulp survival [25]. In contrast, exposure to saliva for 7 days had a negative effect [25]. There is no evidence that size of the exposure has an effect on the outcome.

The long-term success of pulp capping clinically is good [42,57]; however, a lower rate has been found at the histological level. This is attributed to bacterial penetration around the overlying restoration, and through the imperfect dentine bridge [28]. The pulp capping material must be covered by a base; zinc oxide–eugenol cement would seem the most appropriate and has been found to improve the quality of dentine bridges [55].

Zinc oxide–eugenol cement has been an unsuccessful pulp-capping material [41], because of its irritancy [48]. However, when this material is separated from the pulp by a layer of intact dentine, the concentration of eugenol reaching the pulp is sufficiently low to prevent damage.

Mineral trioxide aggregate has been reported to be effective for pulp capping [73].

### Pulpotomy

For treatment of traumatized anterior teeth, an alternative technique of pulpotomy has been used. The traditional method has been to remove the coronal pulp and place calcium hydroxide on the radicular pulp. However, partial pulpotomy has been more widely practised in recent years with a high rate of success [29]. It involves cutting, with a turbine bur under waterspray, a small 2-mm deep cavity into the pulp surrounded by shelf of dentine, placing calcium hydroxide and covering it with a base and restoration. Recent evidence indicates that mineral trioxide aggregate may be an alternative material [54,73].

## TRAUMATIC INJURIES

These may be caused by direct blows to the anterior teeth or indirectly by a blow to the mandible resulting in fracture of cusps, particularly of molars. The extent of damage may range from infraction of enamel through lost cusps to a split tooth that cannot be restored. Direct trauma to the anterior teeth often results in fractures that are horizontal or oblique [1], while with indirect trauma, fractures are generally longitudinal.

Trauma to anterior teeth most commonly affects sound teeth in children. These teeth frequently have large pulps and wide dentinal tubules so any injury which exposes dentine can potentially damage the pulp, therefore early treatment is necessary. Traumatic injuries may damage the blood supply to the pulp, which as a result may calcify or die. The endodontic aspects of traumatic injuries are considered further in Chapter 11.

## CRACKED CUSPS

A patient may complain of poorly localized pain from an unidentified posterior tooth on biting or the application of cold drinks [22,23]. Clinically and radiologically there is often no evidence of caries, and the offending tooth, although it contains a restoration, may not be heavily restored. The affected pulp responds to electrical stimulation. Careful examination of the teeth in that quadrant, particularly with an intraoral light may reveal one with vertical hairline cracks; mandibular molars are the most frequently affected [23]. The pain may be reproduced if the patient is asked to close with an object, e.g. a cotton-wool roll or a tooth slooth placed between that and the opposing teeth. When this fails to pro-

duce a response, cold in the form of ice may be applied to the teeth; a hypersensitive response will indicate the offending tooth. The mechanism of this pain on biting may be explained [9,11,12]: the crack contains bacteria whose toxins pass down the dentinal tubules to cause pulpal inflammation. As the cusp is wedged by chewing there is fluid movement in the crack and the communicating tubules; this elicits pain in an already sensitive tooth.

If there is sufficient evidence to identify the cracked cusp, treatment should be carried out. The form of treatment will depend on whether there have been symptoms of reversible or irreversible pulpitis. In the case of reversible pulpitis and if there is a loose cusp, any restoration should be removed together with the loose cusp; the tooth is restored as appropriate for the shape and size of cavity. If no loose cusp is detected, the tooth may be crowned, initially with a temporary crown. Following placement of the temporary crown, relief from pain is normally achieved. Where there have been symptoms of irreversible pulpitis, pulpal extirpation and root canal filling will be required. During root canal treatment it is advisable to place a band (e.g. stainless steel orthodontic band) around the tooth to stop it splitting, and to reduce the tooth out of occlusion other than in the intercuspal position.

## PULP RESPONSE TO PERIODONTAL DISEASE AND TREATMENT

Periodontal disease does not cause pathological change in the pulp until major lateral canals become contaminated by plaque [30]. The normality of the pulp is maintained because of the intact layer of cementum on the root surface. If this layer is destroyed then pulpal inflammation under the affected tubules occurs [6]. The pulp responds to the stimuli by formation of tubular sclerosis and irritation dentine [43].

It has been shown that scaling or root planing procedures, which remove cementum, may cause pulpal inflammation, and frequently the formation of irritation dentine [6,43]. However, the response to scaling is not severe and does not adversely affect pulp vitality. Following scaling, dentinal tubules become opened and the teeth are hypersensitive;

after several weeks the sensitivity decreases, presumably as the tubules become blocked by mineral deposits [12].

## PULP RESPONSE TO INTRA-ALVEOLAR SURGERY

It has usually been considered that pulp necrosis and abscess formation will follow surgical cutting or severance of a root near its apex. However, orthognathic surgery has led to the roots of some teeth being cut without undesirable sequelae. The effect on the remaining pulp of severing roots in the apical region has been investigated [45]. It was found that if all the roots of a tooth were severed, the coronal pulp underwent necrosis but inflammation did not occur. After one year there was no evidence of inflammation, and cementum had formed on the cut root surface and on the root canal walls near the cut surface. Where several roots of a multirooted tooth were cut through but one root remained intact the entire coronal pulp maintained its vitality. The cut surface of the apical fragment became covered by cementum, while its pulp remained normal. It appears from this study that accidental surgical damage to the roots of healthy teeth causes far less injury than was previously considered. The situation might not be so favourable if the teeth lack a complete covering of enamel, which is necessary to exclude infection, or if at a later date enamel or cementum is breached.

## REFERENCES

1. Andreasen JO, Andreasen FM (1994) *Textbook and Color Atlas of Traumatic Injuries to The Teeth*, 3rd edn. Copenhagen, Denmark: Munksgaard.
2. Attalla MN, Noujaim AA (1969) Role of calcium hydroxide in the formation of reparative dentine. *Journal of the Canadian Dental Association* **35**, 267–269.
3. Bender IB, Landau MA, Fonseca S, Trowbridge HO (1989) The optimum placement-site of the electrode in electric pulp testing of the 12 anterior teeth. *Journal of the American Dental Association* **118**, 305–310.
4. Bergenholtz G (1991) Iatrogenic injury to the pulp in dental procedures: aspects of pathogenesis, management and preventive measures. *International Dental Journal* **41**, 99–110.
5. Bergenholtz G, Cox CF, Loesche WJ, Syed SA (1982) Bacterial leakage around dental restorations: its effect on the pulp. *Journal of Oral Pathology* **11**, 439–450.
6. Bergenholtz G, Lindhe J (1978) Effect of experimentally induced marginal periodontitis and periodontal scaling on the dental pulp. *Journal of Clinical Periodontology* **5**, 59–73.
7. Bjorndal L, Thylstrup A (1998) A practice-based study on stepwise excavation of deep carious lesions in permanent teeth. *Community Dentistry and Oral Epidemiology* **26**, 122–128.
8. Brännström M (1968) The effect of dentin desiccation and aspirated odontoblasts on the pulp. *Journal of Prosthetic Dentistry* **20**, 165–171.
9. Brännström M. (1982) *Dentin and Pulp in Restorative Dentistry*. London, UK: Wolfe Medical Publications.
10. Brännström M (1984) Communication between the oral cavity and the dental pulp associated with restorative treatment. *Operative Dentistry* **9**, 57–68.
11. Brännström M (1986) The hydrodynamic theory of dentinal pain: sensation in preparations, caries and the dentinal crack syndrome. *Journal of Endodontics* **12**, 453–457.
12. Brännström M (1986) The cause of postrestorative sensitivity and its prevention. *Journal of Endodontics* **12**, 475–481.
13. Brännström M (1996) Reducing the risk of sensitivity and pulpal complications after the placement of crowns and fixed partial dentures. *Quintessence International* **27**, 673–678.
14. Brännström M, Garberoglio R (1972) The dentinal tubules and the odontoblast processes. A scanning electron microscopic study. *Acta Odontologica Scandinavica* **30**, 291–311.
15. Brännström M, Nordenvall KJ (1978) Bacterial penetration, pulpal reaction and the inner surface of Concise Enamel Bond. Composite fillings in etched and unetched cavities. *Journal of Dental Research* **57**, 3–10.
16. Brännström M, Nyborg H (1971) The presence of bacteria in cavities filled with silicate cement and composite resin materials. *Swedish Dental Journal* **64**, 149–155.
17. Brännström M, Vojinovic O (1976) Response of the dental pulp to invasion of bacteria around three filling materials. *Journal of Dentistry for Children* **43**, 83–89.
18. Brännström M, Vojinovic O, Nordenvall KJ (1979) Bacteria and pulpal reactions under silicate cement restorations. *Journal of Prosthetic Dentistry* **41**, 290–295.
19. Browne RM (1988) The in vitro assessment of the cytotoxicity of dental materials – does it have a role? *International Endodontic Journal* **21**, 50–58.
20. Browne RM, Tobias RS (1986) Microbial microleakage and pulpal inflammation: a review. *Endodontics and Dental Traumatology* **2**, 177–183.
21. Browne RM, Tobias RS, Crombie IK, Plant CG (1983) Bacterial microleakage and pulpal inflammation in experimental cavities. *International Endodontic Journal* **16**, 147–155.
22. Cameron CE (1964) Cracked-tooth syndrome. *Journal of the American Dental Association* **68**, 405–411.

23. Cameron CE (1976) The cracked tooth syndrome: additional findings. *Journal of the American Dental Association* **93**, 971–975.

24. Cotton WR (1974) Bacterial contamination as a factor in healing of pulp exposures. *Oral Surgery, Oral Medicine, Oral Pathology* **38**, 441–450.

25. Cox CF, Bergenholtz G, Fitzgerald M, Heys DR, Heys RJ, Avery JK, Baker JA (1982) Capping of the dental pulp mechanically exposed to the oral microflora – a 5-week observation of wound healing in the monkey. *Journal of Oral Pathology* **11**, 327–339.

26. Cox CF, Bergenholtz G, Heys DR, Syed SA, Fitzgerald M, Heys RJ (1985) Pulp capping of the dental pulp mechanically exposed to the oral microflora: a 1–2 year observation of wound healing in the monkey. *Journal of Oral Pathology* **14**, 156–168.

27. Cox CF, Keall CL, Keall HJ, Ostro E, Bergenholtz G (1987) Biocompatibility of surface-sealed dental materials against exposed pulps. *Journal of Prosthetic Dentistry* **57**, 1–8.

28. Cox CF, Suzuki S (1994) Re-evaluating pulp protection: calcium hydroxide liners vs. cohesive hybridization. *Journal of the American Dental Association* **125**, 823–831.

29. Cvek M (1978) A clinical report on partial pulpotomy and capping with calcium hydroxide in permanent incisors with complicated crown fracture. *Journal of Endodontics* **4**, 232–237.

30. Czarnecki RT, Schilder H (1979) A histological evaluation of the human pulp in teeth with varying degrees of periodontal disease. *Journal of Endodontics* **5**, 242–253.

31. Dummer PMH, Hicks R, Huws D (1980) Clinical signs and symptoms in pulp disease. *International Endodontic Journal* **13**, 27–35.

32. Dummer PMH, Tanner M (1986) The response of caries-free, unfilled teeth to electrical excitation: a comparison of two new pulp testers. *International Endodontic Journal* **19**, 172–177.

33. Dummer PMH, Tanner M, McCarthy JP (1986) A laboratory study of four electric pulp testers. *International Endodontic Journal* **19**, 161–171.

34. Edwardsson S (1974) Bacteriological studies on deep areas of carious dentine. *Odontologisk Revy* **25**, Supplement 32, 1–143.

35. Fairbourn DR, Charbeneau GT, Loesche WJ (1980) Effect of Improved Dycal and IRM on bacteria in deep carious lesions. *Journal of the American Dental Association* **100**, 547–552.

36. Felton D, Bergenholtz G, Cox CF (1989) Inhibition of bacterial growth under composite restorations following GLUMA pretreatment. *Journal of Dental Research* **68**, 491–495.

37. Fisher FJ (1981) The treatment of carious dentine. *British Dental Journal* **150**, 159–162.

38. Frank RM (1975) Reactions of dentin and pulp to drugs and restorative materials. *Journal of Dental Research* **54**, B176–187.

39. Fusayama T (1979) Two layers of carious dentin: diagnosis and treatment. *Operative Dentistry* **4**, 63–70.

40. Gazelius B, Olgart L, Edwall B, Edwall L (1986) Non-invasive recording of blood flow in human dental pulp. *Endodontics and Dental Traumatology* **2**, 219–221.

41. Glass RL, Zander HA (1949) Pulp healing. *Journal of Dental Research* **28**, 97–107.

42. Haskell EW, Stanley HR, Chellimi J, Stringfellow H (1978) Direct pulp capping treatment: a long-term follow-up. *Journal of the American Dental Association* **97**, 607–612.

43. Hattler AB, Listgarten MA (1984) Pulpal response to root planing in a rat model. *Journal of Endodontics* **10**, 471–476.

44. Heyeraas KJ (1984) Pulpal, microvascular, and tissue pressure. *Journal of Dental Research* **64**, 585–589.

45. Hitchcock R, Ellis E, Cox CF (1985) Intentional vital root transection: a 52-week histopathologic study in Macaca Mulatta. Oral Surgery, *Oral Medicine, Oral Pathology* **60**, 2–14.

46. Hoshino E (1985) Predominant obligate anaerobes in human carious dentin. *Journal of Dental Research* **64**, 1195–1198.

47. Hoshino E, Ando N, Sato M, Kota K (1992) Bacterial invasion of non-exposed dental pulp. *International Endodontic Journal* **25**, 2–5.

48. Hume WR (1988) *In vitro* studies on the local pharmacodynamics, pharmacology and toxicology of eugenol and zinc oxide–eugenol. *International Endodontic Journal* **21**, 130–134.

49. Jukic S, Anic I, Koba K, Najzar-Fleger D, Matsumoto K (1997) The effect of pulpotomy using $CO_2$ and Nd:YAG lasers on dental pulp tissue. *International Endodontic Journal* **30**, 175–180.

50. Kidd EA, Joyston-Bechal S, Beighton D (1993) The use of a caries detector dye during cavity preparation: a microbiological assessment. *British Dental Journal* **174**, 245–248.

51. Kim S (1984) Regulation of pulpal blood flow. *Journal of Dental Research* **64**, 590–596.

52. Kim S (1986) Ligamental injection: a physiological explanation of its efficacy. *Journal of Endodontics* **12**, 486–491.

53. King JB, Crawford JJ, Lindahl RL (1965) Indirect pulp capping: a bacteriologic study of deep carious dentine in human teeth. *Oral Surgery, Oral Medicine, Oral Pathology* **20**, 663–671.

54. Koh ET, Pitt Ford TR, Kariyawasam SP, Chen NN, Torabinejad M (2001) Prophylactic treatment of dens evaginatus using mineral trioxide aggregate. *Journal of Endodontics* **27**, 540–542.

55. Langer M, Ulmansky M, Sela J (1970) Behaviour of human dental pulp to Calxyl with or without zinc oxide–eugenol. *Archives of Oral Biology* **15**, 189–194.

56. Lundy T, Stanley HR (1969) Correlation of pulpal histopathology and clinical symptoms in human teeth subjected to experimental irritation. *Oral Surgery, Oral Medicine, Oral Pathology* **27**, 187–201.

57. McWalter GM, El-Kafrawy AH, Mitchell DF (1976) Long-term study of pulp capping in monkeys with three agents. *Journal of the American Dental Association* **93**, 105–110.

58. Magnusson BO, Sundell SO (1977) Stepwise excavation of deep carious lesions in primary molars. *Journal of the International Association of Dentistry for Children* **8**, 36–40.

59. Massler M, Pawlak J (1977) The affected and infected pulp. *Oral Surgery, Oral Medicine, Oral Pathology* **43**, 929–947.

60. Meryon SD (1988) The model cavity method incorporating dentine. *International Endodontic Journal* **21**, 79–84.

61. Miserendino LJ, Levy GC, Abt E, Rizoiu IM (1994) Histologic effects of a thermally cooled Nd:YAG laser on the dental pulp and supporting structures of rabbit teeth. *Oral Surgery, Oral Medicine, Oral Pathology* **78**, 93–100.

62. Mjör IA, Tronstad L (1972) Experimentally induced pulpitis. *Oral Surgery, Oral Medicine, Oral Pathology* **34**, 102–108.

63. Mjör IA, Tronstad L (1974) The healing of experimentally induced pulpitis. *Oral Surgery, Oral Medicine, Oral Pathology* **38**, 115–121.

64. Morrant GA (1977) Dental instrumentation and pulpal injury. Part II clinical considerations. *Journal of the British Endodontic Society* **10**, 55–63.

65. Odor TM, Pitt Ford TR, McDonald F (1996) Effect of wavelength and bandwidth on the clinical reliability of laser Doppler recordings. *Endodontics and Dental Traumatology* **12**, 9–15.

66. Odor TM, Pitt Ford TR, McDonald F (1998) Use of laser Doppler flowmetry for pulp testing – preliminary findings. *International Endodontic Journal* **31**, 189–220 (Abstract).

67. Odor TM, Watson TF, Pitt Ford TR, McDonald F (1996) Pattern of transmission of laser light in teeth. *International Endodontic Journal* **29**, 228–234.

68. Olgart L, Gazelius B, Lindh-Strömberg U (1988) Laser Doppler flowmetry in assessing vitality in luxated permanent teeth. *International Endodontic Journal* **21**, 300–306.

69. Pameijer CH, Stanley HR (1998) The disastrous effects of the 'total etch' technique in vital pulp capping in primates. *American Journal of Dentistry* **11**, Supplement, 45-54.

70. Pashley DH (1986) Dentin permeability, dentin sensitivity and treatment through tubule occlusion. *Journal of Endodontics* **12**, 465–474.

71. Paterson RC (1974) Management of the deep cavity. *British Dental Journal* **137**, 250–252.

72. Pitt Ford TR, Roberts GJ (1991) Immediate and delayed direct pulp capping with the use of a new visible light-cured calcium hydroxide preparation. *Oral Surgery, Oral Medicine, Oral Pathology* **71**, 338–342.

73. Pitt Ford T, Torabinejad M, Abedi H, Bakland LK, Kariawasam SP (1996) Using mineral trioxide aggregate as a pulp-capping material. *Journal of the American Dental Association* **127**, 1491–1494.

74. Plant CG, Anderson RJ (1978) The effect of cavity depth on the pulpal response to restorative materials. *British Dental Journal* **144**, 10–13.

75. Plant CG, Jones DW (1976) The damaging effects of restorative materials. Part 1 – Physical and chemical properties. *British Dental Journal* **140**, 373–377.

76. Plant CG, Jones DW (1976) The damaging effects of restorative materials. Part 2 – Pulpal effects related to physical and chemical properties. *British Dental Journal* **140**, 406–412.

77. Reeves R, Stanley HR (1966) The relationship of bacterial penetration and pulpal pathosis in carious teeth. *Oral Surgery, Oral Medicine, Oral Pathology* **22**, 59–65.

78. Rowe AHR, Pitt Ford TR (1990) The assessment of pulpal vitality. *International Endodontic Journal* **23**, 77–83.

79. Seltzer S, Bender IB, Ziontz M (1963) The dynamics of pulp inflammation: correlations between diagnostic data and actual histologic findings in the pulp. *Oral Surgery, Oral Medicine, Oral Pathology* **16**, 846–871, 969–977.

80. Shovelton DS (1968) A study of deep carious dentine. *International Dental Journal* **18**, 392–405.

81. Smith AJ, Murray PE, Lumley PJ (2002) Preserving the vital pulp in operative dentistry: 1. A biological approach. *Dental Update* **29**, 64–69.

82. Stanley HR (1961) Traumatic capacity of high-speed and ultrasonic dental instrumentation. *Journal of the American Dental Association* **63**, 749–766.

83. Stanley HR, Lundy T (1972) Dycal therapy for pulp exposures. *Oral Surgery, Oral Medicine, Oral Pathology* **34**, 818–827.

84. Stanley HR, Pereira JC, Spiegal E, Broom C, Schultz M (1983) The detection and prevalence of reactive and physiologic sclerotic dentin, reparative dentin and dead tracts beneath various types of dental lesions according to tooth surface and age. *Journal of Oral Pathology* **12**, 257–289.

85. Stanley HR, Swerdlow H, Buonocore MG (1967) Pulp reactions to anterior restorative materials. *Journal of the American Dental Association* **75**, 132–141.

86. Stenvik A, Iversen J, Mjör IA (1972) Tissue pressure and histology of normal and inflamed tooth pulps in Macaque monkeys. *Archives of Oral Biology* **17**, 1501–1511.

87. Swerdlow H, Stanley HR (1959) Reaction of the human dental pulp to cavity preparation. Part II at 150,000 rpm with an air-water spray. *Journal of Prosthetic Dentistry* **9**, 121–131.

88. Takamori K (2000) A histopathological and immunohistochemical study of dental pulp and pulpal nerve fibers in rats after the cavity preparation using Er:YAG laser. *Journal of Endodontics* **26**, 95–99.

89. Tanabe K, Yoshiba K, Yoshiba N, Iwaku M, Ozawa H (2002) Immunohistochemical study on pulpal response in rat molars after cavity preparation by Er:YAG laser. *European Journal of Oral Sciences* **110**, 237–245.

90. Tobias RS, Plant CG, Browne RM (1982) Reduction in pulpal inflammation beneath surface-sealed silicates. *International Endodontic Journal* **15**, 173–180.

91. Torstenson B, Nordenvall KJ, Brännström M (1982) Pulpal reaction and microorganisms under Clearfil composite resin in deep cavities with acid etched dentin. *Swedish Dental Journal* **6**, 167–176.

92. Tronstad L (1974) Reaction of the exposed pulp to Dycal treatment. *Oral Surgery, Oral Medicine, Oral Pathology* **38**, 945–953.

93. Trowbridge H0 (1981) Pathogenesis of pulpitis resulting from dental caries. *Journal of Endodontics* **7**, 52–60.

94. Van Hassel HJ (1971) Physiology of the human dental pulp. *Oral Surgery, Oral Medicine, Oral Pathology* **32**, 126–134.

95. Watts A (1979) Bacterial contamination and the toxicity of silicate and zinc phosphate cements. *British Dental Journal* **146**, 7–13.

96. White JM, Goodis HE, Setcos JC, Eakle WS, Hulscher BE, Rose CL (1993) Effects of pulsed Nd:YAG laser energy on human teeth: a three-year follow-up study. *Journal of the American Dental Association* **124**, 45–51.

97. White KC, Cox CF, Kanka J, Dixon DL, Farmer JB, Snugs HM (1994) Pulpal response to adhesive resin systems applied to acid-etched vital dentin: damp versus dry primer application. *Quintessence International* **25**, 259–268.

98. Zander HA (1939) Reaction of the pulp to calcium hydroxide. *Journal of Dental Research* **18**, 373–379.

99. Zander HA (1946) The reaction of dental pulps to silicate cements. *Journal of the American Dental Association* **33**, 1233–1243.

# Basic instrumentation in endodontics

## B. S. Chong

Introduction 51

Basic instrument pack 51

Rubber dam 51

Instruments for access cavity preparation 56
  Burs 56

Instruments for root canal preparation 57
  Hand instruments 57
  Newer instrument design and technology 59
  Power-assisted root canal instruments 60

Devices to determine working length 63
  Measuring devices 65

Irrigant delivery devices 65

Instruments for retrieving broken instruments and posts 66

Instruments for filling root canals 68
  Lateral condensation 68
  Vertical condensation 68
  Thermomechanical compaction 69
  Thermoplasticized injectable gutta-percha 70
  Gutta-percha carrier devices 70

Storage and sterilization of endodontic instruments 71
  Instrument stands and storage systems 71
  Sterilization of endodontic instruments 72

Loupes, fibre-optic lights and operating microscopes 73

References 74

available. Some of the instruments are common to all branches of dentistry while others have been modified or are specifically designed for endodontics.

## BASIC INSTRUMENT PACK

For convenience, a basic selection of instruments should be packaged or set-up in a tray, ready to use (Fig. 5.1). A front-surfaced mouth mirror produces an undistorted image for good visibility deep within the pulp chamber. The endodontic explorer is a double-ended, extra-long, sharp instrument designed to help in the location of canal entrances and for detecting fractures. A long spoon excavator is required to remove pulpal contents and soft caries where present. Locking tweezers are ideal for handling paper points, gutta-percha points, cotton wool pellets and root canal instruments. Both Briault and periodontal probes are necessary for the initial assessment of the tooth for caries and the localized periodontal condition. A flat plastic instrument and an amalgam plugger are needed for placement of an inter-appointment restoration. A millimetre ruler or other measuring device should be available for measuring purposes. A surgical haemostat may be used to position X-ray films, for radiography during treatment.

## INTRODUCTION

The principles of root canal treatment consist of thorough cleaning, adequate shaping and complete filling of the root canal system. In order to accomplish these objectives, many different instruments are

## RUBBER DAM

It is a prerequisite that the tooth being treated must be isolated and this is effectively and efficiently achieved by the use of rubber dam. There are many good reasons for using rubber dam:

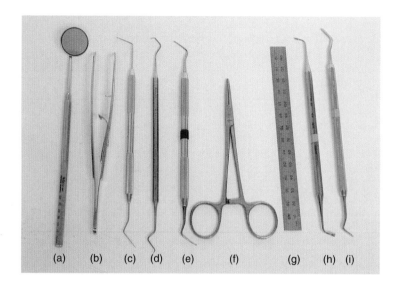

**Figure 5.1** (**a**) Front surface mirror; (**b**) endodontic locking tweezers; (**c**) DG16 endodontic explorer; (**d**) Briault probe; (**e**) long-shank excavator; (**f**) surgical haemostat; (**g**) millimetre ruler; (**h**) amalgam plugger; (**i**) flat plastic.

- It protects the patient from inhalation or ingestion of instruments, medicaments and debris.
- It prevents infection by providing a clean, dry, aseptic working field, free from salivary contamination.
- It allows retraction of soft tissues and the tongue so as not to obstruct the operating field and also protects them from injury.
- It enhances access thereby improving the efficiency of treatment.
- It provides better patient comfort without the oral cavity being flooded with water and/or debris.

Rubber dam is available in pre-cut (commonly 150 mm) squares and also in a roll. The sheets come in different colours and thickness (thin, medium, heavy, extra heavy and special heavy); some are even scented. The thicker material has the advantage of a tighter fit around the neck of the tooth, thus providing a more hermetic seal, so floss ligatures may not be required. It is also less likely to tear [68] and offers better protection for the underlying soft tissues. If there is a small amount of seepage around the margins between the tooth and the rubber dam, temporary filling material (e.g. Cavit, 3M ESPE, Seefeld, Germany) or a non-setting silicone putty (Oraseal, Ultradent, Salt Lake City, UT, USA) (Fig. 5.2) may be placed as a caulking agent to seal off the leakage. For patients allergic to latex, non-latex rubber dam, made of silicone (Roeko, Langenau, Germany) is also obtainable.

The other items for the application of rubber dam include the following.

*Rubber dam punch*

A punch is used to make the required numbers of holes depending on the teeth to be isolated. Usually single tooth isolation is all that is required for endodontic treatment. Single-hole punches (Ash Dentsply, Weybridge, Surrey, UK) are available which will cut a neat hole (1.63 or 1.93 mm), while those with a rotatable table (Ainsworth pattern) will cut different sized holes ranging in diameter from 0.5 to 2.5 mm (Fig. 5.3). Whichever is chosen, it is important to ensure that the punch is sharp, so as to produce a clean hole without any residual tags on the rubber dam. Otherwise, the rubber dam will

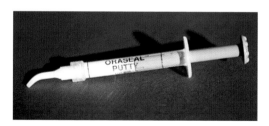

**Figure 5.2** Oraseal caulking agent, a non-setting silicone putty.

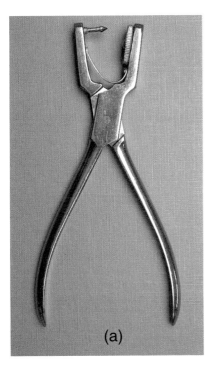
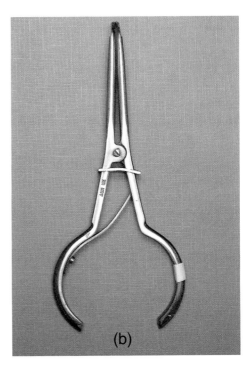

(a)       (b)

**Figure 5.3** (**a**) Rubber dam punch and (**b**) clamp forceps.

tear when stretched and applied to the tooth. The size of hole that is punched is also important; the ease of application with a larger hole must be balanced by the quality of the seal at the cervical margin.

*Rubber dam clamp*

There are many different designs of rubber dam clamp to cater for every possible situation. However, there are no standards governing the manufacture of rubber dam clamps [67].

Clamps have two uses: first, they anchor the rubber dam to the tooth, and second, they retract the gingivae. In endodontics, anchorage is the main requirement. Most clamps are made from stainless steel; some are made from plated steel, which may be susceptible to corrosion by sodium hypochlorite. Clamps are winged or wingless, retentive or bland (Fig. 5.4). A winged clamp allows the attachment of the rubber dam to the clamp so that both clamp and rubber dam may be applied to the tooth together. Retentive clamps are designed to make a four-point contact with the tooth; they have narrow, curved

and slightly inverted jaws, which may displace gingival tissue to grip the tooth below the level of greatest circumference; they are very useful on partly erupted teeth. Bland clamps are less likely to impinge on the gingivae as they have flat jaws, which grip the tooth around its entire circumference. However, they can only be used where a tooth is fully erupted and has a cervical constriction that prevents the clamp from slipping off.

A basic assortment of clamps may consist of the following (Fig. 5.5): Ivory pattern 00, 0, 1, 2A, 9, W8A, 14 and 14A. The winged 14A and the wingless W8A are for molars, the 2A and 1 for premolars, and the 9 for incisors. A range of lettered Ash clamps, which are generally smaller, may also be used; the winged K and E for molars and premolars respectively, and the wingless EW for incisors and broken down premolars. The EW clamp gives better access than the 9.

In anterior teeth, it is sometimes possible to secure the rubber dam without the use of clamps. The interproximal spaces may be wedged with wooden wedges, strips of rubber dam or short lengths of specially made rubber cords (Wedjets, Hygenic, Akron, OH, USA).

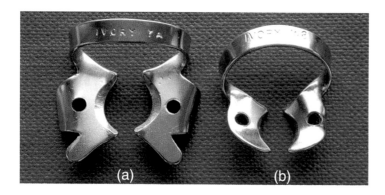

**Figure 5.4** Rubber dam clamps: (a) winged clamp with bland jaws (7A); (b) wingless clamp with retentive jaws (W8).

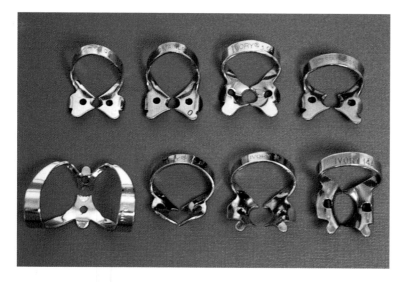

**Figure 5.5** A basic assortment of clamps. Top row, left to right: Ivory patterns 00, 0, 1, 2A. Bottom row: Ivory patterns 9, W8A, 14, 14A.

## Clamp forceps

Several types are available and the choice is a matter of personal preference (Fig. 5.3). The forceps are used to place, adjust and remove the rubber dam clamp. Some forceps may require adjustment to their working ends prior to first use. If the ends are too large, they need to be reshaped so that it is less difficult to disengage the clamp on the tooth.

## Rubber dam frame

The corners of the rubber dam are held apart on a frame, stretched over the patient's mouth, so as not to obscure the operator's vision and not to be uncomfortable for the patient. Rubber dam frames come in various sizes and designs; they are shaped so that they do not impinge on the patient's face. Rubber dam frames are made from either metal or

plastic; the latter is lighter, more comfortable and being radiolucent, removal is unnecessary when taking radiographs (Fig. 5.6).

## Methods of application

Basically, there are three methods of application. In the first method, the rubber dam is attached to the clamp, with or without the frame beforehand, and the whole assembly placed onto the tooth. In this method, only winged clamps can be used. Once the clamp is firmly seated, a plastic instrument is used to lift the rubber off the wings to fit against the side of the tooth (Fig. 5.7).

In the second method, winged or wingless clamps may be used. The clamp is placed on the tooth and the dam is then stretched over the clamp. If this technique is used, the clamp should be wrapped in dental floss as a precaution against

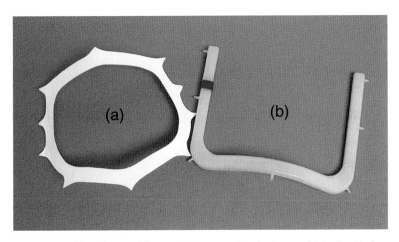

**Figure 5.6** Rubber dam and frames: **(a)** Nygaard-Ostby frame; **(b)** Starlite Visiframe.

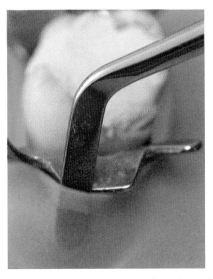

**Figure 5.7** After the clamp is positioned on the tooth, the rubber is lifted off the wings with a flat plastic instrument.

clamp fracture or dislodgement. A length of floss should be tied to one of the holes in the jaw of the clamp and then knotted; it is then wound around the bow of the clamp, threaded through the other hole in the opposite jaw and tied again.

In the third method, the dam is stretched over the tooth and the clamp, winged or wingless, then placed on the tooth. The assistance of a dental nurse is normally required for this method of application.

If more than one tooth is to be isolated, the rubber is knifed through each succeeding contact point.

The rubber is stretched, positioned vertically above the contact point and gently forced through the point. It is important that the rubber remains as a single layer and does not fold over on contact with the teeth. Sometimes knifing is insufficient and the rubber must be forced through the contacts using dental floss. Techniques for placing rubber dam have been reviewed [2,20–22,51]. The use of a lubricant on the undersurface of the dam will aid placement; brushless shaving cream or water-soluble tasteless gels are suitable lubricants.

If a tooth is broken-down and there is insufficient tooth structure for clamp placement, there are several ways of managing the problem. It is normally possible to cement an orthodontic band onto the tooth; this transforms a tooth that is difficult to isolate into one that is straightforward. It may alternatively be possible to remove enough soft tissue surgically, or by electrosurgery, to allow a clamp to be placed. Another method is the 'split-dam' technique in which clamps are placed on the teeth mesial and distal to it. Three holes are punched in the rubber dam and these holes are joined by cutting through with a pair of scissors. The dam is then stretched over both the mesial and distal clamps, isolating the broken-down tooth. Protection against salivary contamination is aided by the use of a cotton-wool roll placed beneath the dam buccally and an aspirator lingually, plus a caulking agent to stop any seepage. This technique may also be used for cases where bridgework is present.

## INSTRUMENTS FOR ACCESS CAVITY PREPARATION

The first stage of root canal treatment is to gain entry into the pulp chamber. Several types of bur will be required for access cavity preparation (Fig. 5.8).

### Burs

*Friction grip burs*

Friction grip tapered or cylindrical fissure burs, ISO 010 or ISO 012, are used in the initial stages of access preparation to establish the correct outline form. For penetrating ceramic or composite materials, diamond-coated burs are needed.

*Round burs*

Round burs, normal and extra-long, sizes ISO 010, 014 and 018, in a contra-angle handpiece are used to lift the roof off the pulp chamber and eliminate overhanging dentine. If a standard length bur is too short, burs with longer shanks, up to 28 mm, are available. So as not to obstruct vision when in use, some long neck burs have a slender shank (Hager & Meisinger, Düsseldorf, Germany). The longer and smaller sizes of burs may be used to remove dentine when opening calcified canals.

*Safe-ended burs*

Following initial access to the pulp space, a safe-ended or non-cutting tip, tapered diamond or tungsten-carbide bur (Endo Z bur, Dentsply Maillefer, Ballaigues, Switzerland) (Fig. 5.8), can be used to remove the entire roof of the pulp chamber. The non-cutting tip prevents 'gouging' of the pulpal floor.

*Gates-Glidden burs*

The Gates-Glidden bur has a slender shank with a cutting bulb and a pilot-tip (Fig. 5.9). It is designed so that if it fractures, this will occur near the hub rather than between the shank and the cutting bulb. Gates-Glidden burs are made of stainless steel and the set of six different sizes of burs have cutting bulbs with diameter ranging 0.5–1.5 mm. They also available in different lengths, a standard 32 mm, a shorter 24 mm and a longer 36 mm. The Gates-Glidden bur is operated at low-speed and may be used for coronal root canal enlargement. In retreatment cases, Gates-Glidden burs are also used to remove gutta-percha in the coronal part of the root canal. The properties of Gates-Glidden drills have been extensively studied [8,40,42,43].

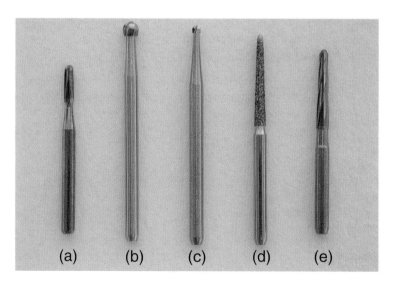

(a)   (b)   (c)   (d)   (e)

**Figure 5.8** Access cavity burs (left to right): (**a**) FG 557 ISO 010 (TC); (**b**) FG ISO round 018 (long); (**c**) FG ISO round 010 (long); (**d**) FG safe-ended diamond 332 ISO 018; (**e**) FG safe-ended TC, Endo Z (Dentsply Maillefer).

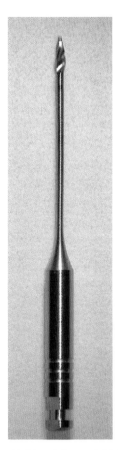

**Figure 5.9** Gates-Glidden drill size 3 (ISO 090).

**Table 5.1** Nominal sizes, diameters, and colour of root canal files and reamers

| Size | $d_1$ (mm) | Colour |
| --- | --- | --- |
| 008 | 0.08 | Grey |
| 010 | 0.10 | Purple |
| 015 | 0.15 | White |
| 020 | 0.20 | Yellow |
| 025 | 0.25 | Red |
| 030 | 0.30 | Blue |
| 035 | 0.35 | Green |
| 040 | 0.40 | Black |
| 045 | 0.45 | White |
| 050 | 0.50 | Yellow |
| 055 | 0.55 | Red |
| 060 | 0.60 | Blue |
| 070 | 0.70 | Green |
| 080 | 0.80 | Black |
| 090 | 0.90 | White |
| 100 | 1.00 | Yellow |
| 110 | 1.10 | Red |
| 120 | 1.20 | Blue |
| 130 | 1.30 | Green |
| 140 | 1.40 | Black |

size; $d_3$ represents a point at 16 mm from $d_1$ where the cutting part of the instrument ends. The taper is a constant 0.02 mm per mm of cutting flute. The shape of the tip is variable. The lengths of instruments available are normally 21, 25 and 31 mm. Root canal instruments have been reviewed [55].

## INSTRUMENTS FOR ROOT CANAL PREPARATION

### Hand instruments

Hand instruments are grouped according to usage and to the classification established by the International Organization for Standardization (ISO). The terminology, dimensions, physical properties, measuring systems and quality control of endodontic instruments and materials are defined by these standards. As a result, endodontic hand instruments, i.e. files, reamers and barbed broaches, are standardized in relation to size, colour coding and physical properties [34]. Table 5.1 lists the relevant information on sizing and colour coding for files and reamers; $d_1$ is an assessment of the diameter of the working part at the tip end, and is its nominal

### Barbed broaches

Barbed broaches are used mainly for the removal of pulp tissue from wide root canals, and cotton wool dressings from the pulp chamber. Provided the instrument is loose within the canal and is used to engage soft tissue, the risk of fracture is minimal. Barbed broaches are made from soft steel wire (Fig. 5.10). The barbs are formed by cutting into the metal and distending the cut portion away from the shaft. The cuts are made eccentrically around the shaft so that it is not weakened excessively at any one point.

### Reamers

Reamers (Fig. 5.10) are manufactured by twisting a tapered stainless steel blank to form an instrument with sharp cutting edges along the spiral. They are used with a half-turn twist and pull action, which

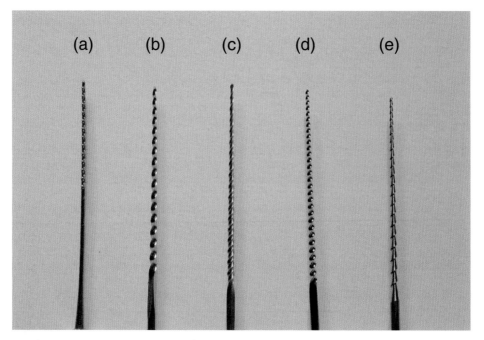

**Figure 5.10** Hand instruments: (**a**) barbed broach; (**b**) reamer; (**c**) K-flex file; (**d**) Flexofile; (**e**) Hedstrom file.

shaves the canal wall, removing dentine chips from the root canal. Nominally they have a triangular cross-section, but the smaller sizes may be manufactured from a square blank.

*Files*

There are various types of root canal file, and they are mostly made from stainless steel. Files are predominantly used with a filing or rasping action, in which there is little or no rotation of the instrument in the root canal. The properties of different files are related to their design features [28,56,57,59]. The common types of files on the market are:

- K-file;
- K-flex file;
- Flexofile;
- Hedstrom file.

*K-file*. This file (Fig. 5.10) is so named as it was introduced by the Kerr Company. These files are made, like reamers, by twisting a triangular or square blank, but into a tighter series of spirals to produce from 0.9 to 1.9 cutting edges per millimetre length. They will work either in a reaming or a push-and-pull filing motion.

*K-flex file*. The K-flex file (Fig. 5.10) was developed in an effort to improve on the original K-file design. It has a rhomboid-shaped cross-section. As a result, when the blank is twisted to form the instrument, it has a series of cutting flutes with alternate sharp (<60°) cutting edges and obtuse non-cutting edges. The high and low flute configuration is designed to endow the instrument with greater flexibility [12], and provide a reservoir for the dentinal debris. A disadvantage of the K-Flex file is that it tends to lose its cutting efficiency quicker.

*Flexofile*. This file (Fig. 5.10) is manufactured by Dentsply Maillefer in the same way as the K-file but using a more flexible stainless steel alloy. The alloy used in file manufacture has a bearing on its cutting efficiency [9] and resistance to fracture [15]. The Flexofile has a non-cutting (Batt) tip and a triangular cross-section so the cutting flutes are sharper and there is more room for debris removal; it was reported to produce good instrumentation results [60].

*Hedstrom file*. The Hedstrom file (Fig. 5.10) is made by a milling process from a steel blank of round cross-section to produce elevated cutting edges. The tapering effect appears to form a series of intersecting cones. Although the design leads to a sharp and flexible instrument, the file is inherently weaker due to the reduced shaft diameter and is therefore slightly more prone to breakage. It is most effective when used in a pull motion [70]. With sharp cutting flutes, it is also used to engage and remove retained instruments, gutta-percha and silver points.

## Newer instrument design and technology

There have been a number of new developments in instrument design and technology.

### Nickel-titanium files

Instead of stainless steel, nickel-titanium (Ni-Ti) alloys have been introduced in the manufacture of endodontic instruments [73]. The Ni-Ti alloys have many interesting properties: a shape memory effect (ability to return perfectly to its original shape), superelasticity (low modulus of elasticity), good biocompatibility and high corrosion resistance. The concept of using Ni-Ti for endodontic instruments came from orthodontics, where its properties have been utilized in the archwires of fixed appliances. The Ni-Ti alloy used in root canal instruments is known generically as Nitinol (*Ni* for nickel, *ti* for titanium and *nol* for Naval Ordinance Laboratory). The manufacture of Ni-Ti endodontic instruments is more complicated than that of stainless steel; the instruments are machined rather than twisted [62].

Compared with stainless steel, files manufactured from Ni-Ti alloy have greater elastic flexibility in bending and greater resistance to torsional fracture [13,53,72,74]; Ni-Ti files have a non-cutting tip and they cannot easily be precurved. Their cutting efficiency is dependent on cross-sectional shape [14], but is less compared with stainless steel files [58,71]. The Ni-Ti files tend to straighten curved root canals less than stainless steel files [26], producing a more centered, tapered and acceptable preparation [6,82]. The files also have different wear characteristics compared with stainless steel files [7].

### GT hand files

The GT (Greater Taper) files (Dentsply Tulsa Dental, Tulsa, OK, USA) were designed by Buchanan [11];

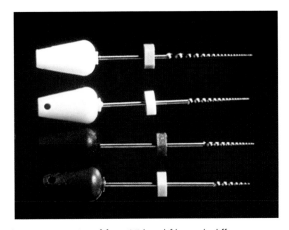

**Figure 5.11** Set of four GT hand files with different tapers.

and are made from Ni-Ti. The set of four hand files of varying tapers (see section on variable taper instruments), 0.12–0.06, all have a tip size of ISO 20. They have pear-shaped handles (Fig. 5.11) and each file is designed for different areas and types of canals. For example, the 0.12 GT file is suited to canal orifices and deeper in relatively straight canals of large apical diameter, while the 0.06 GT file is suited to the apical third in a thin or curved canal. They are intended to allow the creation of a predetermined funnel-shaped canal with fewer instruments than using the ISO series. Operated using a sequence of counterclockwise and clockwise rotations to engage and cut dentine, each rotation is meant to take the GT file closer to the apex, without the need to employ a stepback preparation technique.

### Series 29 Files

In accordance with ISO specifications for traditional hand instrument sizes, the measurement $d_1$ increases by 0.02 mm for sizes 06–10, 0.05 mm for sizes 10–60 and 0.1 mm for sizes 60–130. The percentage difference between tip diameters of sizes 10–15 is 50%, whilst between sizes 55 and 60 the difference is only 9%. The variable percentage changes appear illogical and have been blamed for procedural errors, such as ledging, during apical root canal preparation. Another problem is the difficulty in negotiating narrow and curved canals, since the size increment from one instrument to the next is not uniform and there are insufficient instruments between ISO sizes 10 and 35.

Instruments based on a constant percentage change of diameter at $d_1$ instead of the variable linear dimensional changes have been developed. The Series 29 instruments (Dentsply Tulsa Dental) are made with a constant 29% increase in tip diameter between successive sizes. Therefore, in the critical smaller sizes, there are more instruments than in the ISO range.

## Power-assisted root canal instruments

Many different power-assisted root canal instruments have been developed over the years in the hope of making root canal preparation quicker and to reduce operator fatigue.

### Reciprocating handpieces

These handpieces impart a mechanical action to the root canal instrument to cut dentine. An early example is the Giromatic, a mechanized handpiece in which the continuous rotation of the driveshaft is transformed into an alternating quarter-turn movement of the file. A later example is the M4 Safety handpiece (Kerr) (Fig. 5.12). This handpiece

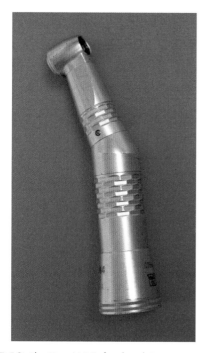

**Figure 5.12** The Kerr M4 Safety handpiece.

has a push button-type chuck mechanism to accommodate plastic handled root canal instruments. The handpiece imparts a watch-winding oscillatory movement to the attached root canal instrument.

### Ultrasonic instrumentation (Endosonics)

The concept of using ultrasonic energy to prepare root canals was first described by Richman [46,52]. The dentine-removing characteristics of ultrasonic devices are dependent on how the ultrasound is generated [27] and the load applied [44].

The Cavi-Endo (Dentsply, Weybridge, UK) was the first ultrasonic device specifically designed for endodontic use (Fig. 5.13). It is a modified Cavitron scaling unit with an irrigant reservoir to deliver a continuous flow of sodium hypochlorite through the handpiece onto the energized file. The ultrasonic energy is generated by magnetostriction, in which electromagnetic energy is converted to mechanical energy. Another means of generating ultrasound is by crystal deformation, the piezo-electric effect. These ultrasonic units (e.g. Piezon-Master 400, EMS, Le Sentier, Switzerland) are supplied with a multifunctional handpiece, into which different tips may be fitted (Fig. 5.14). A file-holding tip is used for ultrasonic instrumentation. Other tips are also available for controlled removal of dentine during the location of calcified canals, to break up the cement lute when removing cemented posts, and for root-end cavity preparation during periradicular surgery (Fig. 5.15).

### Rotary Instruments

With the advent of instruments made from Ni-Ti, the endodontic market has become dominated by many new rotary root canal instrument systems (Table 5.2). It is impossible to detail all the different systems but many new and unique design features have been incorporated by manufacturers.

*Variable taper.* The concept of taper variation is to maximize the cutting efficiency by minimizing the contact area between the surface of the instrument and the canal wall. Instead of having to flare a canal using different sizes of standard 0.02 taper files to achieve the desired taper, the preparation is produced by using files of the desired taper straight-

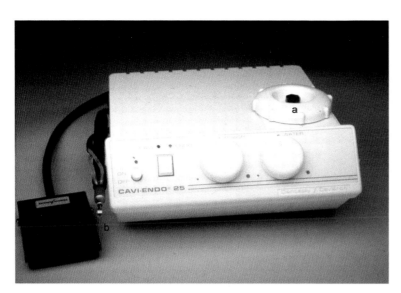

**Figure 5.13** The Cavi-Endo unit which can be used as a scaler or for endosonic use. The reservoir (**a**) supplies a constant flow of irrigant through the special handpiece (**b**).

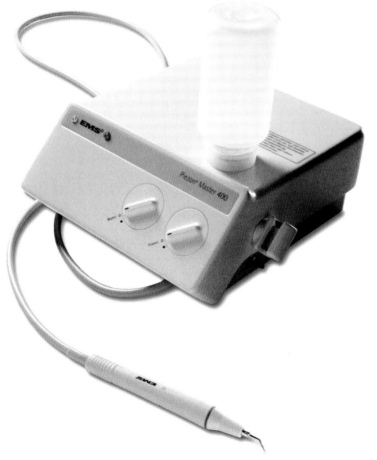

**Figure 5.14** The Piezon-Master 400 unit; the ultrasonic vibration is generated piezo-electrically.

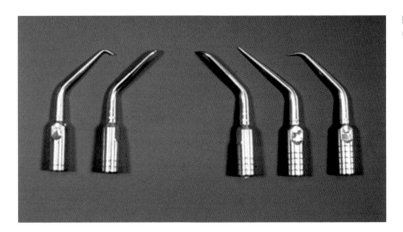

**Figure 5.15** A set of specially designed ultrasonic micro-tips for endodontic surgery.

**Table 5.2** Rotary instrument systems

ProFile (Dentsply Maillefer, Ballaigues, Switzerland)
GT Rotary (Dentsply Maillefer)
Quantec (Analytic Endodontics, Orange, CA, USA)
Lightspeed (Lightspeed Technology, San Antonio, TX, USA)
Hero 642 (Micro-Mega, Besançon, France)
K3 (Kerr Europe, Potters Bar, Herts, UK)
ProTaper (Dentsply Maillefer)

away. The larger the taper, the more conical the shape of the instrument (Fig. 5.16). For ease of use, many rotary instrument systems have matching variable taper paper points and gutta-percha points.

*Flute design.* The shape of the flutes in cross-section determines cutting efficiency and the ability to remove debris. A design incorporating a reservoir for the dentine debris, for example, a U-shaped

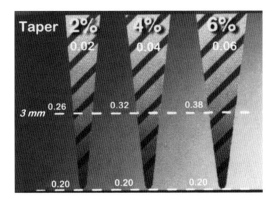

**Figure 5.16** Taper of root canal instruments.

cross-section, will help effective evacuation of the debris through the cutting flutes.

*Rake angle.* The rake or cutting angle of most conventional instruments is negative so the cutting blade scrapes rather than cuts the dentine, and this is inefficient. A positive rake angle results in more effective cutting but if the rake angle is excessively positive, the cutting blade will dig into the dentine substrate. Therefore the rake angle should be only slightly positive.

*Helical flute angle.* This is the angle at which the cutting flutes spiral around the shaft of the instrument. If there are too few spirals, the dentine debris will accumulate quickly before being removed, and the instrument will become clogged. On the other hand, if there are too many spirals, the dentine debris has too great a distance to travel before being evacuated, and frictional resistance may trap and compress the debris. The ideal helical flute angle allows efficient removal of dentinal debris without clogging the instrument. Also, increasing the helical flute angle along the length of the file, from tip to handle, assists in debris removal.

*Core diameter/flute depth.* The core strength and flexibility of an instrument is dependent on its core cross-sectional diameter; the larger the core diameter, the more robust and rigid the instrument. The core diameter is inversely related to the flute depth. The proportion of the core diameter to the outside diameter should be greatest at the tip, where strength is most important. By uniformly decreasing

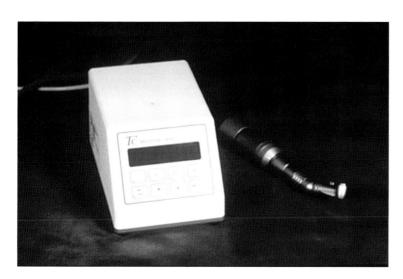

**Figure 5.17** Electric motor and handpiece for rotary root canal instruments.

this proportion as the fluting moves up the taper, resulting in greater flute depth, the flexibility increases while the strength of the instrument is maintained. An additional advantage is that dentine debris is also removed more efficiently.

*Non-cutting tip.* A non-cutting, safe-ended or Batt tip, helps to pilot the instrument down the canal so that it follows the canal shape. Rather than gouging into the canal wall, the tip will help guide the instrument and this reduces the risk of apical transportation.

*Radial lands.* A radial land is a flat, radial surface designed to provide cutting blade support, so as to prevent crack propagation and hence instrument fracture. The larger the amount of metal behind the cutting edge, the more blade support and the greater the instrument's resistance to torsional or rotational stresses. Radial lands also act to centre the instrument to help prevent canal transportation.

### Rotary handpiece and motor

Rotary instruments are normally operated at low torque and low speed (150–350 rpm). Therefore, these instruments must be used with a speed-reducing handpiece, which is driven by either an air or electric motor (Fig. 5.17). Handpieces driven by electric motors have the advantage of being smoother, vibration-free and maintaining the selected speed. To improve access, some of these handpieces are available with a reduced size head. Many rotary files are also made in shorter lengths to facilitate access in posterior teeth.

Some rotary handpieces and motors, particularly electric motors, have control units, which allow for different speed and torque settings. The risk of instrument breakage can be reduced by selecting lower speeds [80] and setting the torque to the limit of elasticity of each instrument [25]. The control units may also have a built-in auto-reverse feature so that the instrument will run in reverse when a pre-set torque is exceeded. Some sophisticated units have programmable memory, for storing different instrumentation protocols that will automatically alter the speed and torque settings depending on the type, size and brand of rotary file used.

Instrument fracture is also related to the degree of canal curvature and instrument taper [29]. It was found that torsional failures caused by using too much apical force during instrumentation occur slightly more frequently than flexural failures, which may result from usage in curved canals [54].

## DEVICES TO DETERMINE WORKING LENGTH

The objectives of endodontic treatment cannot be achieved without knowing the canal length, therefore, the accurate determination of root canal length is important to ensure success of root canal treatment. The two commonest ways of verifying canal

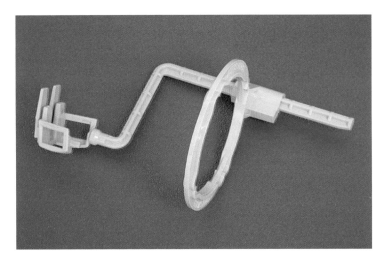

**Figure 5.18** Endoray II beam-aiming device used for taking working length radiographs.

length are by radiography and by the use of an electronic apex locator.

### Radiographic method

In this method of verifying canal length, an instrument is placed into the root canal and then a radiograph taken. The length of the instrument, marked with a rubber/silicone stop, is recorded. Depending on whether the desired depth is reached, as shown radiographically, adjustments are made accordingly. When determining the working length using this method, the X-ray film must be positioned and kept in place. This is achieved with the aid of a surgical haemostat rather than the patient's finger. Alternatively, specially designed film holders are available (e.g. Endoray II, Rinn, Elgin, IL, USA) (Fig. 5.18).

### Electronic apex locators

A method of estimating root canal length based on the different electrical conductivity in a root canal and the oral mucosa has been reported [66] and developed [65]. The operation of electronic apex locators (EALs) has evolved from measuring the electrical resistance with direct, alternating or high frequency currents, to measuring the voltage gradients and calculating the ratio between impedances [38].

A typical EAL has a meter or digital display and two electrodes. One electrode, the ground electrode, is fashioned into a hook and placed into the oral cavity. The other electrode, in the form of a spring-loaded clip

or probe is attached to the endodontic instrument, which is inserted into the root canal. As the instrument is advanced apically, a visual display will show, and often an audio signal will also be emitted, to indicate when the apical foramen is reached. The depth is marked on the instrument and the length measured following its removal from the root canal.

There are two main types on the market – absolute and gradient impedance EALs. Absolute impedance EALs measures impedance using an electric current of one frequency. They have a fixed impedance, range 4.7–9.2 k $\Omega$, and the canal must be dried before taking a measurement. Gradient impedance EALs employ two or more frequencies and the canal does not need to be dry. An example, the Root ZX (Morita, Kyoto, Japan) works on the feedback variation impedance of two frequencies (Fig. 5.19) while the Apex Finder AFA (Analytic Endodontics, Orange, CA, USA) uses five frequencies.

While these devices are useful in determining root canal length, they must be used carefully to avoid errors [17]. A major influencing factor is the size of the apical foramen; when this is large, the apex locator may give a reading short of the apex. However when the apex is small, an accurate reading within 0.5 mm of the apical foramen is likely. Newer generations of EALs are less susceptible to inaccuracies [19] caused by the presence of fluid (blood, exudate or hypochlorite irrigant) in the root canal. The Root ZX was reported to be reliable when tested in the presence of a variety of irrigants commonly used in endodontics [35] and even when the anatomical constriction was eliminated by

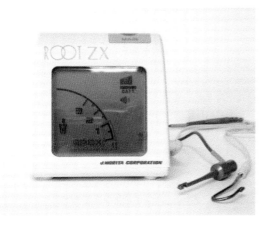

**Figure 5.19** Root ZX apex locator with a digital visual display.

intentional enlargement [49]. The use of an EAL is invaluable in assessing the root canal working length; combined with radiographic confirmation, this should reduce the number of X-ray exposures [24].

A combined, cordless, motorized handpiece and EAL (Tri Auto ZX, Morita) that will measure root canal length and also drive rotary instruments for canal preparation is available (Fig. 5.20). Powered by a rechargeable battery, the motor is capable of a speed

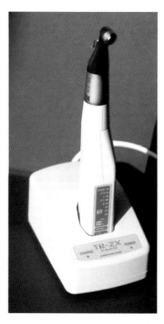

**Figure 5.20** Tri Auto ZX, a combined, cordless, motorized handpiece and electronic apex locator.

of up to 400 rpm without load and one of eight speed settings may be selected. Other features of this dual-function handpiece/EAL include the following:

- auto start/stop – the handpiece will run automatically when the rotary instrument is inserted into the root canal and stop when it is withdrawn;
- auto-apical reverse – the motor drives the rotary instrument in reverse when it reaches the apical constriction;
- auto-torque reverse – if too much torque is applied, the rotation is automatically reversed [39].

## Measuring devices

Devices for measuring file lengths range from a simple metal ruler, obtainable from a hardware shop, to specially designed gauges and measuring blocks. Silicone stops, as markers, are usually already placed on hand instruments by most manufacturers. The ruler incorporated into combination devices like a silicone stop dispenser and a file-bending instrument may also be used for measuring.

## IRRIGANT DELIVERY DEVICES

Irrigants are used to wash out canal debris, dissolve pulpal remnants and lubricate the canal, thus improving the efficiency of canal preparation. Irrigants may be delivered into the root canal using either a needle and syringe or an ultrasonic device. Endodontic irrigation needles are blunt-ended with either a hole or the side cut out (Fig. 5.21). They come in different gauges and are secured to the syringes using a Luer-lock, twist mechanism so the needle will not be dislodged when the plunger of the syringe is depressed.

Ultrasonic devices to irrigate root canals can be very effective, as large volumes of irrigant can be dispensed with ease, to flush out the root canal system thoroughly; the irrigant cleans by acoustic microstreaming [1]. There are two main types of ultrasonic devices on the market depending on whether the ultrasound is generated by the piezo-electric effect or by magnetostriction (see Figs 5.13 and 5.14).

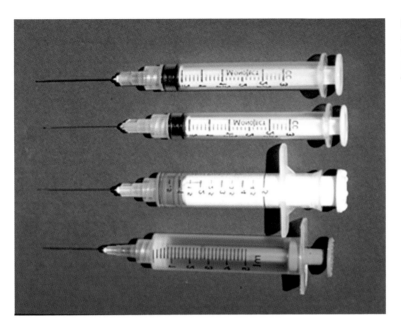

**Figure 5.21** Endodontic irrigating syringes and needles from different manufacturers; the blunt-ended, notched needles are attached to the syringes using a Luer-lock mechanism.

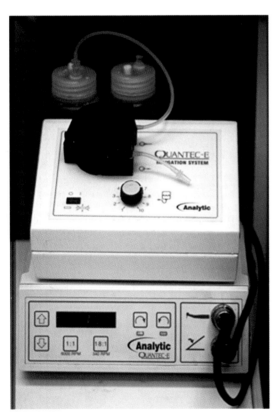

**Figure 5.22** Quantec irrigation system, a self-contained unit designed to sit on top of the electric motor console; irrigant flows through the handpiece during canal instrumentation.

To complement rotary root canal instrumentation, there is a portable self-contained irrigation system (Quantec Irrigation System, Analytic Endodontics) (Fig. 5.22). The peristaltic pump delivers irrigant via the handpiece as the root canal is being prepared with rotary files.

## INSTRUMENTS FOR RETRIEVING BROKEN INSTRUMENTS AND POSTS

All root canal instruments should be used with care to prevent breakage. However, if breakage does occur it may be possible to remove the fragment with one of a number of different devices and techniques.

### Forceps

Fine-beaked haemostats or Steiglitz forceps (Hu-Friedy, Chicago, IL, USA) can be used to remove a broken instrument (Fig. 5.23). However, this is only possible if the end of the fractured instrument is accessible and not jammed firmly within the canal.

### Cancellier kit

If the fractured file is loose but not free, a Cancellier extractor (Analytic Endodontics) may be used. The

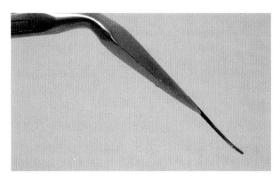

**Figure 5.23** Steiglitz forceps, fine-beaked, for removal of retained instruments or metal filling points.

extractors are a set of hollow tubes, which fit into a handle; the assembly resembles a hollow plugger. The appropriately sized extractor is chosen to fit over the file. A drop of cyanoacrylate glue is placed into the hollow end of the extractor so that it adheres when fitted over the file. A drop of acrylic monomer liquid is then used to accelerate the setting of the cyanoacrylate glue so that the file is retrieved when the extractor is removed. The Cancellier extractors can be cleaned with a solvent, e.g. Xylol, and reused.

### Masserann kit

The technique using the Masserann instrument (Micro-Mega, Besançon, France) (Fig. 5.24) to remove a broken post or retained instrument is well documented [47,79]. A hollow trepan bur is chosen whose internal diameter corresponds to the diameter of the obstruction. The principle of the technique is

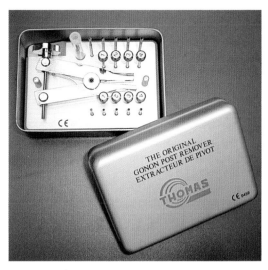

**Figure 5.25** The Gonon post remover system.

to create a trough around the top of the post or instrument to be removed using the trepans, which are rotated in an anticlockwise direction; this action frees the obstruction around its periphery enabling its removal.

### Post removal devices

Many techniques have been devised to remove cemented posts [18]. These include the use of ultrasound to disrupt the cement lute and loosen the post or simple drilling with burs. There are also dedicated post removal devices; examples are the Post Puller [75], the Eggler post remover [64] and the Gonon post removal system [45] (Fig. 5.25). The

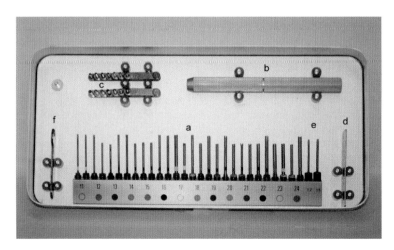

**Figure 5.24** Masserann kit (Micro-Mega) containing a range of trepans (**a**), handle (**b**), gauges (**c, d**), extractor (**e**) and spanner (**f**).

principle behind all these devices is the same and is akin to a corkscrew in which opposing forces are created to extract the post from the root canal. The Ruddle Post Removal System (Analytic Endodontics) is an improved version of the Gonon system.

## INSTRUMENTS FOR FILLING ROOT CANALS

The instruments needed depend on the technique employed to fill the root canal.

### Lateral condensation

In this technique, a well-fitting master gutta-percha point is chosen and combined with sealer to fill the root canal. A finger spreader (Fig. 5.26), designed with a pointed tip, is used to condense the gutta-percha, creating space for placement of accessory gutta-percha points. The gutta-percha is added sequentially until the canal is completely filled. Spreaders are available in a variety of different lengths and widths; they are usually made of stainless steel but there are also Ni-Ti versions. The Ni-Ti fingers spreaders are reported to penetrate to a significantly greater depth in curved canals [5,61] compared with stainless steel spreaders. Depending on the manufacturer, spreaders are available with matching sizes of non-standardized (Fig. 5.26),

standardized and variable taper accessory gutta-percha points. However, there may be a degree of variation between sizes of finger spreaders and their corresponding accessory gutta-percha points [10,84].

### Vertical condensation

In this technique, hand or finger pluggers (Fig. 5.26), which have blunt, flat ends, are used to apply vertical pressure to condense the gutta-percha and sealer. Hand pluggers of different diameters are usually marked with reference lines to allow the assessment of plugger depth. In the classic Schilder technique, small segments of gutta-percha are added, heat is applied using heat carriers to soften the gutta-percha and then condensed with the aid of a series of different sized pluggers; the sequence is repeated until the canal is completely filled. Double-ended instruments, with one end a heat carrier and the other a plugger, are available. Electrically heated carriers (Fig. 5.27) fitted with spreaders or pluggers have been developed for warm gutta-percha filling techniques (Touch 'n Heat and System B, Analytic Endodontics, Orange, CA, USA). The tips of these carriers are heated rapidly and internally so that the heat is concentrated at the tip. A contact spring on the front of the handle acts as a switch to activate the heater. Different temperatures may be chosen for different stages of the filling sequence; with the System B, the chosen temperature will be maintained

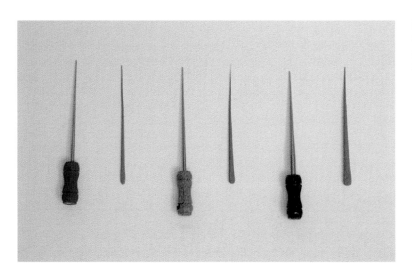

**Figure 5.26** Finger spreaders with corresponding non-standardized accessory gutta-percha points (Kerr medium fine, fine and medium).

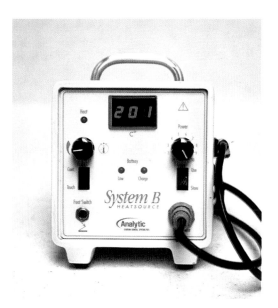

**Figure 5.27** Analytic Technology System B heat source for vertical condensation of gutta-percha.

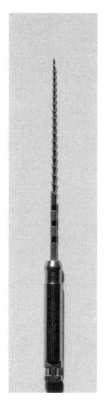

**Figure 5.28** Dentsply Maillefer Gutta-Condensor for thermomechanical compaction of gutta-percha.

throughout when activated. The System B is used for the Buchanan 'Continuous Wave' filling technique, which is a modification of the Schilder technique. The root surface temperature produced varies depending on the heat source and technique used [41,63].

## Thermomechanical compaction

In this technique, an engine-operated compactor, e.g. Gutta Condensor (Dentsply Maillefer) (Fig. 5.28), designed with reverse turning screw threads, is rotated in a forward direction alongside a fitted gutta-percha point, or several points. The heat created by the friction plasticizes the gutta percha and, at the same time, the centrifugal forces generated compacts the gutta-percha onto the canal walls. The higher the speed of rotation the greater the heat generated [48]. As the bulk of gutta-percha in the canal builds up, the compactor is forced out of the canal. The result can be a well-condensed root canal filling that is more homogeneous compared with lateral condensation [83]. If the compactor is used accidentally in reverse, it screws into the root canal and will break. Another disadvantage is that it is possible to extrude gutta-percha through the

apex with this technique; to prevent this, the hybrid technique was developed, in which an apical gutta-percha plug is first created by lateral condensation prior to thermomechanical compaction [69].

A modified technique of thermomechanical compaction involves coating the condenser with already plasticized gutta-percha of a different viscosity (e.g. Microseal, Analytic Endodontics, Orange, CA, USA). The ultra-low fusing gutta-percha for this technique comes in cartridges, which are heated in an oven and delivered with a syringe. A master gutta-percha point is placed beforehand and as previously, when the coated condensor is operated in the canal, plasticized gutta-percha is compacted onto the canal walls. Without the reliance on friction to plasticize the gutta-percha, the condensor can be operated at a lower speed lessening the risk of instrument fracture and potential heat damage to the periodontium.

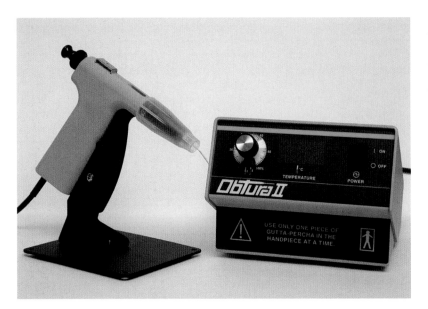

**Figure 5.29** Obtura II thermoplasticized injectable gutta-percha system. The heated delivery gun extrudes gutta-percha through the fine needle; the temperature is controlled by the main unit.

## Thermoplasticized injectable gutta-percha

The concept of injecting softened gutta-percha into the root canal was introduced many years ago [81] as a development of vertical condensation. An example is the Obtura II (Obtura/Spartan, Fenton, MO, USA), a second generation high temperature system capable of taking the temperature of gutta-percha in the heating chamber to 200°C. It consists of a delivery unit with an electrical cord connected to a temperature control box with a digital display (Fig. 5.29). The gutta-percha is loaded into the heating chamber. When the trigger of the delivery unit is squeezed, the softened gutta-percha is extruded through a 20 or 23 gauge needle; the needles are reusable, bendable and sterilizable. Thermal protectors are used to insulate the heating unit and to prevent burning the patient's lip. This technique is useful when filling large and irregular canals. The root filling produced is well adapted to the prepared canal [76]. It is also used for back filling canals after an apical plug has been established.

Concern has been expressed about the heat generated by the Obtura system. However, there is more than a 100°C decrease in temperature as the gutta-percha is extruded [77]; any rise in intra-radicular temperature is below the critical level and should not cause damage to the periodontal ligament [78].

## Gutta-percha carrier devices

The Thermafil system (Dentsply Tulsa Dental) is an example of a gutta-percha carrier device. This commercial product originated from a technique of moulding heated gutta-percha to a root canal file, which was then used to fill the root canal [36].

The current generation Thermafil obturators have a 0.04 taper, V-shaped cross-section plastic core, which is coated with alpha-phase gutta-percha that has excellent flow properties (Fig. 5.30). The obturators are colour-coded and come in ISO sizes 20–140. The size of the Thermafil obturator required is first determined with the aid of a set of Verifier files, made of nickel-titanium. The chosen obturator is warmed by placement in a special oven (ThermaPrep Plus oven). When heated, the obturator is removed from the oven and inserted, with force, into the root canal. After cooling, the handle, if already pre-notched is twisted off; otherwise it is cut off with a bur. A Thermafil Post Space bur is available if post space preparation is required.

The Thermafil system is intended to make filling easier and faster [4], however a minor disadvantage of leaving a plastic core filling material in the root canal is the problem of removing it, should retreatment be required. The retained obturator is not easy to remove [23,33].

## STORAGE AND STERILIZATION OF ENDODONTIC INSTRUMENTS

### Instrument stands and storage systems

Root canal hand instruments such as files may be sterilized and stored in small boxes with stands (Fig. 5.31), or in Pyrex glass test tubes with different coloured covers for instrument identification (Fig. 5.32). Complete sets of instruments can be pre-arranged, sterilized and kept, ready for use. Metal or plastic boxes with lids, in a variety of sizes are available. Some can house all the basic instruments required for endodontic treatment; there is also a file stand, a medicament dish and a cotton wool pellet container. Alternatively, instruments can be sterilized and stored in transparent autoclave bags and laid out on an open plastic tray, with a sponge for files.

Another instrument-holding device, the Endoring II system (Jordco, Beaverton, OR, USA) comprises a triangular disposable sponge for root canal instruments, which is inserted into an autoclavable thermoplastic resin sponge holder, with a snap-on finger ring handle (Fig. 5.33). Disposable wells (Gelwells) for medicaments and canal lubricants, may be attached to the sponge holder; there is also a ruler incorporated. The Endoring II system allows easy access to root canal instruments within the operating field as they can be placed, stored, measured and cleaned, eliminating the time-consuming action of picking up instruments from the bracket table.

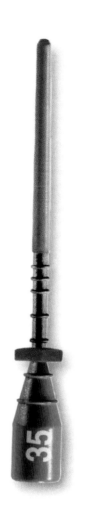

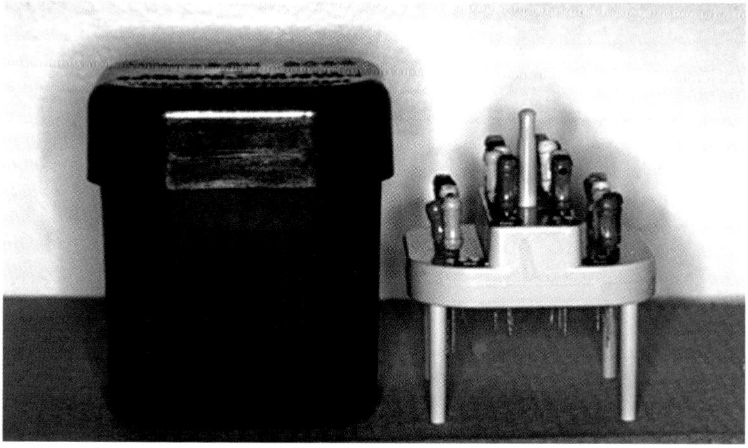

**Figure 5.30** Thermafil obturator. The plastic carrier is coated with gutta-percha.

**Figure 5.31** Autoclavable box with stand for root canal instruments.

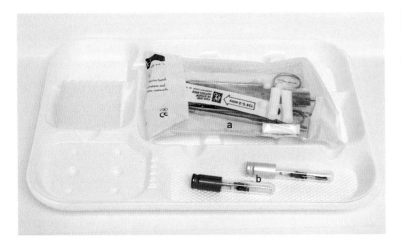

**Figure 5.32** (a) Plastic tray containing instruments in a transparent sterile bag; (b) files can be stored and sterilized in Pyrex glass test tubes.

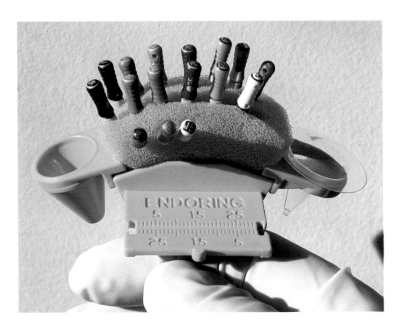

**Figure 5.33** Endoring II, comprising a sponge for instruments in a plastic holder incorporating a ruler and two Gelwells.

## Sterilization of endodontic instruments

The control of infection is the responsibility of every dentist. Adequate, universal methods of infection control must be employed to prevent the risk of transmission of infection within the dental surgery. All instruments and equipment must be cleaned thoroughly prior to sterilization for reuse [50]. Small items like burs and root canal hand instruments must be placed in an ultrasonic bath to remove any debris. The method of choice for sterilization is autoclaving.

Depending on the alloy used in manufacture, the cutting efficiency and some of the mechanical properties of root canals files may be altered by different cleaning, disinfection and sterilization procedures [30]. However, their properties still meet the relevant standards [16,31].

For convenience, and if available, single-use, disposable items are recommended. Sterile packs of files, burs and blister packs of paper points are produced by many manufacturers. These meet requirements for infection control and avoid the use of damaged instruments.

*Glass bead or salt heater*

The glass bead or salt heater is not suitable for sterilizing instruments [32]. It may be used to heat finger spreaders for warm lateral condensation. Glass bead heaters have also been criticized because it is relatively easy to carry a glass bead into the root canal and cause an obstruction; salt, on the other hand, can be dissolved out.

## LOUPES, FIBRE-OPTIC LIGHTS AND OPERATING MICROSCOPES

Endodontic procedures are often performed in areas of limited access and reduced visibility. The use of magnification and better illumination can certainly be extremely helpful in these situations. Magnifying binocular loupes (e.g. Orascoptic telescopes, Orascoptic Research Inc., Madison, WI, USA) (Fig. 5.34) can help enhance vision while fibre-optic lighting provides better illumination. Dedicated dental operating microscopes (e.g. Global Microscope, Global Surgical Corp., St. Louis, MO, USA) (Fig. 5.35) provide the combined benefits of magnification and illumination [37]. They allow greater magnification and facilitate canal orifice location in difficult cases; they are widely used by specialist practitioners. A

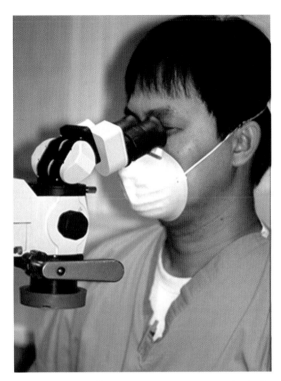

**Figure 5.35** Dental operating microscope provides both magnification and improved illumination.

fibre-optic endoscope, to provide magnified intra-canal visualization has also been developed for use in endodontics [3].

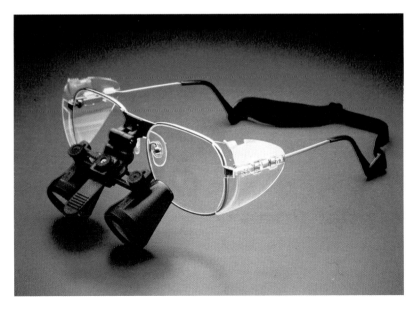

**Figure 5.34** Orascoptic telescopes attached to spectacles for enhanced vision.

# REFERENCES

1. Ahmad M, Pitt Ford TR, Crum LA (1987) Ultrasonic debridement of root canals: acoustic streaming and its possible role. *Journal of Endodontics* **13**, 490–499.
2. Antrim DD (1983) Endodontics and the rubber dam: a review of techniques. *General Dentistry* **31**, 294–299.
3. Bahcall JK, Barss JT (2001) Fiberoptic endoscope usage for intracanal visualization. *Journal of Endodontics* **27**, 128–129.
4. Becker TA, Donnelly JC (1997) Thermafil obturation: a literature review. *General Dentistry* **45**, 46–55.
5. Berry KA, Loushine RJ, Primack RD, Runyan DA (1998) Nickel-titanium versus stainless-steel finger spreaders in curved canals. *Journal of Endodontics* **24**, 752–754.
6. Bishop K, Dummer PMH (1997) A comparison of stainless steel Flexofiles and nickel-titanium NiTiFlex files during the shaping of simulated canals. *International Endodontic Journal* **30**, 25–34.
7. Bonetti Filho I, Miranda Esberard R, De Toledo Leonardo R, Del Rio CE (1998) Microscopic evaluation of three endodontic files pre- and postinstrumentation. *Journal of Endodontics* **24**, 461–464.
8. Brantley WA, Luebke NH, Luebke FL, Mitchell JC (1994) Performance of engine-driven rotary endodontic instruments with a superimposed bending deflection: V. Gates Glidden and Peeso drills. *Journal of Endodontics* **20**, 241–245.
9. Brau-Aguade E, Canalda-Sahli C, Berastegui-Jimeno E (1996) Cutting efficiency of K-files manufactured with different metallic alloys. *Endodontics and Dental Traumatology* **12**, 286–288.
10. Briseno Marroquin B, Wolter D, Willershausen-Zönnchen B (2001) Dimensional variability of nonstandardized greater taper finger spreaders with matching gutta-percha-points. *International Endodontic Journal* **34**, 23–28.
11. Buchanan LS (2001) The standardized-taper root canal preparation – Part 1. Concepts for variably tapered shaping instruments. *International Endodontic Journal* **34**, 411–413.
12. Camps JJ, Pertot WJ (1994) Relationship between file size and stiffness of stainless steel instruments. *Endodontics and Dental Traumatology* **10**, 260–263.
13. Camps JJ, Pertot WJ (1995) Torsional and stiffness properties of nickel-titanium K files. *International Endodontic Journal* **28**, 239–243.
14. Camps JJ, Pertot WJ (1995) Machining efficiency of nickel-titanium K-type files in a linear motion. *International Endodontic Journal* **28**, 279–284.
15. Canalda-Sahli C, Brau-Aguade E, Berastegui-Jimeno E (1996) A comparison of bending and torsional properties of K-files manufactured with different metallic alloys. *International Endodontic Journal* **29**, 185–189.
16. Canalda-Sahli C, Brau-Aguade E, Sentis-Vilalta J (1998) The effect of sterilization on bending and torsional properties of K-files manufactured with different metallic alloys. *International Endodontic Journal* **31**, 48–52.
17. Chong BS, Pitt Ford TR (1994) Apex locators in endodontics: which, when and how? *Dental Update* **21**, 328–330.
18. Chong BS, Pitt Ford TR (1996) Endodontic retreatments. 2: Methods. *Dental Update* **23**, 384–387.
19. Czerw RJ, Fulkerson MS, Donnelly JC, Walmann JO (1995) In vitro evaluation of the accuracy of several electronic apex locators. *Journal of Endodontics* **21**, 572–575.
20. Elderton RJ (1971) A modern approach to the use of rubber dam. Part 1. *Dental Practitioner and Dental Record* **21**, 187–193.
21. Elderton RJ (1971) A modern approach to the use of rubber dam. Part 2. *Dental Practitioner and Dental Record* **21**, 226–232.
22. Elderton RJ (1971) A modern approach to the use of rubber dam. Part 3. *Dental Practitioner and Dental Record* **21**, 267–273.
23. Frajlich SR, Goldberg F, Massone EJ, Cantarini C, Artaza LP (1998) Comparative study of retreatment of Thermafil and lateral condensation of endodontic fillings. *International Endodontic Journal* **31**, 354–357.
24. Fouad AF, Reid LC (2000) Effect of using electronic apex locators on selected endodontic treatment parameters. *Journal of Endodontics* **26**, 364–367.
25. Gambarini G (2000) Rationale for the use of low-torque endodontic motors in root canal instrumentation. *Endodontics and Dental Traumatology* **16**, 95–100.
26. Glosson CR, Haller RH, Dove SB, Del Rio CE (1995) A comparison of root canal preparations using Ni-Ti hand, Ni-Ti engine-driven, and K-Flex endodontic instruments. *Journal of Endodontics* **21**, 146–151.
27. Gulabivala K, Briggs P, Setchell DJ (1993) A comparison of the dentine-removing characteristics of two endosonic units. *International Endodontic Journal* **26**, 26–36.
28. Haikel Y, Gasser P, Allemann C (1991) Dynamic fracture of hybrid endodontic hand instruments compared with traditional files. *Journal of Endodontics* **17**, 217–220.
29. Haikel Y, Serfaty R, Bateman G, Senger B, Allemann C (1999) Dynamic and cyclic fatigue of engine-driven rotary nickel-titanium endodontic instruments. *Journal of Endodontics* **25**, 434–440.
30. Haikel Y, Serfaty R, Bleicher P, Lwin TT, Allemann C (1996) Effects of cleaning, disinfection, and sterilization procedures on the cutting efficiency of endodontic files. *Journal of Endodontics* **22**, 657–661.
31. Haikel Y, Serfaty R, Bleicher P, Lwin TT, Allemann C (1997) Effects of cleaning, chemical disinfection, and sterilization procedures on the mechanical properties of endodontic instruments. *Journal of Endodontics* **23**, 15–18.
32. Hurtt CA, Rossman LE (1996) The sterilization of endodontic hand files. *Journal of Endodontics* **22**, 321–322.
33. Ibarrola JL, Knowles KI, Ludlow MO (1993) Retrievability of Thermafil plastic cores using organic solvents. *Journal of Endodontics* **19**, 417–418.

34. International Organization for Standardization (ISO) (1992) *Dental Root Canal Instruments – Part 1: Specification for Files, Reamers, Barbed Broaches, Rasps, Paste Carriers, Explorers and Cotton Broaches.* ISO 3630-1: 1992. London, UK: British Standards Institution.

35. Jenkins JA, Walker WA, Schindler WG, Flores CM (2001) An in vitro evaluation of the accuracy of the Root ZX in the presence of various irrigants. *Journal of Endodontics* **27**, 209–211.

36. Johnson WB (1978) A new gutta-percha technique. *Journal of Endodontics* **4**, 184–188.

37. Kim S (1997) Principles of endodontic microsurgery. *Dental Clinics of North America*. **41**, 481–497.

38. Kobayashi C (1995) Electronic canal length measurement. *Oral Surgery, Oral Medicine, Oral Pathology, Oral Radiology, Endodontics* **79**, 226–231.

39. Kobayashi C, Yoshioka T, Suda H (1997) A new engine-driven canal preparation system with electronic canal measuring capability. *Journal of Endodontics* **23**, 751–754.

40. Lausten LL, Luebke NH, Brantley WA (1993) Bending and metallurgical properties of rotary endodontic instruments. IV. Gates-Glidden and Peeso drills. *Journal of Endodontics* **19**, 440–447.

41. Lee FS, Van Cura JE, BeGole E (1998) A comparison of root surface temperatures using different obturation heat sources. *Journal of Endodontics* **24**, 617–620.

42. Luebke NH, Brantley WA (1990) Physical dimensions and torsional properties of rotary endodontic instruments. I. Gates-Glidden drills. *Journal of Endodontics* **16**, 438–441.

43. Luebke NH, Brantley WA (1991) Torsional and metallurgical properties of rotary endodontic instruments. II. Stainless steel Gates-Glidden drills. *Journal of Endodontics* **17**, 319–323.

44. Lumley PJ, Walmsley AD, Thomas A (1994) An *in vitro* investigation into the cutting ability of ultrasonic K files. *Endodontics and Dental Traumatology* **10**, 264–267.

45. Machtou P, Sarfati P, Cohen AG (1989) Post removal prior to retreatment. *Journal of Endodontics* **15**, 552–554.

46. Martin H (1976) Ultrasonic disinfection of the root canal. *Oral Surgery, Oral Medicine, Oral Pathology* **42**, 92–99.

47. Masserann J (1979) Entfernen metallischer Fragmente aus Wurzelkanälen. *Journal of the British Endodontic Society* **5**, 55–59.

48. McCullagh JJ, Biagioni PA, Lamey PJ, Hussey DL (1997) Thermographic assessment of root canal obturation using thermomechanical compaction. *International Endodontic Journal* **30**, 191–195.

49. Nguyen HQ, Kaufman AY, Komorowski RC, Friedman S (1996) Electronic length measurement using small and large files in enlarged canals. *International Endodontic Journal* **29**, 359–364.

50. Reams GJ, Baumgartner JC, Kulild JC (1995) Practical application of infection control in endodontics. *Journal of Endodontics* **21**, 281–284.

51. Reuter JE (1983) The isolation of teeth and the protection of the patient during endodontic treatment. *International Endodontic Journal* **16**, 173–181.

52. Richman MJ (1957) Use of ultrasonics in root canal therapy and root resection. *Journal of Dental Medicine* **12**, 12–18.

53. Rowan MB, Nicholls JI, Steiner J (1996) Torsional properties of stainless steel and nickel-titanium endodontic files. *Journal of Endodontics* **22**, 341–345.

54. Sattapan B, Nervo GJ, Palamara JE, Messer HH (2000) Defects in rotary nickel-titanium files after clinical use. *Journal of Endodontics* **26**, 161–165.

55. Schafer E (1997) Root canal instruments for manual use: a review. *Endodontics and Dental Traumatology* **13**, 51–64.

56. Schafer E (1999) Relationship between design features of endodontic instruments and their properties. Part 1. Cutting efficiency. *Journal of Endodontics* **25**, 52–55.

57. Schafer E (1999) Relationship between design features of endodontic instruments and their properties. Part 2. Instrumentation of curved canals. *Journal of Endodontics* **25**, 56–59.

58. Schafer E, Tepel J (1996) Cutting efficiency of Hedstrom, S and U files made of various alloys in filing motion. *International Endodontic Journal* **29**, 302–308.

59. Schafer E, Tepel J (2001) Relationship between design features of endodontic instruments and their properties. Part 3. Resistance to bending and fracture. *Journal of Endodontics* **27**, 299–303.

60. Schafer E, Tepel J, Hoppe W (1995) Properties of endodontic hand instruments used in rotary motion. Part 2. Instrumentation of curved canals. *Journal of Endodontics* **21**, 493–497.

61. Schmidt KJ, Walker TL, Johnson JD, Nicoll BK (2000) Comparison of nickel-titanium and stainless-steel spreader penetration and accessory cone fit in curved canals. *Journal of Endodontics* **26**, 42–44.

62. Serene TP, Adams JD, Saxena A (1995) *Nickel-Titanium Instruments: Applications in Endodontics*. St. Louis MO, USA: Ishiyaku Euro America, Inc.

63. Silver GK, Love RM, Purton DG (1999) Comparison of two vertical condensation obturation techniques: Touch 'n Heat modified and System B. *International Endodontic Journal* **32**, 287–295.

64. Stamos DE, Gutmann JL (1991) Revisiting the Post Puller. *Journal of Endodontics* **17**, 466–468.

65. Sunada I (1962) New method of measuring the length of the root canal. *Journal of Dental Research* **41**, 375–387.

66. Suzuki K (1942) Experimental study on iontophoresis. *Japanese Journal of Stomatology* **16**, 411–417.

67. Svec TA, Powers JM, Ladd GD (1997) Hardness and stress corrosion of rubber dam clamps. *Journal of Endodontics* **23**, 397–398.

68. Svec TA, Powers JM, Ladd GD, Meyer TN (1996) Tensile and tear properties of dental dam. *Journal of Endodontics* **22**, 253–256.

69. Tagger M, Tamse A, Katz A, Korzen BH (1984) Evaluation of the apical seal produced by a hybrid root canal filling method, combining lateral condensation and thermatic compaction. *Journal of Endodontics* **10**, 299–303.

70. Tepel J, Schafer E (1997) Endodontic hand instruments: cutting efficiency, instrumentation of curved canals,

bending and torsional properties. *Endodontics and Dental Traumatology* **13**, 201–210.

71. Tepel J, Schafer E, Hoppe W (1995) Properties of endodontic hand instruments used in rotary motion. Part 1. Cutting efficiency. *Journal of Endodontics* **21**, 418–421.

72. Tepel J, Schafer E, Hoppe W (1997) Properties of endodontic hand instruments used in rotary motion. Part 3. Resistance to bending and fracture. *Journal of Endodontics* **23**, 141–145.

73. Thompson SA (2000) An overview of nickel-titanium alloys used in dentistry. *International Endodontic Journal* **33**, 297–310.

74. Walia HM, Brantley WA, Gerstein H (1988) An initial investigation of the bending and torsional properties of Nitinol root canal files. *Journal of Endodontics* **14**, 346–351.

75. Warren SR, Gutmann JL (1979) Simplified method for removing intraradicular posts. *Journal of Prosthetic Dentistry* **42**, 353–356.

76. Weller RN, Kimborough WF, Anderson RW (1997) A comparison of thermoplastic obturation techniques: adaptation to the canal walls. *Journal of Endodontics* **23**, 703–706.

77. Weller RN, Koch KA (1994) *In vitro* temperatures produced by a new injectable gutta-percha system. *International Endodontic Journal* **27**, 299–303.

78. Weller RN, Koch KA (1995) *In vitro* radicular temperatures produced by injectable thermoplasticized gutta-percha. *International Endodontic Journal* **28**, 86–90.

79. Williams VD, Bjorndal AM (1983) The Masserann technique for the removal of fractured posts in endodontically treated teeth. *Journal of Prosthetic Dentistry* **49**, 46–48.

80. Yared GM, Bou Dagher FE, Machtou P (2001) Influence of rotational speed, torque and operator's proficiency on Profile failures. *International Endodontic Journal* **34**, 47–53.

81. Yee FS, Marlin J, Krakow AA, Gron P (1977) Three-dimensional obturation of the root canal using injection molded thermoplasticized dental gutta-percha. *Journal of Endodontics* **3**, 168–174.

82. Zmener O, Balbachan L (1995) Effectiveness of nickel-titanium files for preparing curved root canals. *Endodontics and Dental Traumatology* **11**, 121–123.

83. Zmener O, Gimenes Frias J (1991) Thermomechanical compaction of gutta-percha: a scanning electron microscope study. *Endodontics and Dental Traumatology* **7**, 153–157.

84. Zmener O, Hilu R, Scavo R (1996) Compatibility between standardized endodontic finger spreaders and accessory gutta-percha cones. *Endodontics and Dental Traumatology* **12**, 237–239.

# Preparation of the root canal system

J. D. Regan and J. L. Gutmann

Introduction  77

Preoperative assessment  78

Preparation of the clinical crown  80

Access cavity  81

Root canal orifices  83

Working length determination  84

Root canal irrigation  85

Instrumentation techniques  86
Crowndown technique  87
Stepback technique  88
Calcified canals  89

Nickel-titanium instruments  90

Controversies in root canal cleaning and shaping  90
Where should the preparation end?  90
When should the preparation end?  90
Should apical patency filing be performed?  91
Should treatment be completed in one or multiple
visits?  91

References  91

## INTRODUCTION

The key factor in the development of pulpal inflammation and apical periodontitis is the presence of bacteria [42]. It has been widely accepted that bacteria and/or their products are the main aetiological factors in the initiation and progress of these diseases [10]. Consequently, the central focus of root canal treatment has been directed towards the elimination of bacteria and their substrates from the pulp canal system. This may involve removal of necrotic pulp and tissue debris, removal of an inflamed pulp or, in elective treatment, the removal of healthy tissue. Retreatment of failing cases is addressed in Chapter 13.

Historically, a mechanistic approach to root canal treatment was frequently adopted, but in recent years a greater awareness of the complexities of the root canal system (Fig. 6.1) has led to the development of newer techniques, instruments and materials. These new developments have greatly enhanced the clinician's ability to achieve the biologically-based objectives of root canal treatment, which include:

1. Removal of all tissue, bacteria and bacterial products and substrates from the root canal system.

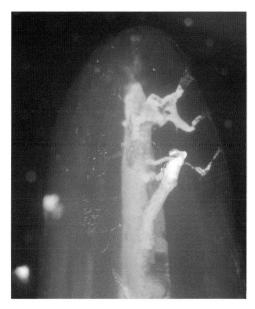

**Figure 6.1** A root end which has been made transparent showing two lateral canals.

2. Shaping of the root canal system to facilitate placement of a root canal filling.
3. filling of the shaped canal system coupled with an adequate and timely coronal restoration.

Traditionally the *'endodontic triad'* concept of cleaning, shaping and filling has been promulgated widely. However, considering that a major goal of root canal treatment is removal of microorganisms from the complex root canal system, it would therefore appear that *'shaping to facilitate cleaning and filling'* might be a more appropriate concept. These objectives must be achieved while ensuring conservation of tooth structure and maintaining canal shape.

## PREOPERATIVE ASSESSMENT

Once a diagnosis has confirmed the need for root canal treatment, then a treatment plan that includes the marginal periodontal status and restorability of the tooth is essential before treatment commences. In addition to the clinical examination this assessment includes radiological evaluation of the tooth.

Good quality preoperative radiographs (preferably from two different angles) are indicated (Fig. 6.2). These films must not be distorted, and must be processed properly to ensure a permanent record. Alternatively, digital radiographs should be filed and a permanent copy stored. Use of a paralleling technique and a film-holder (Fig. 6.3) will minimize distortion of the radiograph and facilitate accurate preoperative, postoperative and review comparisons.

Periapical films are the radiographic views most frequently used during root canal treatment. However, other intraoral and extraoral views can often contribute to the overall preoperative assessment and to diagnosis. These additional films include bitewing, panoramic and occlusal films. For example, a supplemental bitewing radiograph may be useful in detecting suspected caries not readily visible on the periapical radiograph or to determine the relationship of the pulp chamber to the external surface of the tooth (Fig. 6.4).

The tooth to be treated should be located centrally on the periapical film with at least 2 mm of periradicular tissue visible beyond and around the apex. A subsequent film should be exposed with the X-ray beam angled 15°–20° to the original exposure. This shift in angulation results in an apparent change in the position of the roots and is called the parallax effect. Both horizontal and vertical parallax techniques can be used. A good quality film (Fig. 6.2) will provide information concerning the general tooth form and the relationship of the tooth to the surrounding structures. Furthermore it will reveal evidence about the number of roots, their length, and the relationship of the roots to the crown of the tooth. Moreover, it can provide details of previous dental disease and treatment, as well as the resultant pulp reactions such as narrowing of the pulp

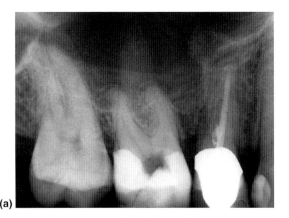
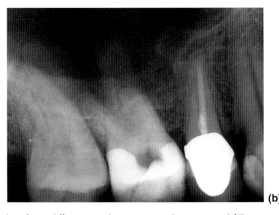

(a)  (b)

**Figure 6.2** Two radiographs of the maxillary second premolar taken from different angles: (**a**) a single root canal filling is observed in the buccal root canal; (**b**) the two root canals are superimposed on each other but the periapical radiolucency is clearly seen.

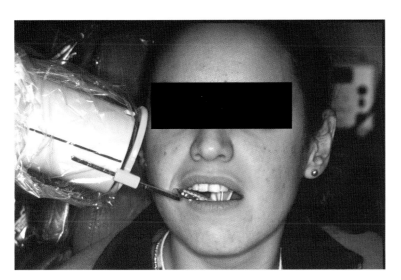

**Figure 6.3** Use of a paralleling technique and film-holder minimize distortion of the radiograph.

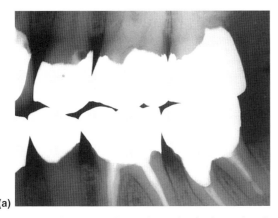

(a)

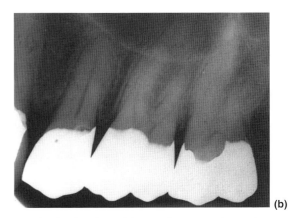

(b)

**Figure 6.4** A bitewing radiograph (**a**) clearly shows dental caries on the distal surface of the maxillary second premolar, whereas it is far less clear on the periapical radiograph (**b**).

chamber and root canals or presence of pulp calcifications. However, interpretation of radiographs can be misleading if certain concepts are not understood; for example, teeth with irreversibly inflamed or necrotic pulps frequently show no radiological changes. Likewise radiological evidence of periradicular lesions may not become obvious until the dense cortical plate of bone has undergone some resorption [8,9].

The radicular anatomy of teeth is variable, as is the relationship of the roots to the surrounding bone. A number of anatomical structures overlie the roots such as the zygomatic arch, mandibular and maxillary tori and the maxillary sinus; they frequently confuse radiological interpretation of the

image. It must be appreciated that a radiograph is merely a two-dimensional shadow of a three-dimensional object. In addition, interpretation of radiographs has been shown to be highly subjective [29,30,31,72].

During the preoperative assessment it may become evident that a tooth requires coronal build-up, crown lengthening or extrusion before a rubber dam clamp can be placed and root canal treatment started. Localized periodontal surgical procedures or electrosurgery are recommended frequently when caries or fractures extend more than 2–3 mm subgingivally. Before the tooth can be restored adequately, a sound dentine margin should protrude at least 1 mm above the free gingival margin that is normally 1–2 mm from the sulcus depth. This implies that the dentine margin should be approximately 3 mm above the crestal bone. The combined connective tissue and epithelial attachment from the crest of the alveolar bone to the base of the gingival sulcus is called the biological width. It is important that restorations do not encroach on this normal soft tissue attachment.

## PREPARATION OF THE CLINICAL CROWN

Preliminary procedures involve isolation of the tooth and removal of all dental caries. Existing restorations may need to be removed completely especially if defective [1]. Even if dental caries does not dictate the complete removal of the restoration, it is often beneficial to do so as hidden fracture lines in the proximal areas become visible (Fig. 6.5). If cast restorations are present, it is important to assess the integrity of the restoration and its cement lute, and to decide whether to retain or to remove the restoration. If the tooth is at risk of fracture, a provisional crown or an orthodontic band should be placed prior to treatment. Orthodontic bands provide an excellent option when there has been extensive loss of coronal tooth tissue. These bands are supplied in a wide variety of sizes and are readily adjusted and cemented to the existing tooth structure.

Failure to prepare the crown adequately prior to root canal treatment can result in:

- bacterial contamination from saliva or caries during or between treatments;
- displacement of restorative materials into the canal;
- fracture of unsupported tooth structure between visits or after treatment.

Isolation of the tooth with rubber dam is a necessary prerequisite for endodontic treatment. It is essential for protection of the airway. The inhalation or swallowing of instruments by a patient in the absence of rubber dam is a serious but preventable accident and is indefensible.

The rubber dam application technique is a matter of choice for the individual clinician. A wide variety

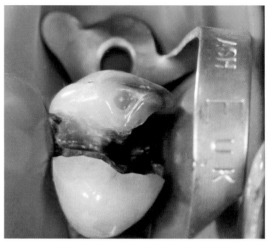

(a)

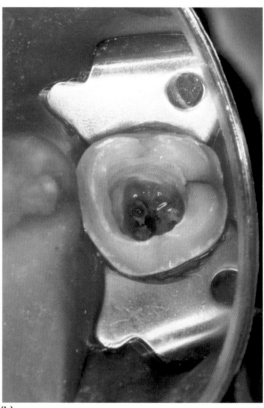

(b)

**Figure 6.5** The maxillary premolar (**a**) shows a crack in the floor of the mesial box after removal of the restoration and staining; (**b**) the mandibular molar shows a crack on the distal aspect after removal of the crown and staining.

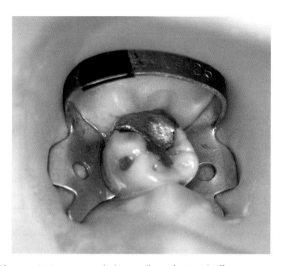

**Figure 6.6** A winged clamp allows fast and efficient placement of rubber dam, in this case on a mandibular molar.

of clamps are available but a skilled clinician will normally use a limited range. Winged clamps are most suitable for the fast and efficient placement of rubber dam (Fig. 6.6). These winged clamps allow the dentist to place the clamp, dam and frame in one action. In recent years an increasing number of reports of allergies to latex have been reported and therefore non-latex rubber dam has been developed. A complete dam placement kit should include:

- rubber dam;
- rubber dam punch;
- clamp forceps;
- selection of clamps;
- dental floss;
- caulking agent.

Occasional improvization is necessary when routine rubber dam placement proves difficult. Examples include cases where the tooth in question has undergone extensive coronal tissue loss or where the tooth to be treated is the abutment for a fixed bridge. These situations frequently necessitate clamping an adjacent tooth and stretching the dam over the tooth to be treated, using a 'split-dam' technique (Fig. 6.7). Following placement, minor defects in the adaptation of the dam can be corrected with a caulking agent such as OraSeal (Ultradent, Salt Lake City, UT, USA) or cyanoacrylate [67].

Excellent reviews of rubber dam placement have been published [50,65,66]. In general, rubber dam application prior to endodontic treatment should be a simple procedure and will enhance both treatment and patient comfort.

## ACCESS CAVITY

The main function of the access cavity is to create an unimpeded pathway to the pulp space and the apical foramen of the tooth. Many problems encountered during root canal treatment can be

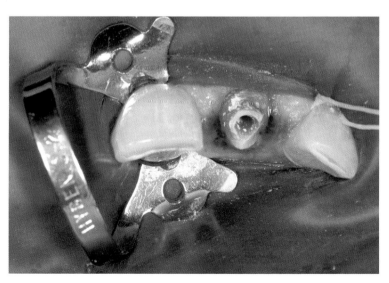

**Figure 6.7** In the split-dam technique the right central incisor has been clamped and the dam stretched over the left lateral incisor to allow isolation of the left central incisor.

81

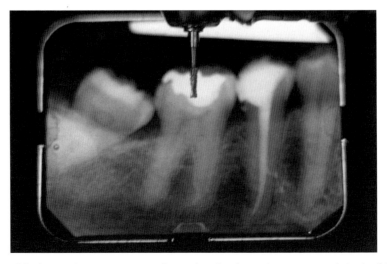

**Figure 6.8** Alignment of the bur on the preoperative radiograph will indicate the position and depth of the restoration and pulp chamber.

avoided or eliminated by a properly designed access opening. The major consideration in all access openings is that conservation of coronal tooth structure should never preclude the proper design and purpose of the access opening [36].

The design of the access cavity to the pulp chamber should reflect the anticipated position of the underlying root canal orifices. The relationship between the pulp chamber and external anatomical outlines must be assessed on the preoperative radiographs. Careful analysis of the radiographs and careful alignment of the bur will reduce the possibility of mishaps during access preparation (Fig. 6.8). Inadvertent overextension of a bur either vertically through the floor of the chamber into the furcation or laterally can be prevented by taking these precautions. Occasionally, in cases where an extracoronal restoration is severely tilted relative to the roots or in cases with sclerosed root canal systems, access to the pulp canal chamber may best be created prior to placing rubber dam to permit more accurate orientation of the rotary instruments to the root outline.

The pulp chamber must be completely unroofed. The pulp chamber dimensions can vary enormously and reflect the nature of the 'insults' that the tooth suffered since eruption. In addition, mineralized deposits are frequently found in the chamber and root canal system (Fig. 6.9).

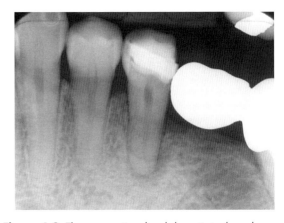

**Figure 6.9** There are mineralized deposits in the pulp chambers of the canine and first premolar.

A well-designed access cavity (Fig. 6.10) permits:

- complete debridement of the pulp chamber;
- visualization of its floor;
- unimpeded placement of instruments into the root canals;
- conservation of tooth tissue.

Coronal and cervical obstructions that may have a restrictive effect on canal exploration and instrumentation need to be eliminated [47].

Irrigation of the pulp chamber with sodium hypochlorite (NaOCl) during access cavity

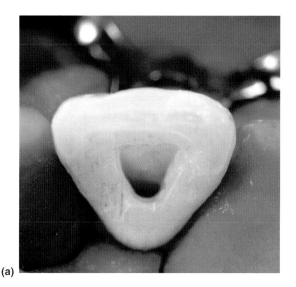

(a)

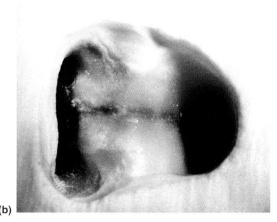

(b)

**Figure 6.10** A well-designed access cavity conserves tooth tissue (**a**), and facilitates visualization of the floor of the pulp chamber in a molar (**b**).

preparation is used to dissolve tissue and aid in debridement of the chamber. This will also reduce the opportunity for the inadvertent inoculation of microorganisms from the pulp chamber into the root canal system. Ultrasonically energized tips (Fig. 6.11) are useful adjuncts during debridement of the pulp chamber to break up calcific masses with relative safety and to facilitate removal of debris. These instruments are contra-angled to enhance access.

## ROOT CANAL ORIFICES

A sound knowledge of the anatomy of the tooth is very important to the practice of predictable and successful endodontics. The number of canals and their approximate positions can be predicted from a knowledge of dentinogenesis and the nature of root formation. No technological advances or innovations can fully compensate for a lack of understanding of the anatomical features of the pulp chamber, which along with the root canal space are always located in the cross-sectional centre of the crown and root respectively [36]. The location of canal orifices is best achieved with good illumination and a dry pulp floor. Magnification with either loupes or a microscope is usually considered beneficial; however the microscope is better for detecting orifices [91]. Careful inspection of the floor will usually reveal anatomical 'guidelines' (Fig. 6.10) that will facilitate identification of the orifices even in calcified cases. If the orifice is not immediately apparent,

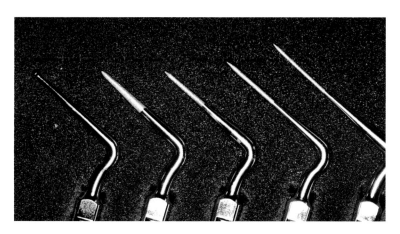

**Figure 6.11** Ultrasonically energized tips are used to break up calcific masses in canal orifices.

a sharp DG 16 probe can be used to explore along the anatomical landmarks on the pulp floor. Re-assessment of the relationship of the internal anatomical features to the external outlines will also help with orientation during a search for orifices that are difficult to locate.

In extensively calcified canals transillumination or the use of dye may provide some guidance for orifice identification and instrument progression. Even extensively calcified canals may contain pulp tissue and judicious use of a variety of instruments usually facilitates entry into the canal system. A number of ultrasonically energized instruments have been designed for this purpose. Despite being relatively safe, care must be taken if perforation of the root is to be avoided. Radiographs taken with radiopaque markers in the chamber can help confirm the direction of instrumentation (Fig. 6.12). When using rotary instruments such as Müller burs or long-shank small round high-speed tungsten-

carbide burs, frequent re-evaluation of bur position visually and/or radiographically will reduce procedural errors. The direction of search can then be adjusted if necessary and the procedure continued. Furthermore, enlargement of the canal orifices prior to instrumentation facilitates mid-root and apical instrumentation, and enhances irrigation.

## WORKING LENGTH DETERMINATION

Planning a final point for instrumentation and filling depends on the philosophy of treatment, while establishment of this point can be determined in a number of ways. It is necessary to establish the length of the tooth accurately during root canal treatment [12,13,18,33,37,46]. The most widely accepted method for establishing working length has been the use of radiographs. In this method

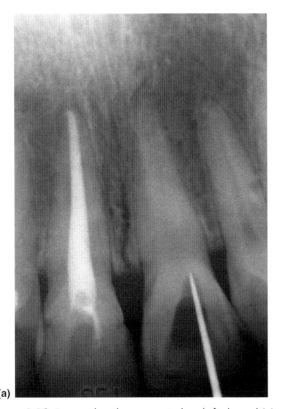
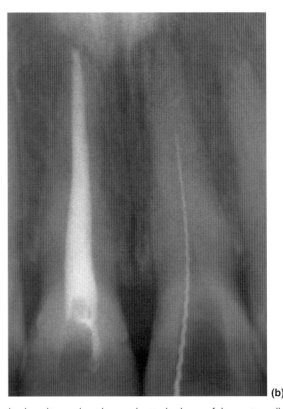

**(a)** **(b)**

**Figure 6.12** In a tooth with an extensively calcified canal (a) a check radiograph with a probe in the base of the cavity will provide guidance for instrument progression. (b) A later radiograph confirms that the file is in the root canal.

[40], an estimated working length is initally established by measuring from an accurate, non-distorted, preoperative radiograph. A file, preferably ISO size 15 or greater, is then placed to the estimated working length and a second radiograph is exposed. If the tip of the file is within 1 mm of the ideal location then the radiograph can be accepted as an accurate representation of the tooth length. If adjustments of 2 mm or more need to be made, working length should be reconfirmed with a new radiograph [19]. This method usually provides acceptable results. However, radiographs are frequently difficult to interpret especially in posterior teeth. In addition it is widely accepted that the apical foramen may be distant from the radiographic apex further confusing interpretation.

Electronic apex locators work on the principle that the impedance between the periodontal membrane and the oral mucosa is constant at 6.5 k $\Omega$ [82]. Recent apex locators (Root ZX, AFA, Justy, Endex-Plus) have been reported to be accurate to within 0.5 mm in >90% of cases [20,74]. The apex locator is significantly more reliable than the radiograph for determining working length [62]. As a consequence of their accuracy, apex locators allow for a reduction in the number of radiographs necessary to determine the working length especially in teeth where the apex is difficult to visualize on the radiograph. These findings indicate that apex locators should be regarded as the primary means of determining the working length during endodontic procedures. Moreover, in a recent long-term retrospective study in which an apex locator was the sole determinant of working length in infected root canals with periradicular lesions, a high success rate was achieved [57].

## ROOT CANAL IRRIGATION

Regardless of the instrumentation technique or system used, the use of irrigants is essential for debridement of the canal system [15,80]. Consequently the preparation of root canal systems involves both mechanical and chemical components; hence the concept of 'chemomechanical' preparation. Irrigation with appropriate solutions contributes to the cleaning of the canal system in several ways including:

- rinsing of debris;
- lubrication of the canal system which facilitates instrumentation;
- dissolution of remaining organic matter;
- antibacterial properties;
- softening and removing the smear layer;
- penetrating into areas inaccessible to instruments thereby extending the cleaning processes.

Ideally the irrigant should be non-toxic and have a low surface tension in addition to being stable, inexpensive and easy to use.

A plethora of irrigants have been used. Currently, the most widely used irrigant is NaOCl, which has both antibacterial and tissue-dissolving properties. The effectiveness of this irrigant has been shown to depend on its concentration and time of exposure. Higher concentrations of NaOCl have greater tissue-dissolving properties [38]. However, the greater the concentration, the more severe the potential reaction should some of the irrigant be inadvertently forced into the tissues; hence, various concentrations of NaOCl, varying from 0.5% to 5.25%, have been recommended [54]. Those using the lower concentrations are attempting to minimize the postoperative sequelae should irrigant be inadvertently introduced into the tissues, whilst those using the higher concentrations are attempting to maximize the tissue-dissolving and antibacterial properties of the NaOCl. Accidental extrusion of NaOCl into the periradicular tissues may result is tissue damage accompanied by varying degrees of pain, swelling and bruising. To prevent procedural errors with NaOCl:

- avoid forceful injection of the irrigant;
- use specially designed side-venting needles;
- use carefully in the presence of resorbed or open apices and perforations.

The use of calcium hydroxide as an intracanal medicament between visits has been shown to enhance disinfection following use of NaOCl. This synergism has beneficial effects for the chemomechanical preparation of the canal system. Other irrigants used in root canal chemomechanical preparation include chlorhexidine [48], iodine potassium iodide (IKI) [70] and electrolytically activated water [49].

During root canal preparation a layer of 'sludge' is formed by the action of the instruments against the canal walls. This material is deposited on the canal wall and is called the 'smear layer'. The smear layer has both organic and inorganic components and exists as a superficial loosely bound layer and a deeper adherent layer [51]. Considerable debate has occurred as to whether or not the smear layer should be removed. Complete removal of the smear layer may open up dentinal tubules to the passage of microorganisms from the root canal into the body of the dentine. On the other hand, failure to remove the smear layer will possibly allow bacteria to remain in the canal system and impairs the adaptation of the root filling to the dentine wall by preventing the movement of filling material into the dentine tubules. Removal of the smear layer is beneficial to root canal sealing [43], and significantly less micro-leakage occurs when these 'smear-free' canals are filled with thermoplasticized gutta-percha [86]. A very close adaptation of thermoplasticized gutta-percha to the dentine wall has been shown following smear layer removal [35].

Removal of the smear layer is best achieved by irrigating the canal system with NaOCl throughout the preparation procedure to prevent accumulation of debris on the canal walls and to flush out the canal system. A final rinse with 17.5% ethylene diamine tetra-acetic acid (EDTA) is recommended for removal of the inorganic component [7]; EDTA is also produced commercially in a paste form for lubrication during the instrumentation procedure. The effects of chelating agents such as EDTA are self-limiting.

Delivery of the irrigant is usually achieved by placing a side-venting needle 1–2 mm short of the working length of the canal. Alternatively, ultra-sonically energized files can be used. Their effectiveness is due to the creation of acoustic microstreaming and to the effective delivery of irrigant to the apical part of the root canal system [3,4].

## INSTRUMENTATION TECHNIQUES

Access to the apical part of the root canal will largely depend on adequate coronal preparation. All root canal systems are curved in one or more planes with the degree and extent of curvature varying from root to root. Elimination of coronal obstructions will greatly enhance the instrumentation procedures in the apical part of the root. Irrespective of the instrumentation technique used, the apical part of the canal system is invariably the least well-cleaned and prepared part of the root canal system. Contrary to the idealized picture depicted in many texts, the morphology of the apical canal system is complex and highly variable. Five major apical morphological forms have been described [22] (Fig. 6.13). Experimental clearing of roots has confirmed these variations and underscores the importance of a chemomechanical approach to preparation especially in the apical third of the canal system.

Preparation of the root canal system requires considerable skill, particularly in cases with more severely curved canals or complex anatomical features. Despite advances in instrument design, the experience and tactile skills of the operator

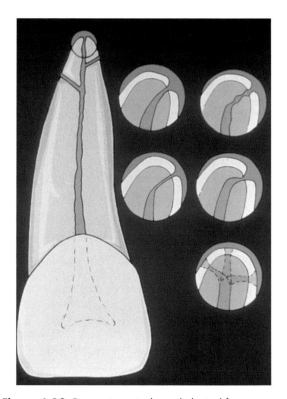

**Figure 6.13** Five major apical morphological forms are shown.

remain important [34]. Considerable efforts have been devoted to the study of instrument design and metallurgy in an attempt to produce an ideal instrument. The advances in design have been driven, in part by development of new alloys, and in part by an increase in understanding of the anatomy of the root canal system.

Regardless of the instrumentation procedure or instrument type used, the goals of shaping and cleaning of the root canal systems are:

- debridement of the root canal system;
- development of a continuously tapering preparation;
- avoidance of procedural errors.

Maintaining the anatomy of the apical constriction (Fig. 6.14) during canal shaping is essential for predictable healing of the apical tissues, in addition to mechanically retaining the filling material within the confines of the canal system. Long-term studies have shown improved success rates when instrumentation and filling procedures are maintained within the canal system approximately at the level of the cemento-dentinal junction [90].

Historically, canal preparation techniques have included the standardized and serial preparation techniques that focus on achieving a round apical preparation with either a small or minimal taper from apex to coronal aspect of the preparation. In recent decades the concept of the ideal preparation has altered to take into consideration a greater understanding of the natural anatomy of the root canal system moving away from the more rigid mechanistic approach.

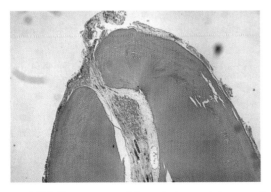

**Figure 6.14** The anatomy of the apical constriction must be maintained during canal preparation.

Canal preparation techniques can be broadly divided into those that adopt an 'apical to coronal' preparation procedure and those that adopt a 'coronal to apical' approach.

## Crowndown technique

Most recently many clinicians have used coronal to apical techniques to clean and shape root canals. There are several advantages:

- elimination of debris and microorganisms from the more coronal parts of the root canal system thereby preventing inoculation of apical tissues with contaminated debris;
- elimination of coronally placed interferences that might adversely influence instrumentation;
- early movement of large volumes of irrigant and lubricant to the apical part of the canal;
- facilitation of accurate working length determination as coronal curvature is eliminated early in the preparation.

The crowndown and stepback techniques of preparations aim to produce a similar result, i.e. a flared preparation with small apical enlargement.

The essentials of the coronal to apical approach to root canal cleaning and shaping are as follows:

- development of straight-line access from the occlusal or lingual surface into the pulp chamber;
- removal of all overhanging ledges from the pulp chamber roof;
- removal of lingual ledges or cervical bulges that form due to the deposition of dentine in the cervical part of the tooth;
- development of divergent walls in the pulp chamber from the cavosurface margin to the chamber floor;
- cutting of a funnel-shaped preparation, with its narrowest part located in the tooth apically, in a stepwise manner in the coronal, middle and apical parts of the root canal.

The benefits of using the crowndown technique are multiple and greatly influence the achievement of predictable success with root canal treatment. The clinical benefits of the crowndown technique are:

- ease of removal of pulp stones;
- enhanced tactile feedback with instruments by removal of coronal interferences;

- enhanced apical movement of instruments into the canal;
- enhanced working length determination due to minimal tooth contact in the coronal third;
- increased space for irrigant penetration and debridement;
- rapid removal of pulp tissue located in the coronal third;
- straight-line access to root curves and canal junctions;
- enhanced movement of debris coronally;
- decreased deviation of instruments in canal curvatures by reducing root wall contact;
- decrease in canal blockages;
- minimization of instrument separation by reducing contact with canal walls;
- predictable quality of canal shaping;
- predictable quality of canal cleaning;
- faster preparation which may allow one-visit root canal treatment.

The biological benefits of the crowndown technique are:

- rapid removal of contaminated, infected tissue from the root canal system;
- removal of tissue debris coronally, thereby minimizing pushing debris apically;
- reduction in postoperative pain that may occur with apical extrusion of debris;
- better dissolution of tissue with increased irrigant penetration;
- easier smear layer removal because of better contact with chelating agents;
- enhanced disinfection of canal irregularities due to irrigant penetration.

The basic steps common to all 'crown to apical' techniques involve early coronal and mid-root flaring and enlargement before proceeding to the apical part of the canal. The initial coronal flaring can be completed most efficiently with either Gates-Glidden burs or with rotary NiTi instruments, such as orifice shapers (Dentsply Tulsa Dental, Tulsa, OK, USA) designed specifically for this purpose. Early coronal flaring significantly reduces the change in working length during canal preparation [21]. As an instrument initially moves into the coronal third of the canal, the pathway is enlarged; the approach permits rapid irrigant penetration

and facilitates further movement of small instruments deeper into the root canal. This entire process is continued until the working length can be determined easily. This then allows unimpeded placement of instruments to the middle and apical parts of the canal system. Irrigants and lubricants will penetrate more easily and will facilitate passage of instruments in an apical direction.

'Crown to apical' instrumentation techniques that have been proposed include the crown-down pressureless technique, the Roane technique [68], the 'double flare' technique [25], and the modified double-flare technique [71]. Numerous protocols have been detailed for use with a crown-down preparation technique. A composite protocol for use with a 'coronal to apical' preparation is:

1. Access development to remove cervical bulges in posterior teeth or lingual bulges in anterior teeth.
2. Eliminate pulp chamber obstructions.
3. Gates-Gliddens sizes 4, 3, 2, or orifice shapers to enlarge canal orifices; irrigate.
4. Coronal to mid-root enlargement using instruments from large to small; irrigate.
5. Explore canal and establish working length with small instrument (size 10 or 15) using apex locator and/or radiograph; irrigate.
6. Sizes 10, 15, 20 hand instruments to working length; irrigate.
7. Introduce large files to coronal part of canal; when apical resistance is met the file is removed and cleaned; irrigate.
8. Introduce progressively smaller files deeper into the canal again until resistance is encountered; irrigate.
9. Establish apical preparation size; irrigate.
10. Complete preparation to achieve desired taper.

### Stepback technique

The most widely used preparation technique until recently has been the stepback or telescope technique first described in the 1960s [17] and later modified [56]. It replaced earlier non-tapering preparation techniques and aimed to reduce instrument transportation in the apical part. It has been effectively superseded by crowndown techniques. The following are the stages of a stepback preparation.

*Stage 1*

1. Access.
2. Establish working length with a pathfinder instrument.
3. Lubricate a fine instrument and place to length with a 'watch-winding' motion (a watch-winding motion implies a gentle clockwise and anti-clockwise rotation of a file with minimal apical pressure); irrigate.
4. Place the next larger size file to length; instrument circumferentially; irrigate.
5. Repeat the process until a size 25 K-file (or a file two to three sizes larger than the first file that binds at the apex) reaches working length. Recapitulate between files by placing a small file to working length.

This completes the apical preparation; stage 2 involves flaring of the preparation.

*Stage 2*

1. Place the next file in the series to a length 1 mm short of the working length; instrument circumferentially, irrigate and recapitulate.
2. Repeat this process placing the next larger file in the series to 2 mm short of the working length; instrument circumferentially, irrigate and recapitulate.
3. Repeat the process with successively larger files at 1 mm increments from the preceding file. It is important not to omit any instrument in the sequence.
4. Complete the coronal preparation with Gates-Glidden burs.

Variations to the classic technique include:

- initial enlarging of the coronal aspect with Gates-Glidden drills;
- use of small Gates-Glidden burs in the mid-root level;
- use of Hedstrom files to flare the preparation.

The stepback approach allowed creation of a small apical preparation with larger instruments used at successively decreasing lengths to create a taper. The taper could be altered by changing the interval between the stepback positions. In other words, the taper of the final preparation could be increased by

reducing the stepback intervals from 1 to 0.5 mm between each file. The stepback technique has been considered to minimize procedural errors, such as transportation, ledging and apical perforation, over previous techniques [88].

However despite the advances of the stepback preparation over the standardized preparation in producing a tapered preparation, these 'apex to coronal' techniques tended to result in significant apical extrusion of debris [6,22,52,64,69]. Apical blockage, canal deviation and alteration of working length have also been frequently encountered with the stepback technique. In addition, apical extrusion of debris during root canal instrumentation has been associated with postoperative pain or discomfort [73,85].

## Calcified canals

The basic principles apply to preparation of calcified canals. As with patent canals, once the access cavity to a calcified canal is completed, the pulp chamber is rinsed with NaOCl. If the orifices are identified as being calcified, an ultrasonically energized tip (Fig. 6.11) can be used to loosen debris in the orifice. The tip of the ultrasonic instrument can be used either to activate the solution in the chamber or it can be placed into the calcified orifice in an attempt to provide some initial patency. The use of either a NaOCl or EDTA soak for up to 10 minutes along with the use of an ultrasonic tip in these cases may remove some of the mineralized or partially mineralized tissue in the orifices. A small K-file, or a specific file designed for canal penetration (e.g. Pathfinder, Kerr Sybron), can be used to begin canal penetration. At this point, a small orifice shaper can be used to provide a tapered orifice penetration that facilitates further irrigant penetration and allows for the continued use of small K-files, or in some cases a size 15 0.04 tapered instrument, to penetrate further into the canal. The clinician can return to a small ultrasonic tip to penetrate further into the canal. Gates-Glidden burs will not be beneficial as they have a non-cutting tip. This procedure will take time and patience, and the clinician should resist the temptation to try to drill a canal into the root, as this invariably leads to deviation and potential root perforation.

## NICKEL-TITANIUM INSTRUMENTS

Following the introduction of nickel-titanium (NiTi) alloy to endodontic instrument design [87], many new NiTi hand and rotary instruments have become available. The clinical and mechanical properties of these NiTi instruments have been compared with those of stainless-steel instruments; various aspects of instrument performance in canal preparation such as the efficacy of canal preparation, cleanliness of the canals after preparation, the shaping ability of the instruments and fracture properties of the instruments have been examined [2,11,24,28,41,44,63,75,76,83,84]. There is a general acceptance that rotary NiTi instruments produce well-shaped canals in an efficient manner with the creation of fewer iatrogenic problems than stainless-steel files. However, direct comparison between stainless-steel and NiTi instruments is difficult unless the instrument design is identical [45]. In addition, most testing procedures have been done *in vitro*, frequently in plastic simulated canals, and long-term clinical evidence of the superiority of one instrument type is unavailable.

## CONTROVERSIES IN ROOT CANAL CLEANING AND SHAPING

A number of issues remain unresolved concerning endodontic treatment procedures; these include:

- Where should the preparation end?
- When should the preparation end?
- Should apical patency filing be performed?
- Should treatment be completed in one or multiple visits?

### Where should the preparation end?

This question was addressed succinctly in a short paper entitled 'Where should the root filling end?' [39]. Current treatment protocols used by many clinicians are frequently based on opinion rather than fact. An illogical belief exists that the quality of treatment provided is determined by the presence of sealer 'puffs' visible on a postoperative radiograph: *the more the better*! There is little or no evidence to support this belief; in fact there is considerable evidence for maintaining all instrumentation procedures and filling material within the root canal system [32,53,78,81]. There should be differentiation between vital teeth, those with infected canals, and retreatment cases, when deciding where to terminate the instrumentation and filling [90]. Based on biological principles and experimental evidence instrumentation should terminate 2–3 mm from the radiographic apex in vital cases. In cases where canals are infected, the position should be 0–2 mm from the apex, while in retreatment cases the ideal termination should be at the apical foramen. However, irrespective of the preoperative condition of the canal system, it is recommended that all instrumentation and filling procedures should not extend beyond the apical foramen.

Discussion on the ideal termination of the preparation and filling procedures presupposes the existence of the '*ideal*' root apex as described by Kuttler [46]; however it has been found that this ideal apical terminus exists in less than half of teeth [22]. Instead, a number of apical anatomical configurations have been described. No apical constriction may be present especially in the presence of any resorptive process [18,77]. Consequently, it is often very difficult or even impossible to locate either the apical constriction or the apical foramen.

### When should the preparation end?

Removal of all microorganisms, tissue and debris is the aim of root canal treatment and hence this can be taken to be the end point of preparation. However, determining when this has been achieved remains difficult clinically [16]. Historically instrumentation procedures have taken little account of canal anatomy, such as fins, webs, anastamoses or apical ramifications. Outdated standardized preparation techniques aimed to enlarge the canal to a predetermined size and circular cross-sectional shape. The presence of white dentine chips has been used as a sign of canal cleanliness; however, a lack of correlation between their presence and the cleanliness of the canal has been demonstrated [88].

Because of the complexities of canal anatomy, the emphasis has shifted to chemomechanical preparation of the canal system [16]. Removal of the smear layer improves disinfection [16]. The importance of an intracanal dressing of calcium hydroxide has been demonstrated as canals can be rendered bacteria-free [14]. An unanswered question is how long should the irrigant be left in the canal system to achieve adequate disinfection of the canal. This concern has fuelled a further controversy; namely can root canal treatment be completed in one visit or should it be done in multiple visits?

## Should apical patency filing be performed?

There are two concepts of patency filing. The first and original concept aimed to remove debris collected during instrumentation from the apical part of the canal. This involved sequentially rotating files two to four sizes larger than the initial apical file at working length, then rotating the largest apical file again after a final irrigation and drying. This was called 'apical clearing' [59], and aimed to achieve:

- better debridement;
- enhanced filling;
- a more defined apical stop.

Apical clearing is recommended in canals which have been prepared with an apical stop. Further, apical clearing in teeth without an apical stop would increase the chances of overpreparation and overfilling.

The second concept of patency filing refers to the placement of small files to and through the apical constriction [56]. The aim is to allow for creation of a preparation and filling extending fully to the periodontal ligament. Evidence to support this concept is unavailable.

## Should treatment be completed in one or multiple visits?

One-visit root canal treatment has assumed a position of controversy for many reasons. Clinical studies have addressed the advantages and disadvantages. The advantages of one-visit treatment are:

- reduced number of appointments;
- no risk of intra-appointment microbial recontamination;
- use of canal space for immediate post-retention.

The disadvantages are:

- longer appointments may cause patient fatigue;
- inability to control exudates may prevent completion of the procedure.

Those studies concerning postoperative pain [5,23,26,27,55,58,60] as well as effective healing rates [61,79,89] have shown that outcomes are similar, whether completed in one or multiple visits. Many of these studies have used older preparation techniques, which have the potential for less effective canal cleaning. There are some indications and contraindications that should be considered when contemplating this approach to treatment. The indications are:

- uncomplicated teeth with vital pulps;
- fractured teeth where aesthetics is important and extensive restoration is indicated;
- patient unable to return for appointments;
- patient requires antibiotic prophylaxis or sedation.

Contraindications are:

- patients with acute apical periodontitis;
- teeth with severe anatomical anomalies;
- molars with necrotic pulps and periradicular radiolucencies;
- root canal retreatment [78].

One-visit treatment does not sit easily with evidence on canal disinfection in infected cases [14,16].

## REFERENCES

1. Abou-Rass M (1982) Evaluation and clinical management of previous endodontic therapy. *Journal of Prosthetic Dentistry* **47**, 528–534.
2. Ahlquist M, Henningsson O, Hultenby K, Ohlin J (2001) The effectiveness of manual and rotary techniques in the cleaning of root canals: a scanning electron microscopy study. *International Endodontic Journal* **34**, 533–537.
3. Ahmad M (1989) Effect of ultrasonic instrumentation on *Bacteroides intermedius. Endodontics and Dental Traumatology* **5**, 83–86.
4. Ahmad M, Pitt Ford TR, Crum LA (1987) Ultrasonic debridement of root canals: an insight into the mechanisms involved. *Journal of Endodontics* **13**, 93–101.

5. Alaçam T (1985) Incidence of postoperative pain following the use of different sealers in immediate root canal filling. *Journal of Endodontics* **11**, 135–137.

6. Al-Omari MA, Dummer PM (1995) Canal blockage and debris extrusion with eight preparation techniques. *Journal of Endodontics* **21**, 154–158.

7. Behrend GD, Cutler CW, Gutmann JL (1996) An in-vitro study of smear layer removal and microbial leakage along root-canal fillings. *International Endodontic Journal* **29**, 99–107.

8. Bender IB (1997) Factors influencing the radiographic appearance of bony lesions. *Journal of Endodontics* **23**, 5–14.

9. Bender IB, Seltzer S (1961) Roentgenographic and direct observation of experimental lesions in bone. *Journal of the American Dental Association* **62**, 708–716.

10. Bergenholtz G (1990) Pathogenic mechanisms in pulpal disease. *Journal of Endodontics* **16**, 98–101.

11. Bishop K, Dummer PM (1997) A comparison of stainless steel Flexofiles and nickel-titanium NiTiFlex files during the shaping of simulated canals. *International Endodontic Journal* **30**, 25–34.

12. Blaney JR (1927) The biologic aspect of root canal therapy. *Dental Items of Interest* **49**, 681–708.

13. Bramante CM, Berbert A (1974) A critical evaluation of some methods of determining tooth length. *Oral Surgery, Oral Medicine, Oral Pathology* **37**, 463–473.

14. Byström A, Claesson R, Sundqvist G (1985) The antibacterial effect of camphorated paramonochlorophenol, camphorated phenol and calcium hydroxide in the treatment of infected root canals. *Endodontics and Dental Traumatology* **1**, 170–175.

15. Byström A, Sundqvist G (1981) Bacteriologic evaluation of the efficacy of mechanical root canal instrumentation in endodontic therapy. *Scandinavian Journal of Dental Research* **89**, 321–328.

16. Byström A, Sundqvist G (1985) The antibacterial action of sodium hypochlorite and EDTA in 60 cases of endodontic therapy. *International Endodontic Journal* **18**, 35–40.

17. Clem WH (1969) Endodontics: the adolescent patient. *Dental Clinics of North America* **13**, 482–493.

18. Coolidge ED (1929) Anatomy of the root apex in relation to treatment problems. *Journal of the American Dental Association* **16**, 1456–1465.

19. Cox VS, Brown CE, Bricker SL, Newton CW (1991) Radiographic interpretation of endodontic file length. *Oral Surgery, Oral Medicine, Oral Pathology* **72**, 340–344.

20. Czerw RJ, Fulkerson MS, Donnelly JC, Walmann JO (1995) In vitro evaluation of the accuracy of several electronic apex locators. *Journal of Endodontics* **21**, 572–575.

21. Davis RD, Marshall JG, Baumgartner JC (2002) Effect of early coronal flaring on working length change in curved canals using rotary nickel-titanium versus stainless steel instruments. *Journal of Endodontics* **28**, 438–442.

22. Dummer PM, McGinn JH, Rees DG (1984) The position and topography of the apical canal constriction and apical foramen. *International Endodontic Journal* **17**, 192–198.

23. Eleazer PD, Eleazer KR (1998) Flare-up rate in pulpally necrotic molars in one-visit versus two-visit endodontic treatment. *Journal of Endodontics* **24**, 614–616.

24. Fabra-Campos H. Rodriguez-Vallejo J (2001) Digitization, analysis and processing of dental images during root canal preparation with Quantec Series 2000 instruments. *International Endodontic Journal* **34**, 29–39.

25. Fava LR (1983) The double-flared technique: an alternative for biomechanical preparation. *Journal of Endodontics* **9**, 76–80.

26. Fava LR (1994) A clinical evaluation of one and two-appointment root canal therapy using calcium hydroxide. *International Endodontic Journal* **27**, 47–51.

27. Fox J, Atkinson JS, Dinin AP et al (1970) Incidence of pain following one-visit endodontic treatment. *Oral Surgery, Oral Medicine, Oral Pathology* **30**, 123–130.

28. Gambarini G (2000) Rationale for the use of low-torque endodontic motors in root canal instrumentation. *Endodontics and Dental Traumatology* **16**, 95–100.

29. Goldman M, Pearson AH, Darzenta N (1972) Endodontic success – who's reading the radiograph? *Oral Surgery, Oral Medicine, Oral Pathology* **33**, 432–437.

30. Goldman M, Pearson AH, Darzenta N (1974) Reliability of radiographic interpretations. *Oral Surgery, Oral Medicine, Oral Pathology* **38**, 287–293.

31. Goldstein IL, Mobley WH, Chellemi SJ (1971) The observer process in the visual interpretation of radiographs. *Journal of Dental Education* **35**, 485–491.

32. Grahnen H, Hansson L (1961) The prognosis of pulp and root canal therapy. A clinical and radiographic follow-up examination. *Odontolgisk Revy* **12**, 146–165.

33. Grove CJ (1921) Nature's method of making perfect root fillings following pulp removal, with a brief consideration of the development of secondary cementum. *Dental Cosmos* **63**, 968–982.

34. Gulabivala K, Abdo S, Sherriff M, Regan JD (2000) The influence of interfacial forces and duration of filing on root canal shaping. *Endodontics and Dental Traumatology* **16**, 166–174.

35. Gutmann JL (1993) Adaptation of injected thermoplasticized gutta-percha in the absence of the dentinal smear layer. *International Endodontic Journal* **26**, 87–92.

36. Gutmann JL, Dumsha TC, Lovdahl PE, Hovland EJ (1997) *Problem Solving in Endodontics. Prevention, Identification and Management*, 3rd. edn. St Louis, MO, USA: Mosby-Year Book, p. 47.

37. Gutmann JL, Leonard JE (1995) Problem solving in endodontic working-length determination. *Compendium of Continuing Education in Dentistry* **16**, 288–294.

38. Hand RE, Smith ML, Harrison JW (1978) Analysis of the effect of dilution on the necrotic tissue dissolution property of sodium hypochlorite. *Journal of Endodontics* **4**, 60–64.

39. Hasselgren G (1994) Where shall the root filling end? *New York State Dental Journal* **60**, 34–35.

40. Ingle JI (1957) Endodontic instruments and instrumentation. *Dental Clinics of North America* **1**, 805–822.

41. Jardine SJ, Gulabivala K (2000) An in vitro comparison of canal preparation using two automated rotary nickel-titanium instrumentation techniques. *International Endodontic Journal* **33**, 381–391.

42. Kakehashi S, Stanley HR, Fitzgerald RJ (1965) The effects of surgical exposures of dental pulps in germ-free and conventional laboratory rats. *Oral Surgery, Oral Medicine, Oral Pathology* **20**, 340–349.

43. Karagöz-Kücükay I, Bayirli G (1994) An apical leakage study in the presence and absence of the smear layer. *International Endodontic Journal* **27**, 87–93.

44. Kavanagh D, Lumley PJ (1998) An in-vitro evaluation of canal preparation using Profile .04 and .06 taper instruments. *Endodontics and Dental Traumatology* **14**, 16–20.

45. Kazemi RB, Stenman E, Spangberg L (2000) A comparison of stainless steel and nickel-titanium H-type instruments of identical design: torsional and bending tests. *Oral Surgery, Oral Medicine, Oral Pathology, Oral Radiology and Endodontics* **90**, 500–506.

46. Kuttler Y (1955) Microscopic investigation of root apexes. *Journal of the American Dental Association* **50**, 544–552.

47. Leeb J (1983) Canal orifice enlargement as related to biomechanical preparation. *Journal of Endodontics* **9**, 463–470.

48. Leonardo MR, Tanomaru Filho M, Silva LA, Nelson Filho P, Bonifacio KC, Ito IY (1999) In vivo antimicrobial activity of 2% chlorhexidine used as a root canal irrigating solution. *Journal of Endodontics* **25**, 167–171.

49. Marais JT, Williams WP (2001) Antimicrobial effectiveness of electro-chemically activated water as an endodontic irrigation solution. *International Endodontic Journal* **34**, 237–243.

50. Marshall K (1990) Rubber dam. *British Dental Journal* **184**, 218–219.

51. McComb D, Smith DC (1975) A preliminary scanning electron microscopic study of root canals after endodontic procedures. *Journal of Endodontics* **1**, 238–242.

52. McKendry DJ (1990) Comparison of balanced forces, endosonic, and step-back filing instrumentation techniques: quantification of extruded apical debris. *Journal of Endodontics* **16**, 24–27.

53. Molven O (1974) The frequency, technical standard and results of endodontic therapy. Dr Odont thesis. Bergen, Norway: University of Bergen.

54. Moorer WR, Wesselink PR (1982) Factors promoting the tissue dissolving capability of sodium hypochlorite. *International Endodontic Journal* **15**, 187–196.

55. Mulhern JM, Patterson SS, Newton CW, Ringel AM (1982) Incidence of postoperative pain after one-appointment endodontic treatment of asymptomatic pulpal necrosis in single-rooted teeth. *Journal of Endodontics* **8**, 370–375.

56. Mullaney TP (1979) Instrumentation of finely curved canals. *Dental Clinics of North America* **23**, 575–592.

57. Murakami M, Inoue S, Inoue N (2002). Clinical evaluation of audiometric control root canal treatment: a retrospective study. *Quintessence International* **33**, 465–474.

58. Oliet S (1983) Single-visit endodontics: a clinical study. *Journal of Endodontics* **9**, 147–152.

59. Parris J, Wilcox L, Walton R (1994) Effectiveness of apical clearing: histological and radiographical evaluation. *Journal of Endodontics* **20**, 219–224.

60. Pekruhn RB (1981) Single-visit endodontic therapy: a preliminary clinical study. *Journal of the American Dental Association* **103**, 875–877.

61. Pekruhn RB (1986) The incidence of failure following single-visit endodontic therapy. *Journal of Endodontics* **12**, 68–72.

62. Pratten DH, McDonald NJ (1996) Comparison of radiographic and electronic working lengths. *Journal of Endodontics* **22**, 173–176.

63. Pruett JP, Clement DJ, Carnes DL (1997) Cyclic fatigue testing of nickel-titanium endodontic instruments. *Journal of Endodontics* **23**, 77–85.

64. Reddy SA, Hicks LM (1998) Apical extrusion of debris using two hand and two rotary instrumentation techniques. *Journal of Endodontics* **24**, 180–183.

65. Reid JS, Callis PD, Patterson CJW (1991) Rubber dam in clinical practice. London, UK: Quintessence, pp. 1–108.

66. Reuter JE (1983) The isolation of teeth and the protection of the patient during endodontic treatment. *International Endodontic Journal* **16**, 173–181.

67. Roahen JO, Lento CA (1992) Using cyanoacrylate to facilitate rubber dam isolation of teeth. *Journal of Endodontics* **18**, 517–519.

68. Roane J, Sabala CL, Duncanson MG (1985) The 'balanced force' concept for instrumentation of curved canals. *Journal of Endodontics* **11**, 203–211.

69. Ruiz-Hubard EE, Gutmann JL, Wagner MJ (1987) A quantitative assessment of canal debris forced periapically during root canal instrumentation using two different techniques. *Journal of Endodontics* **13**, 554–558.

70. Safavı KE, Spangberg LS, Langeland K (1990) Root canal dentinal tubule disinfection. *Journal of Endodontics* **16**, 207–210.

71. Saunders WP, Saunders EM (1992) Effect of noncutting tipped instruments on the quality of root canal preparation using a modified double-flared technique. *Journal of Endodontics* **18**, 32–36.

72. Saunders MB, Gulabivala K, Holt R, Kahan RS (2000) Reliability of radiographic observations recorded on a proforma measured using inter- and intra-observer variation: a preliminary study. *International Endodontic Journal* **33**, 272–278.

73. Seltzer S (1986) Pain in endodontics. *Journal of Endodontics* **12**, 505–508.

74. Shabahang S, Goon WW, Gluskin AH (1996) An in vivo evaluation of Root ZX electronic apex locator. *Journal of Endodontics* **22**, 616–618.

75. Short JA, Morgan LA, Baumgartner JC (1997) A comparison of canal centering ability of four instrumentation techniques. *Journal of Endodontics* **23**, 503–507.

76. Shuping GB, Ørstavik D, Sigurdsson A, Trope M (2000) Reduction of intracanal bacteria using nickel-titanium rotary instrumentation and various medications. *Journal of Endodontics* **26**, 751–755.

77. Simon JH (1994) The apex: how critical is it? *General Dentistry* **42**, 330–334.

78. Sjögren U, Hägglund B, Sundqvist G, Wing K (1990) Factors affecting the long-term results of endodontic treatment. *Journal of Endodontics* **16**, 498–504.

79. Soltanoff W (1978) A comparative study of the single-visit and the multiple-visit endodontic procedure. *Journal of Endodontics* **4**, 278–281.

80. Stewart GG (1955) The importance of chemomechanical preparation of the root canal. *Oral Surgery, Oral Medicine, Oral Pathology* **8**, 993–997.

81. Strindberg LZ (1956) The dependence of the results of pulp therapy on certain factors. An analytic study based on radiographic and clinical follow-up examinations. *Acta Odontologica Scandinavica* **14**, Suppl. 21, 1–175.

82. Sunada I (1962) New method of measuring the length of the root canal. *Journal of Dental Research* **41**, 375–387.

83. Tepel J, Schafer E, Hoppe W (1995) Properties of endodontic hand instruments used in rotary motion. Part 1. Cutting efficiency. *Journal of Endodontics* **21**, 418–421.

84. Tepel J, Schafer E, Hoppe W (1997) Properties of endodontic hand instruments used in rotary motion. Part 3. Resistance to bending and fracture. *Journal of Endodontics* **23**, 141–145.

85. Torneck CD, Smith JS, Grindall P (1973) Biologic effects of endodontic procedures on developing incisor teeth. 3. Effect of debridement and disinfection procedures in the treatment of experimentally induced pulp and periapical disease. *Oral Surgery, Oral Medicine, Oral Pathology* **35**, 532–540.

86. von Fraunhofer JA, Fagundes DK, McDonald NJ, Dumsha TC (2000) The effect of root canal preparation on microleakage within endodontically treated teeth: an in vitro study. *International Endodontic Journal* **33**, 355–360.

87. Walia HM, Brantley WA, Gerstein H (1988) An initial investigation of the bending and torsional properties of Nitinol root canal files. *Journal of Endodontics* **14**, 346–351.

88. Walton RE (1992) Current concepts of canal preparation. *Dental Clinics of North America* **36**, 309–326.

89. Weiger R, Rosendahl R, Lost C (2000) Influence of calcium hydroxide intracanal dressings on the prognosis of teeth with endodontically induced periapical lesions. *International Endodontic Journal* **33**, 219–226.

90. Wu MK, Wesselink PR, Walton RE (2000) Apical terminus location of root canal treatment procedures. *Oral Surgery, Oral Medicine, Oral Pathology, Oral Radiology and Endodontics* **89**, 99–103.

91. Yoshioka T, Kobayashi C, Suda H (2002) Detection rate of root canal orifices with a microscope. *Journal of Endodontics* **28**, 452–453.

# Intracanal medication

## D. Ørstavik

Introduction 95

History 96

Rationale and overview of applications 96
  Asepsis, antisepsis and disinfection 96
  Secondary functions of medicaments 97

Microbes of the pulp 97

Antimicrobial agents 98
  Antibiotics 98
  Disinfectants 99

Resistance of oral microbes to medicaments 100

Concept of predictable disinfection in endodontics 101
  Mechanical instrumentation 101
  Antibacterial effect of irrigation 101
  Effect of antibacterial dressing 101
  Follow-up studies 102
  The single-visit issue 102
  From controlled to predictable disinfection 102
  Treatment of non-infected teeth 102

Induction of hard tissue formation 103

Pain of endodontic origin 103

Exudation and bleeding 104

Root resorption 104

Tissue distribution of medicaments 105
  Diffusion and solubility 105
  Penetration of dentine 105
  Effect of the smear layer 105

Tissue toxicity and biological considerations 106

Suggested clinical procedures 106
  Mechanical reduction of bacteria 106
  Application of medicaments 107
  Temporary filling 107

References 108

## INTRODUCTION

Endodontic success or failure is related to the absence or presence of signs and symptoms of apical periodontitis [110]. Root canal treatment can therefore be considered the prevention or cure of this disease [76]. Apical periodontitis includes apical granuloma and radicular cyst as well as acute manifestations of inflammation. The aetiology of apical periodontitis is primarily a bacterial infection of the root canal system [58,67,111] (Table 7.1); consequently, the technical and pharmacological aspects of prevention and treatment are mainly aimed at controlling infection. Thus, *preventive* endodontics entails treatment of a tooth without previous signs of apical periodontitis by aseptic pulp extirpation. *Curative endodontics* is the chemomechanical elimination of infection in the pulp canal system and signs of apical periodontitis. Both are completed by the placement of a bacteria-tight filling to prevent (re-)infection.

The use of intracanal medicaments is an adjunct to the prevention or treatment of apical periodontitis.

**Table 7.1** Association of bacteria with apical periodontitis: experimental studies in monkeys. Percentage of teeth with signs of inflammatory apical reactions

| Pulp status | Clinical | Radiological | Histological |
|---|---|---|---|
| Lacerated, non-infected | 0 | 0 | 8 |
| Lacerated, infected | 23 | 90 | 100 |

From Möller et al (1981) [67].

Thus their primary function is to prevent canal infection where none is present, and/or to inactivate bacteria already infecting the root canal. Intracanal *medicaments* would include any agent with intended pharmacological action introduced in the root canal. Antibacterial and other active compounds currently used as irrigating solutions during instrumentation rightly belong in this category. Intracanal *dressings* more concisely describe medicaments left in the root canal to exert their effects over a longer time period.

## HISTORY

The role of microorganisms in pulpless teeth was recognized more than a century ago [62], and strong caustic antiseptics were popular as intracanal medicaments at the turn of the 20th century. Formaldehyde-containing materials, e.g. formocresol [12], and iodoform pastes [126] belong to this category and have remained popular for decades. Formulations with sulphonamides [74] and later antibiotics were tried as intracanal medicaments; Grossman's polyantibiotic paste [40] and Ledermix [94] are examples of these types of dressing.

The reduction of pain through pharmacological control of the inflammatory process has been also attempted in endodontics by the application of eugenol [61], and later corticosteroids and other anti-inflammatory drugs [72], as dressings.

Focus on the possible adverse toxic effects of medicaments [108,131] led to a more systematic selection from the list of disinfectants available for use. Phenol derivatives and iodine formulations gained popularity as medicaments in endodontics; sodium hypochlorite was confirmed as a suitable irrigant.

Calcium hydroxide, while advocated since 1930 [52], has gained popularity in endodontics in the last three decades. Calcium hydroxide has had success in a variety of clinical situations including pulpotomy, root resorption, root-end closure, exudation and canal infection [49]. In recent years, it has become almost a panacea endodontic medicament.

**Table 7.2** Functions of intracanal medicaments

*Primary function: antimicrobial activity*
Antisepsis
Disinfection
*Secondary functions*
Hard tissue formation
Pain control
Exudation control
Resorption control

## RATIONALE AND OVERVIEW OF APPLICATIONS

The primary function of endodontic medicaments is to provide antimicrobial activity. In a few instances, other, secondary functions are desirable (Table 7.2). The rationale for applying intracanal medicaments in various clinical situations has been reviewed [18].

### Asepsis, antisepsis and disinfection

*Asepsis* is the assurance that no pathogenic microorganisms are present in the field of operation. It entails the use not only of clean, but also of sterile or disinfected instruments and utensils, liquids, etc. In the course of treating teeth with no signs of canal infection, maintaining asepsis is the primary means of preserving a bacteria-free canal.

*Antisepsis* is the endeavour to prevent or arrest the growth of microorganisms on living tissue. In vital pulp extirpation, antiseptic measures are necessary to prevent infection in case there is a breach in the chain of asepsis. Irrigating solutions and interappointment dressings need to be antibacterial in action to prevent any microorganisms, which may contaminate the canal system from multiplying and establishing themselves.

*Disinfection* is the elimination of pathogenic microorganisms, usually by chemical or physical means. Disinfection by antiseptic agents is what is attempted in the treatment of infected teeth. Sterilization, on the other hand, implies the use of irradiation or heat to reach a state of complete freedom from live microbes and cannot be applied to root canal treatment. Disinfection entails mechanical removal of tissue and debris containing microbes, irrigation and dressing with antiseptic agents; also, surgical removal of an infected apex contributes to the antiseptic efforts of treatment. The presence of radiologically discernible apical periodontitis is a sign that the root canal system is infected [111]. This state of pre-existing infection also has a negative influence on prognosis [79]. In these cases, bacterial reduction, and if possible disinfection, of the root canal system is a prerequisite for successful treatment.

## Secondary functions of medicaments

Root canal treatment is sometimes associated with clinical features only indirectly related to infection of the canal system. Pain during and after treatment may occur, and the tissue reactions associated with affected root canals include exudation, transudation, swelling and resorption. Each of these phenomena, either singly or in conjunction with infection, has been a target for attempts at medication during, between and after treatment sessions.

### Induction of hard tissue formation

It is often considered desirable to allow hard tissue to form to continue apical root development, to close a wide foramen, or to create a mechanical barrier at a fracture line. Although the mechanism of action is largely unknown, dressings are available with claims of inducing hard tissue formation.

### Pain control

Pain is often associated with infection, and the primary means of pain control in endodontic treatment is infection control. Pharmacological agents that result in pain reduction through a decrease in the tissue responses in inflammation may have a role in further alleviating clinical pain from both infectious and aseptic pulpoperiodontal inflammation.

### Control of exudation or bleeding

Persistent exudation in the root canal may occur, despite apparently successful technical treatment. Exudation reflects inflammation, however, and residual infection should be suspected. Therefore, treatment is aimed at dealing with potential infec-

tion as well as drying or coagulating the exudating surface.

### Control of inflammatory root resorption

Trauma to the teeth may result in various forms of resorptive damage, inflammatory root resorption being the most aggressive and destructive. Inflammatory root resorption is normally associated with infection of the root canal combined with physical damage to the cementum; again, a primary function of treatment is to eliminate infection in the root canal. Secondarily, medicaments may influence the resorption process itself.

## MICROBES OF THE PULP

Following pulpal necrosis, sooner or later the entire pulp canal system will become infected. A long-standing infection will have bacteria not only in the main canal but also in accessory canals and for a distance into the dentinal tubules [97]. If apical periodontitis has progressed to the point where resorption of the cementum occurs, bacteria may be found throughout the length of the tubules [123].

The source of the infecting bacteria may be dental caries, salivary contamination through fractures, cracks or leaking fillings, or contamination of the pulp space during dental, including endodontic, treatment.

With increasing depth and time of pulp infection, the microbial flora changes from a predominantly facultative, Gram-positive flora to an almost completely anaerobic and mainly Gram-negative set of microorganisms [33]. Strains belonging to the genera *Fusobacterium*, *Prevotella*, *Porphyromonas*, *Peptostreptococcus*, *Veillonella* and spirochetes are frequently found in teeth with apical periodontitis [112]. Other microorganisms not found by normal culturing techniques may be present. Facultative streptococci are also common. These same types of microorganisms are found in exacerbations or periapical abscesses [11]. In addition, specific infections involving particular microorganisms, e.g., enterococci [65] and *Actinomyces/Arachnia* [104] may occur.

In most infected teeth, several species are recovered from the root canals [112]. Many of the dominating species, e.g. *Fusobacterium, Prevotella* and *Porphyromonas*, may require the presence of some other synergistic species for their survival and propagation. It may be noteworthy in this context that these same species have not been found in dentinal tubules, which when infected harbour less fastidious microorganisms, such as lactobacilli and streptococci [7].

The microbial flora in retreatment cases has been shown to differ significantly from bacteria in primary apical periodontitis. Typically, retreatment cases show enterococci, streptococci, anaerobic cocci and anaerobic Gram-positive rods in high frequencies [31,66]; enterobacteria and yeasts are relatively more frequent than in primary apical periodontitis [82,101,129].

Infected canals typically contain 2–10 different species, total numbers ranging from $10^3$ to $10^7$ [15]. Exact numbers of microorganisms are unknown as they vary from tooth to tooth, and because of a lack of established quantitative methods of collection.

## ANTIMICROBIAL AGENTS

### Antibiotics

The successful use of various antibiotics, both systemically and topically, in other fields of medicine made them likely candidates for antibacterial action in the root canal. There are three main concerns about the local use of antibiotics in the root canal:

- *Sensitization*. Topical application of an antibiotic increases the risk of the patient becoming allergic to it [124]. Life-threatening anaphylactic reactions may occur from administration of antibiotics to sensitized individuals. Induced allergy to an antibiotic may limit the options for treatment of more severe infections, which would otherwise be curable with that particular drug.
- *Development of bacterial drug resistance*. The drug kinetics of antibiotics applied in the root canal is not well known [4]. Conditions may become favourable for the development of antibiotic-resistant microbial strains, causing an infection, which in turn is more difficult to treat [125].

Moreover, beyond the scope of treatment of the individual patient, the widespread use of antibiotics causes a general increase in pathogenic and indigenous microorganisms that are resistant to a variety of antibiotics [20].

- *Limited spectrum*. No one antibiotic is efficacious against all endodontic microorganisms [6]. Given that most endodontic infections are caused by a combination of species, the chance of one antibiotic achieving effective bacterial inhibition or elimination is small.

### Sulpha preparations

Sulphathiazole as part of a dressing was advocated in the 1950s and 1960s [74]. While irrefutably antibacterial, variable results were shown in comparative clinical studies [37,95]. Moreover, although effective against many Gram-negative and Gram-positive microorganisms, sulpha drugs are ineffective against enterococci and *Pseudomonas aeruginosa*.

### Penicillin

Grossman's polyantibiotic paste contained penicillin as an important ingredient. Beta-lactamase produced by several microbial species found in the root canal makes them resistant to penicillin. This includes *P. aeruginosa* and several anaerobic Gram-negative rods.

### Metronidazole

Metronidazole has good effect against several Gram-negative anaerobic microorganisms [107]. It has been suggested for use in irrigating solutions [91], as an intracanal dressing [53] and for parenteral applications in combination with other antibiotics, particularly penicillin [118]. It has limited activity against enterococci [24].

### Tetracycline

Tetracycline shows affinity for hard tissues and may be retained on tooth surfaces [10]. It is used locally in periodontics with good clinical and bacteriological results [38], and the derivative doxycycline forms the antibiotic ingredient in Ledermix [29]. However, its antimicrobial spectrum is quite narrow, and it may be ineffective against several oral and endodontic pathogens. The fact that resistance to tetracyclines occurs through the formation of transferable R factors also suggests caution in its application.

## Clindamycin

One study has reported on the use of clindamycin as an inter-appointment dressing, but only limited antibacterial efficacy could be demonstrated [64]. An experimental delivery device for clindamycin in the root canal has been reported [39].

## Disinfectants

While antibiotics work through biological interference with essential biochemical processes, disinfectants (Table 7.3) are a group of chemicals that act by direct toxicity to the microbes. Their action is thus quicker and more general, and they usually have a broader antibacterial spectrum than the antibiotic drugs. On the other hand, they may be more toxic to host tissues, and their action is generally more dose dependent.

## Aldehydes

Formaldehyde, paraformaldehyde and glutaraldehyde have been widely used in dentistry including endodontics. They are water-soluble, protein-denaturing agents and are among the most potent disinfectants. Aldehydes have applications in the disinfection of surfaces and medical equipment that cannot be sterilized, but they are quite toxic and allergenic, and some may be carcinogenic.

Formocresol contains formaldehyde as its main ingredient and is still a widely used medicament for pulpotomy procedures in primary teeth [109], but its toxic and mutagenic properties are of concern. These same properties have caused the use of neutral buffered formalin to be discontinued.

Paraformaldehyde is the polymeric form of formaldehyde, best known for its inclusion in some root canal filling materials, e.g. N2 and Endomethasone. It slowly decomposes to give its monomer, formaldehyde; its toxic, allergenic, and genotoxic properties are as for formaldehyde.

**Table 7.3** Root canal disinfectants

*Halogens*
Chlorine
  Irrigating solution: sodium hypochlorite 0.5% in 1% sodium bicarbonate as Dakin's solution; or 0.5 to 5.25% in aqueous solution.
Iodine
  Irrigating solution and short term dressing: 2% $I_2$ in 5% KI aqueous solution; iodophors.
  Field disinfection: 5% $I_2$ in tincture of alcohol.

*Chlorhexidine*
Chlorhexidine gluconate
  Field disinfection and irrigating solution: 0.12–2.0% aqueous solution.
  Irrigation and dressing: 1–5% gel.

Calcium hydroxide
  Dressing: aqueous, viscous or oily suspension/paste with varying amounts of salts added. Other antibacterials (iodine, chlorphenols, chlorhexidine) may be added.

*Aldehydes*
Formocresol
  Dressing: 19% formaldehyde, 35% cresol, 46% water and glycerine.

*Phenols*
Camphorated phenol
  Dressing: 30% phenol, 60% camphor, 10% ethanol.
Paramonochlorphenol (PMCP)
  Irrigating solution: 2% aqueous solution.
  Dressing: camphorated PMCP (CMCP); 65% camphor, 35% PMCP.
Eugenol
  Dressing: full strength.

## Halogens

Halogens include chlorine and iodine, which are both used in various formulations in endodontics. They are potent oxidizing agents with rapid bactericidal effects. Chlorine is released from sodium hypochlorite and from chloramine. The latter releases active chlorine at a lower rate, and has been used for short-term dressing of the root canal. Sodium hypochlorite is the current irrigating solution of choice. It is used clinically in concentrations from 0.5 to 5.25%. Both in vitro and in vivo bacteriological studies support its application. Necrotic tissue and debris are dissolved by sodium hypochlorite [45], a property exploited in bio-mechanical cleansing of root canals [69, 89]. Its toxicity is low; however, its bleaching properties are a nuisance if spilled onto a patient's clothes, its smell is objectionable to some patients, and it may cause severe symptoms if injected beyond the apex [9].

Iodine is used as iodine potassium iodide, and in iodophors, which are organic iodine-containing compounds that release iodine over time. It is also a very potent antibacterial agent of low toxicity, but may stain clothing if spilled. As iodoform it was used in a paste formulation to serve as a permanent root canal filling [126]. Current applications of iodine compounds are as an irrigating solution and short-term dressing in a 2% solution of iodine in 4% aqueous potassium iodide and, more recently, as a constituent in gutta-percha points for filling [87]. Some patients may be allergic to iodine compounds, and their use in these patients is contraindicated.

## Phenols

While phenol itself is no longer used in endodontics because of its high toxicity-to-efficacy ratio, the derivative paramonochlorphenol has been a very popular component of dressings. It has been used as a dressing both in aqueous solution [114] and in combination with camphor (as camphorated mono-chlorphenol, CMCP); it was long recognized as the dressing of choice for infected teeth. Thymol similarly enjoyed widespread popularity, but is less antibacterial than the chlorphenol compounds.

Eugenol is frequently used as a dressing for tem-porary control of pain after vital pulp exposure [48]. It has a well-documented, but limited, antimicrobial effect and is applied primarily for its pain-relieving effect [55].

## Chlorhexidine

Chlorhexidine has been widely used in perio-dontology [57]. Its substantivity (persistence in the area of interest), its relatively broad spectrum of activity, and its low toxicity may make it well suited for irrigation and dressing applications in endodontics. Results of recent studies point to the suitability of chlorhexidine in endodontics [50,51,56,78,122], and some in vivo bacteriological data are emerging [60]. Effective concentrations would be expected to be in the 0.2–2% range. Innovative attempts to utilize the disinfecting properties of chlorhexidine include its inclusion in gutta-percha points for root filling [87].

## Calcium hydroxide

Calcium hydroxide has reached a unique position as a dressing in endodontics. After its successful clinical application for a variety of indications [49], multiple biological functions have been ascribed to calcium hydroxide [36]. Its primary function is probably antibacterial in most clinical situations, with added benefits from its cauterizing activity and high pH, and also from the paste consistency that physically restricts bacterial colonization of the canal space. Calcium hydroxide is applied as a thick, creamy suspension in sterile water, saline, salt solutions, and a variety of other, viscous or oily vehicles [35,100].

## Calcium hydroxide with antimicrobial additives

Complete disinfection by calcium hydroxide cannot be expected in all cases [13]. Moreover, in root filled teeth the flora may contain organisms relatively resistant to its action. Numerous attempts have been made to mix calcium hydroxide with other aqueous and non-aqueous disinfectants. Para-chlorphenol, camphorated parachlorphenol [35], metacresol [130], and iodoform [28] have all been added to calcium hydroxide suspensions. More recently, combinations of calcium hydroxide with chlorhexidine have been tested in vitro [127].

## RESISTANCE OF ORAL MICROBES TO MEDICAMENTS

In some cases, bacteria persist and produce symp-toms of inflammation despite apparently optimal cleansing and disinfection procedures [14]. They may either be inaccessible to the cleaning instruments or to the medicaments, or they may be resistant to the medicaments used [92]. Special interest has recently focussed on enterococci and yeasts in persistent infections; these have been shown to be relatively resistant to calcium hydroxide

[13,43,127,128] and occur in high frequency in retreatment cases [65,82,113].

## CONCEPT OF PREDICTABLE DISINFECTION IN ENDODONTICS

Given the infectious nature of apical periodontitis, any clinical procedure should be based on the ability of each step to prevent contamination and to eliminate infection. A standard procedure should furthermore be based on a worst-case scenario, which would be the infected root canal with associated chronic apical periodontitis. Individual treatment steps have been assessed for their efficacy in eliminating bacteria from infected root canals [13–17,103,105] (Fig. 7.1).

### Mechanical instrumentation

Even in the absence of an antibacterial irrigating solution and subsequent dressing, there is still a

dramatic decrease in bacterial numbers in a root canal from mechanical cleansing alone [15,80]. However, in the majority of cases, bacteria, which are left in the canal, have the potential to multiply between appointments [15] and after filling [86].

### Antibacterial effect of irrigation

The addition of sodium hypochlorite as an anti-bacterial irrigating solution increases the number of bacteria-free canals substantially [16]. The use of 5% rather than 0.5% sodium hypochlorite appears more effective, and the reduction in the number of infected teeth has been shown to be even greater, when ethylene-diamine-tetra-acetate (EDTA) was alternated with sodium hypochlorite [16,17], and when ultrasonic instrumentation of the canal was performed [105].

### Effect of antibacterial dressing

The number of bacteria-free canals may be increased to almost 100% when a dressing of calcium hydroxide

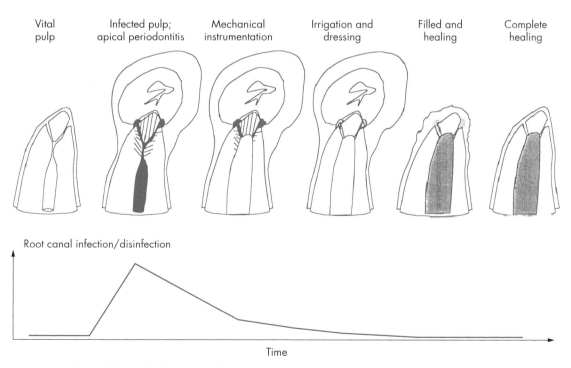

**Figure 7.1** Apical periodontitis develops when the root canal system becomes infected. Treatment entails the reduction of bacteria by mechanical instrumentation and antibacterial irrigation. The antibacterial dressing, when effective, eliminates infection. Total disinfection allows for complete healing of the tooth with apical periodontitis following root canal filling.

is placed in fully instrumented canals between visits [13,21,80,90]. Calcium hydroxide has been found to be more effective than CMCP in comparative experiments [13].

## Follow-up studies

Teeth treated as described above have been followed for periods of up to seven years, and the results have shown successful outcomes (definite signs of healing of apical periodontitis) in more than 90% of cases [14]. While success rates from different studies may be difficult to compare, it appears that these clinical results are better than most, if not all, previous reports.

## The single-visit issue

Single-visit ('one-step') endodontics implies shaping and disinfection of the root canal in the course of one treatment session. This is followed by permanent root filling at the same appointment. Immediate root filling of teeth that are not infected is not controversial and, in principle, probably preferable to treatment in multiple appointments: if asepsis is maintained, there is no need for a disinfecting dressing between appointments. The scientific issue is whether the time and type of medicament that can be applied during one appointment will provide predictable disinfection and healing of infected teeth with apical periodontitis. While it is highly desirable to achieve effective disinfection quickly, data from bacteriological studies show that, with current methods, disinfection in one visit is not as effective and predictable as procedures using an interim dressing. Moreover, clinical follow-up studies show better treatment outcome after dressing-based disinfection compared with single-visit procedures [102,121].

## From controlled to predictable disinfection

Scientific data from clinical studies should be the basis for a rational approach to guidelines for treatment of infected teeth. Clinical experiments have documented *controlled* disinfection by advanced bacteriological techniques. When applied to clinical practice, adherence to the principles of mechanical instrumentation, irrigation with NaOCl and EDTA, and dressing with calcium hydroxide, would be expected to produce *predictable* disinfection (bacteria-free canals) in almost 100% of cases, and in turn to produce clinical and radiological evidence of healing apical periodontitis in over 90% of cases. Indeed, large series of follow-up studies using this treatment regimen for infected teeth have borne out the high success rate [32]. A need for routine chairside bacteriological control of procedures is not implied.

## Treatment of non-infected teeth

None of the steps advocated for the treatment of the infected tooth place in jeopardy the success of treatment of a tooth with an initially non-infected pulp. Vital pulp extirpation followed by instrumentation with NaOCl and a dressing of calcium hydroxide give a clean pulp wound with minimal or no inflammation (Fig. 7.2). Therefore, as a means of securing the absence of microbes in these cases, the same treatment principles should apply. One

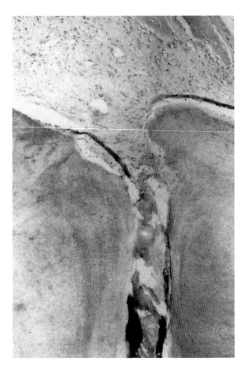

**Figure 7.2** Inflammation-free extirpation wound of a mature monkey central incisor after two weeks of dressing with calcium hydroxide.

exception is when permanent root canal filling is possible at the first appointment; then there is no need to have a period of canal dressing for the purpose of disinfection. Also, it may be questioned whether EDTA serves any purpose in the treatment of non-infected pulps.

Other principles of treatment may have a potential for equal or better efficacy and success rates. However, the extensive documentation with clinical bacteriological control, and clinical and radiological follow-ups makes the above guidelines a standard of reference. Alternative methods and medicaments should be tested and compared with the elements of this method prior to general clinical acceptance.

## INDUCTION OF HARD TISSUE FORMATION

The process of creating a hard tissue barrier at an open apex or at a grossly over-instrumented apex is termed root end closure or apexification [27]. When calcium hydroxide is used in long-term treatment

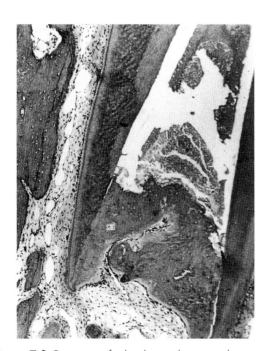

**Figure 7.3** Formation of a hard tissue barrier at the apex of an immature mandibular central incisor (monkey). The pulp was extirpated and a dressing of calcium hydroxide placed for three weeks.

of traumatized young permanent incisors and infection is controlled, a barrier of bone/cementum-like tissue at the apex is formed with a high degree of predictability [22,96] (Fig. 7.3). This barrier allows mechanical compression of the root filling, and any toxic responses of the tissues to the filling materials are minimized by this intervening barrier. While it may not be essential that calcium hydroxide be used as a dressing for this purpose, it has the most extensive clinical documentation. Similar principles apply in the formation of a hard tissue barrier more coronally, e.g. at the line of a horizontal root fracture or at a pulpotomy or pulp-capping wound surface [59].

## PAIN OF ENDODONTIC ORIGIN

Endodontic pain is mainly associated with inflammation, which in turn is usually linked with infection [44,46,47,106]. The inflammatory responses to the trauma of pulp extirpation and instrumentation may elicit pain of lesser magnitude and duration than pain following bacterial activity. The rationale behind pain control by inter-appointment dressings is thus primarily to combat infection. This is reflected also in the finding that interappointment pain is significantly more frequent in infected, necrotic teeth than in vital cases [70,99].

There are strong psychological components to the clinical expression of pain of endodontic origin [63]. Clinical pain is further confounded by the concomitant presence of microbial and iatrogenic and other sources. The quantification of pain clinically is also very difficult to standardize for comparative purposes.

The incidence of inter-appointment or post-treatment pain seems to be very much dependent on the criteria defining pain [75,116]. As an operative definition, the incidence of patients requiring an extra, non-scheduled visit following self-reported pain may have some merit. It would not include the discomfort sometimes or often associated with the practical necessities of the treatment itself (injection, clamp placement, severance and laceration of the pulp). By such criteria, no significant advantage of one medicament over another has been documented [34,88,119].

Due to the lack of precise knowledge of the source of pain in individual cases, the introduction of medicaments in dressings to alleviate inter- and post-treatment pain has been by theoretical considerations, and by trial and error, rather than by clinical research. Most interest has focussed on the use of corticosteroids in the inter-appointment dressing; particularly, the use of Ledermix with triamcinolone has been popular [1,29,94]. Also other commercially available formulations contain corticosteroids. The use of steroids in endodontics was initially criticized as it was felt that they might interfere with the body's reactions to microbial invasion, and because local application could interfere with natural synthesis of steroids. It is doubtful whether these concerns are justified: there is no indication that harmful side-effects are associated with its use in dentistry, and the doses applied are rather small compared with other medical indications [2]. However, while concerns for side effects may have been exaggerated, the clinical benefits, if any, over calcium hydroxide medication remain questionable. Non-steroidal anti-inflammatory drugs have also been tested clinically as intracanal dressings [72], but any clinical advantages again remain obscure.

For the control of pain, little seems to be gained either by the prophylactic addition to dressings or by the routine prescription of parenteral drugs [116]. It seems that endodontic pain may be better dealt with on a case-by-case approach, providing relief in doses of medication and by treatment appropriate for the individual patient.

## EXUDATION AND BLEEDING

Purulent exudate is a clear sign of infection. A serous exudate ('the weeping canal') is a more elusive clinical condition. It may also be associated with a relatively large apical foramen or an over-instrumented, patent foramen. Both conditions are usually controlled by instrumentation and dressing with calcium hydroxide. The application for a few minutes of dry calcium hydroxide packed against the exudating surface may succeed in desiccating or necrotizing that surface to the point where seepage is controlled and treatment may continue. However,

an interim dressing with calcium hydroxide may be necessary to control the exudation.

To the extent that exudation is associated with inflammation, and inflammation may be reduced by local corticosteroids, it would be rational in these cases to include steroid-containing dressings [1]. Given the limited nature of this problem, clinical studies are hard to design and carry out, and data are lacking to support suggested modes of treatment.

Bleeding from the canal is usually easily controlled by simple occlusion of the bleeding surface by paper points, dry or moistened with 3% hydrogen peroxide. Packing of calcium hydroxide onto the bleeding surface also effectively stops bleeding within a few minutes. Bleeding from pulpotomy wounds in primary teeth may be controlled by the application of the formocresol dressing used in the formocresol pulpotomy procedure [115].

## ROOT RESORPTION

Root resorption is a complication of root canal infection and trauma, in some instances with deleterious consequences to the tooth [8]. The apical, external root resorption associated with chronic apical periodontitis is self-limiting and stops when the canal infection is adequately controlled. It is likely that this resorption occurs to eliminate necrotic and/or infected cementum and dentine.

Traumatic tooth injuries, particularly avulsions followed by replantation, frequently lead to resorptive processes. Surface resorption is self-limiting and entails repair of cemental damage induced by the trauma. Ankylosis or replacement resorption, however, may be progressive in nature. Inflammatory resorption of the root surface occurs in response to a necrotic and infected root canal, and may be extremely rapid causing tooth loss in months if left untreated [26]. Root canal treatment is essential when inflammatory root resorption is evident or imminent, and calcium hydroxide is the current medicament of choice for this purpose [120]. Prolonged use of calcium hydroxide with multiple changes of the dressing may lead to necrosis of cells trying to recolonize the cementum surface. While this finding may suggest that the time of treatment with calcium hydroxide in these cases should be kept short (1–2 weeks), long-term placement of calcium hydroxide remains a clinically proven procedure in the treatment of resorption [120].

It has been suggested that because Ledermix inhibits the spread of dentinoclasts [84], it may provide added benefits in the control of inflammatory root resorption [85], particularly when mixed with calcium hydroxide [4]. More experimental is the use of calcitonin, a hormone that inhibits osteoclastic bone resorption, in canal dressings for inflammatory root resorption [83].

# TISSUE DISTRIBUTION OF MEDICAMENTS

There is limited knowledge of the actual distribution, in hard and soft tissues, of medicaments applied to the root canal [5,19,117]. Several barriers limit the penetration of chemical agents from the pulp canal through tooth structures and into the periapical tissues [3,43]. There is also limited knowledge on the localization of microorganisms, inflamed tissues and cells targeted by the medicaments [68,71].

## Diffusion and solubility

The ability of a medicament to dissolve and diffuse in the predominantly aqueous periapical environment may be essential for its action. Lipid soluble substances may have difficulty reaching targets at a distance in the tissues. Amphipathic drugs may have particular benefits; it may not be coincidental that aldehydes and phenol derivatives have had clinical success [132]. Thus aqueous solutions of paramonochlorphenol may penetrate further and have greater antimicrobial activity than the more concentrated lipid solute [114]. The low but significant solubility in water of calcium hydroxide has the dual advantage of limiting its toxic effects while the depot of the compound in suspension at the same time provides continuous release of the agent.

Vaporizing agents have been advocated on the premise that the vapour would be more permeating than liquids [30]. However, limited antibacterial activity might be expected since the gas may or may not be antibacterial, and must still dissolve in tissue fluids to exert its effect.

## Penetration of dentine

Studies in vivo have found the raised pH effect of calcium hydroxide to pervade the width of dentine [117], but to decrease rapidly in the tissues beyond. The application of calcium hydroxide on a dentine surface in turn significantly reduces its permeability [81]. However, it has been shown in vitro that calcium hydroxide is slower than many other medicaments in killing bacteria in experimentally infected dentinal tubules [43]. Similarly, the active ingredients in Ledermix show a gradient in dentine decreasing from the site of application to the cementum surface [4]. Eugenol, which occurs in several root canal sealer formulations, decreases in concentration 100-fold over 1 mm of dentine [55]. Moreover, intact cementum appears to be an effective, if not complete, barrier to medicament penetration [3]. Both the organic and the inorganic components of dentin may also interact with medicaments and reduce their antibacterial properties [42].

## Effect of the smear layer

Bacteriological data, both in vitro [41,78] as well as in vivo [13], indicate that medicaments penetrate to act more effectively when applied in a root canal that has been treated to remove the smear layer. In infected teeth with chronic apical periodontitis one may assume that bacteria are lodged peripheral to the main canal where the medicaments are applied [97,123]. The removal of the smear layer through the use of EDTA seems prudent in these cases. Following complete disinfection, however, or in the treatment of a non-infected tooth, retention or recreation of the smear layer may be advantageous in adding to the sealing off of the canal by the final root filling, although there are conflicting reports on the role of the smear layer in filling root canals [23].

A plug of dentine smear may be formed at the apical part of the instrumented canal (Fig. 7.4). This will obviously impair the ability of any medicament to penetrate through the apex.

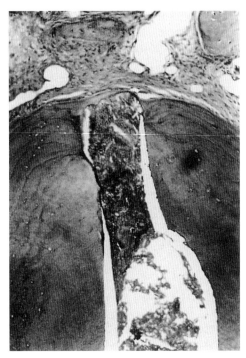

**Figure 7.4** A plug of dentine and pulp debris separates the main canal from the apical orifice.

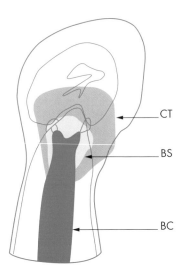

**Figure 7.5** Theoretical zones of bactericidal (BC), bacteriostatic (BS) and cytotoxic (CT) activity from an antiseptic in the root canal.

## TISSUE TOXICITY AND BIOLOGICAL CONSIDERATIONS

Endodontic medicaments can cause tissue damage, which will lead to inflammatory responses in soft tissues. These responses may interfere with the healing of apical periodontitis or serve as a locus for colonization by microorganisms to create a lesion where none existed. Any antiseptic will have a concentration gradient in the tissues with bactericidal and then bacteriostatic activity, but the cytotoxic effects will always be wider-ranging (Fig. 7.5). Experiments with cell-culture techniques and toxicity tests in animals have aided the selection of chemicals and medicaments for endodontic use [108]. Moreover, the allergenic and genotoxic properties of medicaments must form part of the selection criteria [73,77].

The very strong tissue toxicity, as well as the allergenicity and mutagenicity of aldehydes, have been part of the reason why these agents are no longer recommended for routine use. Similarly, phenols are strongly cytotoxic and are hardly recommendable for use by current standards [108]. Although toxicity is reduced by the addition of camphor, the toxicity/efficacy ratio is still very high.

In recommended concentrations, halogen compounds have high antibacterial activity combined with low tissue toxicity. This forms part of the reason why sodium hypochlorite is the irrigating solution of choice and why iodine potassium iodide has been an attractive alternative for short-term intracanal dressing [90]. Cases have been reported, however, of patients having extremely painful reactions to sodium hypochlorite inadvertently placed or injected into the periapical tissues [9,54].

Calcium hydroxide is, by virtue of its extremely high pH, potentially quite toxic. However, applied on vital tissue, the damage is limited to a narrow zone of superficial necrosis with a potential for complete regeneration [93].

## SUGGESTED CLINICAL PROCEDURES

### Mechanical reduction of bacteria

Mechanical instrumentation is the main factor in reducing most bacteria infecting root canals. Rubber dam is essential in preventing the root canal system from salivary infection. All efforts should be made to complete the mechanical phases of cleaning and shaping early in treatment, preferably at the first appointment. Any caries must be completely excavated, defective restorations removed, and the tooth and surrounding rubber dam surface thoroughly disinfected. All instrumentation should be done in the presence of an irrigating solution. The clinical studies with bacteriological control have employed master apical file sizes of ISO 40 or larger, which exceed the general recommendations in many current textbooks. Clinical experiments indicate that more bacteria are removed when larger files are used [80,133], while the type of file or instrumentation technique may not be essential [25,98].

## Application of medicaments

### Irrigation

Sodium hypochlorite has the best clinical and laboratory documentation. It may be applied, as a 1–5% aqueous solution, in a sterile syringe with a short 12–25 mm needle with outer diameter as low as practical (0.4 mm). Every precaution should be taken to keep the needle from wedging in the canal so as to prevent accidental injection of NaOCl into the periapical tissues. Fresh solution is applied and the old suctioned off between each change of files. Syringes of 10 ml capacity are practical for the purpose, but NaOCl may also be used with ultrasonic equipment, and the alternate use of NaOCl and EDTA will further reduce the number of bacteria. Chlorhexidine (0.2–2%) is emerging as a possible substitute for, or supplement to, NaOCl.

### Dressing

Prior to the application of a dressing to disinfect an infected root canal, the canal is flushed with a 15–17% neutral aqueous solution of EDTA. After allowing the chelating agent to act for 1–2 minutes, it is suctioned off and the canal is dried with paper points.

Calcium hydroxide has clearly the best documentation in most, if not all, indications. It may be applied with a Lentulo spiral or a syringe. Care must be taken to avoid overfilling. Paper points may be used to suck up excess water, and root canal

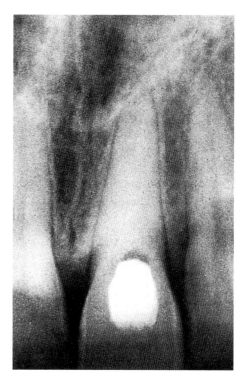

**Figure 7.6** The radiopacity of a thick suspension of calcium hydroxide is close to that of dentine. An effective filling gives the appearance of a completely filled canal.

pluggers of suitable dimensions may be used to make sure that the suspension or paste reaches the apical part of the canal. More material may be added as needed with the lentulo spiral, and the packing procedure repeated until a homogeneous filling is obtained (Fig. 7.6).

Many commercially available products are available. Some have injection syringes for application of calcium hydroxide. In teeth with large pulp canals, as in very young maxillary incisors, the syringe may suffice for placement.

## Temporary filling

The pulp chamber should be free of medicament and cleaned to receive the temporary filling. The dressing should be protected from saliva by a 3–4 mm thick layer of sealing material, typically based on zinc oxide–eugenol (preferably fortified). When the temporary filling is at particular risk of fracture or dislodgement, extra precautions should be considered. A dual filling ('the double seal') is

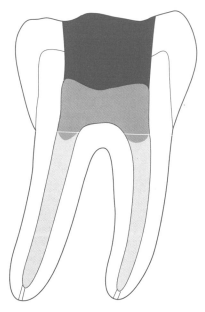

**Figure 7.7** The dressing may be protected by a deeper, self-retained intermediate temporary filling supplemented by a coronal (or aesthetic) superficial part.

then advisable: one internal, sealing the dressing and designed to remain even if the external part breaks off; and one external, designed for occlusal function and/or aesthetical reasons (Fig. 7.7). Should the temporary filling fail, the root canal is at risk of recontamination, so defeating the purpose of placing a medicament.

## REFERENCES

1. Abbott PV (1990) Medicaments: aids to success in endodontics. Part 2. Clinical recommendations. *Australian Dental Journal* **35**, 491–496.
2. Abbott PV (1992) Systemic release of corticosteroids following intra-dental use. *International Endodontic Journal* **25**, 189–191.
3. Abbott PV, Hume WR, Heithersay GS (1989) Barriers to diffusion of Ledermix paste in radicular dentine. *Endodontics and Dental Traumatology* **5**, 98–104.
4. Abbott PV, Hume WR, Heithersay GS (1989) Effects of combining Ledermix and calcium hydroxide pastes on the diffusion of corticosteroid and tetracycline through human tooth roots in vitro. *Endodontics and Dental Traumatology* **5**, 188–192.
5. Abbott PV, Hume WR, Heithersay GS (1989) The release and diffusion through human coronal dentine in vitro of triamcinolone and demeclocycline from Ledermix paste. *Endodontics and Dental Traumatology* **5**, 92–97.
6. Abbott PV, Hume WR, Pearman JW (1990) Antibiotics and endodontics. *Australian Dental Journal* **35**, 50–60.
7. Ando N, Hoshino E (1990) Predominant obligate anaerobes invading the deep layers of root canal dentine. *International Endodontic Journal* **23**, 20–27.
8. Andreasen JO, Andreasen F (1992) Root resorption following traumatic dental injuries. *Proceedings of the Finnish Dental Society* **88**, 95–114.
9. Becker GL, Cohen S, Borer R (1974) The sequelae of accidentally injecting sodium hypochlorite beyond the root apex. *Oral Surgery, Oral Medicine, Oral Pathology* **38**, 633–638.
10. Bjorvatn K (1986) Scanning electron-microscopic study of pellicle and plaque formation on tetracycline-impregnated dentin. *Scandinavian Journal of Dental Research* **94**, 89–94.
11. Brook I, Frazier EH, Gher ME (1991) Aerobic and anaerobic microbiology of periapical abscess. *Oral Microbiology and Immunology* **6**, 123–125.
12. Buckley JP (1906) The rational treatment of putrescent pulps and their sequelae. *Dental Cosmos* **48**, 537–544.
13. Byström A, Claesson R, Sundqvist G (1985) The antibacterial effect of camphorated paramonochlorophenol, camphorated phenol and calcium hydroxide in the treatment of infected root canals. *Endodontics and Dental Traumatology* **1**, 170–175.
14. Byström A, Happonen RP, Sjögren U, Sundqvist G (1987) Healing of periapical lesions of pulpless teeth after endodontic treatment with controlled asepsis. *Endodontics and Dental Traumatology* **3**, 58–63.
15. Byström A, Sundqvist G (1981) Bacteriologic evaluation of the efficacy of mechanical root canal instrumentation in endodontic therapy. *Scandinavian Journal of Dental Research* **89**, 321–328.
16. Byström A, Sundqvist G (1983) Bacteriological evaluation of the effect of 0.5 percent sodium hypochlorite in endodontic therapy. *Oral Surgery, Oral Medicine, Oral Pathology* **55**, 307–312.
17. Byström A, Sundqvist G (1985) The antibacterial action of sodium hypochlorite and EDTA in 60 cases of endodontic therapy. International Endodontic Journal **18**, 35–40.
18. Chong BS, Pitt Ford TR (1992) The role of intracanal medication in root canal treatment. *International Endodontic Journal* **25**, 97–106.
19. Ciarlone AE, Pashley DH (1992) Medication of the dental pulp: a review and proposals. *Endodontics and Dental Traumatology* **8**, 1–5.
20. Cohen ML (1984) Antimicrobial resistance: prognosis for public health. *Trends in Microbiology* **2**, 422–425.
21. Cvek M, Hollender L, Nord CE (1976) Treatment of non-vital permanent incisors with calcium hydroxide. *Odontologisk Revy* **27**, 93–108.
22. Cvek M, Sundström B (1974) Treatment of non-vital permanent incisors with calcium hydroxide. V. Histologic appearance of roentgenographically

demonstrable apical closure of immature roots. *Odontologisk Revy* **25**, 379–391.

23. Czonstkowsky M, Wilson EG, Holstein FA (1990) The smear layer in endodontics. *Dental Clinics of North America* **34**, 13–25.

24. Dahlen G, Samuelsson W, Molander A, Reit C (2000) Identification and antimicrobial susceptibility of enterococci isolated from the root canal. *Oral Microbiology and Immunology* **15**, 309–312.

25. Dalton BC, Ørstavik D, Phillips C, Pettiette M, Trope M (1998) Bacterial reduction with nickel-titanium rotary instrumentation. *Journal of Endodontics* **24**, 763–767.

26. Donaldson M, Kinirons MJ (2001) Factors affecting the time of onset of resorption in avulsed and replanted incisor teeth in children. *Dental Traumatology* **17**, 205–209.

27. Dylewski JJ (1971) Apical closure of nonvital teeth. *Oral Surgery, Oral Medicine, Oral Pathology* **32**, 82–89.

28. Eda S, Kawakami T, Hasegawa H, Watanabe I, Kato K (1985) Clinico-pathological studies on the healing of periapical tissues in aged patients by root canal filling using pastes of calcium hydroxide added iodoform. *Gerodontics* **1**, 98–104.

29. Ehrmann EH (1965) The effect of triamcinolone with tetracycline on the dental pulp and apical periodontium. *Journal of Prosthetic Dentistry* **15**, 144–152.

30. Ellerbruch ES, Murphy RA (1977) Antimicrobial activity of root canal vapors. *Journal of Endodontics* **3**, 189–193.

31. Engström B (1964) The significance of enterococci in root canal treatment. *Odontologisk Revy* **15**, 87–106.

32. Eriksen HM, Ørstavik D, Kerekes K (1988) Healing of apical periodontitis after endodontic treatment using three different root canal sealers. *Endodontics and Dental Traumatology* **4**, 114–117.

33. Fabricius L, Dahlén G, Öhman AE, Möller AJR (1982) Predominant indigenous oral bacteria isolated from infected root canals after varied times of closure. *Scandinavian Journal of Dental Research* **90**, 134–144.

34. Fava LR (1992) Human pulpectomy: incidence of postoperative pain using two different intracanal dressings. *International Endodontic Journal* **25**, 257–260.

35. Fava LR, Saunders WP (1999) Calcium hydroxide pastes: classification and clinical indications. *International Endodontic Journal* **32**, 257–282.

36. Foreman PC, Barnes IE (1990) Review of calcium hydroxide. *International Endodontic Journal* **23**, 283–297.

37. Frank AL, Glick DH, Weichman JA, Harvey H (1968) The intracanal use of sulfathiazole in endodontics to reduce pain. *Journal of the American Dental Association* **77**, 102–106.

38. Genco RJ (1991) Using antimicrobial agents to manage periodontal diseases. *Journal of the American Dental Association* **122**, 31–38.

39. Gilad JZ, Teles R, Goodson M, White RR, Stashenko P (1999) Development of a clindamycin-impregnated fiber as an intracanal medication in endodontic therapy. *Journal of Endodontics* **25**, 722–727.

40. Grossman LI (1951) Polyantibiotic treatment of pulpless teeth. Journal of the *American Dental Association* **43**, 265–278.

41. Guignes P, Faure J, Maurette A (1996) Relationship between endodontic preparations and human dentin permeability measured in situ. *Journal of Endodontics* **22**, 60–67.

42. Haapasalo HK, Siren EK, Waltimo TM, Ørstavik D, Haapasalo MP (2000) Inactivation of local root canal medicaments by dentine: an in vitro study. *International Endodontic Journal* **33**, 126–131.

43. Haapasalo M, Ørstavik D (1987) In vitro infection and disinfection of dentinal tubules. *Journal of Dental Research* **66**, 1375–1379.

44. Hahn CL, Falkler WA, Minah GE (1993) Correlation between thermal sensitivity and microorganisms isolated from deep carious dentin. *Journal of Endodontics* **19**, 26–30.

45. Hand RE, Smith ML, Harrison JW (1978) Analysis of the effect of dilution on the necrotic tissue dissolution property of sodium hypochlorite. *Journal of Endodontics* **4**, 60–64.

46. Hashioka K, Suzuki K, Yoshida T, Nakane A, Horiba N, Nakamura H (1994) Relationship between clinical symptoms and enzyme-producing bacteria isolated from infected root canals. *Journal of Endodontics* **20**, 75–77.

47. Hashioka K, Yamasaki M, Nakane A, Horiba N, Nakamura H (1992) The relationship between clinical symptoms and anaerobic bacteria from infected root canals. *Journal of Endodontics* **18**, 558–561.

48. Hasselgren G, Reit C (1989) Emergency pulpotomy: pain relieving effect with and without the use of sedative dressings. *Journal of Endodontics* **15**, 254–256.

49. Heithersay GS (1975) Calcium hydroxide in the treatment of pulpless teeth with associated pathology. *Journal of the British Endodontic Society* **8**, 74–93.

50. Heling I, Sommer M, Steinberg D, Friedman M, Sela MN (1992) Microbiological evaluation of the efficacy of chlorhexidine in a sustained-release device for dentine sterilization. *International Endodontic Journal* **25**, 15-19.

51. Heling I, Steinberg D, Kenig S, Gavrilovich I, Sela MN, Friedman M (1992) Efficacy of a sustained-release device containing chlorhexidine and Ca(OH)$_2$ in preventing secondary infection of dentinal tubules. *International Endodontic Journal* **25**, 20–24.

52. Hermann BW (1930) Dentinobliteration der Wurzelkanäle nach Behandlung mit Calcium. *Zahnärztliche Rundschau* **39**, 888–899.

53. Hess JC (1986) Germes anaérobies et gangrènes pulpaires. Experience clinique du traitement local au métronidazole. *Journal Dentaire du Quebec* **23**, 15–18.

54. Hülsmann M, Hahn W (2000) Complications during root canal irrigation – literature review and case reports. *International Endodontic Journal* **33**, 186–193.

55. Hume WR (1986) The pharmacologic and toxicological properties of zinc oxide–eugenol. *Journal of the American Dental Association* **113**, 789–791.

56. Jeansonne MJ, White RR (1994) A comparison of 2.0% chlorhexidine gluconate and 5.25% sodium hypochlorite as antimicrobial endodontic irrigants. *Journal of Endodontics* **20**, 276–278.

57. Jolkovsky DL, Waki MY, Newman MG, Otomo-Corgel J, Madison M, Flemmig TF, Nachnani S, Nowzari H (1990) Clinical and microbiological effects of subgingival and gingival marginal irrigation with chlorhexidine gluconate. *Journal of Periodontology* **61**, 663–669.

58. Kakehashi S, Stanley HR, Fitzgerald RJ (1965) The effects of surgical exposures of dental pulp in germ-free and conventional laboratory rats. *Oral Surgery, Oral Medicine, Oral Pathology* **20**, 340–349.

59. Kirk EE, Lim KC, Khan MO (1989) A comparison of dentinogenesis on pulp capping with calcium hydroxide in paste and cement form. *Oral Surgery, Oral Medicine, Oral Pathology* **68**, 210–219.

60. Kuruvilla JR, Kamath MP (1998) Antimicrobial activity of 2.5% sodium hypochlorite and 0.2% chlorhexidine gluconate separately and combined, as endodontic irrigants. *Journal of Endodontics* **24**, 472–476.

61. Markowitz K, Moynihan M, Liu M, Kim S (1992) Biologic properties of eugenol and zinc oxide–eugenol. A clinically oriented review. *Oral Surgery, Oral Medicine, Oral Pathology* **73**, 729–737.

62. Miller WD (1890) *Micro-organisms of the Human Mouth.* Philadelphia, PA, USA: SS White Dental Mfg Co.

63. Mohorn S, Maixner W, Fillingim R, Sigurdsson A, Booker D (1995) Effect of psychological factors on preoperative and postoperative endodontic pain. *Journal of Dental Research* **74**, 43 (abstract 254).

64. Molander A, Reit C, Dahlen G (1990) Microbiological evaluation of clindamycin as a root canal dressing in teeth with apical periodontitis. *International Endodontic Journal* **23**, 113–118.

65. Molander A, Reit C, Dahlen G, Kvist T (1999) Microbiological status of root-filled teeth with apical periodontitis. *International Endodontic Journal* **31**, 1–7.

66. Möller AJR (1966) Microbiological examination of root canals and periapical tissues of human teeth. Methodological studies. *Odontologisk Tidskrift* **74**, 1–380.

67. Möller AJR, Fabricius L, Dahlén G, Öhman AE, Heyden G (1981) Influence on periapical tissues of indigenous oral bacteria and necrotic pulp tissue in monkeys. *Scandinavian Journal of Dental Research* **89**, 475–484.

68. Molven O, Olsen I, Kerekes K (1991) Scanning electron microscopy of bacteria in the apical part of root canals in permanent teeth with periapical lesions. *Endodontics and Dental Traumatology* **7**, 226–229.

69. Moorer WR, Wesselink PR (1982) Factors promoting the tissue dissolving capability of sodium hypochlorite. *International Endodontic Journal* **15**, 187–196.

70. Mor C, Rotstein I, Friedman S (1992) Incidence of interappointment emergency associated with endodontic therapy. *Journal of Endodontics* **18**, 509–511.

71. Nair PN, Luder HU (1985) Wurzelkanal und periapikale Flora: eine licht- und elektronenmikroskopische Untersuchung. *Schweizerische Monatsschrift für Zahnmedizin* **95**, 992–1003.

72. Negm MM (1994) Effect of intracanal use of nonsteroidal anti-inflammatory agents on posttreatment endodontic pain. *Oral Surgery, Oral Medicine, Oral Pathology* **77**, 507–513.

73. Nunn JH, Smeaton I, Gilroy J (1996) The development of formocresol as a medicament for primary molar pulpotomy procedures. *ASDC Journal of Dentistry for Children* **63**, 51–53.

74. Nygaard-Östby B (1971) *Introduction to endodontics.* Oslo, Norway: Universitetsforlaget.

75. Oguntebi BR, DeSchepper EJ, Taylor TS, White CL, Pink FE (1992) Postoperative pain incidence related to the type of emergency treatment of symptomatic pulpitis. *Oral Surgery, Oral Medicine, Oral Pathology* **73**, 479–483.

76. Ørstavik D (1988) Antibacterial properties of endodontic materials. *International Endodontic Journal* **21**, 161–169.

77. Ørstavik D (1988) Endodontic materials. *Advances in Dental Research* **2**, 12–24.

78. Ørstavik D, Haapasalo M (1990) Disinfection by endodontic irrigants and dressings of experimentally infected dentinal tubules. *Endodontics and Dental Traumatology* **6**, 142–149.

79. Ørstavik D, Kerekes K, Eriksen HM (1987) Clinical performance of three endodontic sealers. *Endodontics and Dental Traumatology* **3**, 178–186.

80. Ørstavik D, Kerekes K, Molven O (1991) Effects of extensive apical reaming and calcium hydroxide dressing on bacterial infection during treatment of apical periodontitis: a pilot study. *International Endodontic Journal* **24**, 1–7.

81. Pashley DH, Kalathoor S, Burnham D (1986) The effects of calcium hydroxide on dentin permeability. *Journal of Dental Research* **65**, 417–420.

82. Peciuliene V, Reynaud AH, Balciuniene I, Haapasalo M (2001) Isolation of yeasts and enteric bacteria in root-filled teeth with chronic apical periodontitis. *International Endodontic Journal* **34**, 429–434.

83. Pierce A, Berg JO, Lindskog S (1988) Calcitonin as an alternative therapy in the treatment of root resorption. *Journal of Endodontics* **14**, 459–464.

84. Pierce A, Heithersay G, Lindskog S (1988) Evidence for direct inhibition of dentinoclasts by a corticosteroid/antibiotic endodontic paste. *Endodontics and Dental Traumatology* **4**, 44–45.

85. Pierce A, Lindskog S (1987) The effect of an antibiotic/corticosteroid paste on inflammatory root resorption in vivo. *Oral Surgery, Oral Medicine, Oral Pathology* **64**, 216–220.

86. Pitt Ford TR (1982) The effects on the periapical tissues of bacterial contamination of the filled root canal. *International Endodontic Journal* **15**, 16–22.

87. Podbielski A, Boeckh C, Haller B (2000) Growth inhibitory activity of gutta-percha points containing root canal medications on common endodontic bacterial pathogens as determined by an optimized quantitative in vitro assay. *Journal of Endodontics* **26**, 398–403.

88. Rogers MJ, Johnson BR, Remeikis NA, BeGole EA (1999) Comparison of effect of intracanal use of ketorolac tromethamine and dexamethasone with oral ibuprofen on post treatment endodontic pain. *Journal of Endodontics* **25**, 381–384.

89. Rubin LM, Skobe Z, Krakow AA, Gron P (1979) The effect of instrumentation and flushing of freshly extracted teeth in endodontic therapy: a scanning electron microscope study. *Journal of Endodontics* **5**, 328–335.

90. Safavi KE, Dowden WE, Introcaso JH, Langeland K (1985) A comparison of antimicrobial effects of calcium hydroxide and iodine-potassium iodide. *Journal of Endodontics* **11**, 454–456.

91. Sanjiwan R, Chandra S, Jaiswal JN, Mats AN (1990) The effect of metronidazole on the anaerobic microorganisms of the root canal – a clinical study. *Federation of Operative Dentistry* **1**, 30–36.

92. Sato T, Hoshino E, Uematsu H, Noda T (1993) In vitro antimicrobial susceptibility to combinations of drugs on bacteria from carious and endodontic lesions of human deciduous teeth. *Oral Microbiology and Immunology* **8**, 172–176.

93. Schröder U, Granath LE (1971) Early reaction of intact human teeth to calcium hydroxide following experimental pulpotomy and its significance to the development of hard tissue barrier. *Odontologisk Revy* **22**, 379–396.

94. Schroeder A (1962) Cortisone in dental surgery. *International Dental Journal* **12**, 356–373.

95. Seltzer S, Bender IB, Ehrenreich J (1961) Incidence and duration of pain following endodontic therapy: relationship to treatment with sulfonamides and to other factors. *Oral Surgery, Oral Medicine, Oral Pathology* **14**, 74–82.

96. Sheehy EC, Roberts GJ (1997) Use of calcium hydroxide for apical barrier formation and healing in non-vital immature permanent teeth: a review. *British Dental Journal* **183**, 241–246.

97. Shovelton DS (1964) The presence and distribution of micro-organisms within non-vital teeth. *British Dental Journal* **117**, 101–107.

98. Shuping GB, Ørstavik D, Sigurdsson A, Trope M (2000) Reduction of intracanal bacteria using nickel-titanium rotary instrumentation and various medications. *Journal of Endodontics* **26**, 751–755.

99. Sim CK (1997) Endodontic interappointment emergencies in a Singapore private practice setting: a retrospective study of incidence and cause-related factors. *Singapore Dental Journal* **22**, 22–27.

100. Siqueira JF, De Uzeda M (1997) Intracanal medicaments: evaluation of the antibacterial effects of chlorhexidine, metronidazole, and calcium hydroxide associated with three vehicles. *Journal of Endodontics* **23**, 167–169.

101. Siren EK, Haapasalo MP, Ranta K, Salmi P, Kerosuo EN (1997) Microbiological findings and clinical treatment procedures in endodontic cases selected for microbiological investigation. *International Endodontic Journal* **30**, 91–95.

102. Sjögren U, Figdor D, Persson S, Sundqvist G (1997) Influence of infection at the time of root filling on the outcome of endodontic treatment of teeth with apical periodontitis. *International Endodontic Journal* **30**, 297–306.

103. Sjögren U, Figdor D, Spångberg L, Sundqvist G (1991) The antimicrobial effect of calcium hydroxide as a short-term intracanal dressing. *International Endodontic Journal* **24**, 119–125.

104. Sjögren U, Happonen RP, Kahnberg KE, Sundqvist G (1988) Survival of *Arachnia propionica* in periapical tissue. *International Endodontic Journal* **21**, 277–282.

105. Sjögren U, Sundqvist G (1987) Bacteriologic evaluation of ultrasonic root canal instrumentation. *Oral Surgery, Oral Medicine, Oral Pathology* **63**, 366–370.

106. Skidmore AE (1991) Pain of dental origin. *Clinical Journal of Pain* **7**, 192–204.

107. Slots J, Rams TE (1990) Antibiotics in periodontal therapy: advantages and disadvantages. *Journal of Clinical Periodontology* **17**, 479–493.

108. Spångberg L (1994) Intracanal medication. In: Ingle JI, Bakland LK (eds) *Endodontics*, 4th edn. Malvern, PA, USA: Williams and Wilkins. pp 627–640.

109. Strange DM, Seale NS, Nunn ME, Strange M (2001) Outcome of formocresol/ZOE sub-base pulpotomies utilizing alternative radiographic success criteria. *Pediatric Dentistry* **23**, 331–336.

110. Strindberg LZ (1956) The dependence of the results of pulp therapy on certain factors. An analytic study based on radiographic and clinical follow-up examinations. *Acta Odontologica Scandinavica* **14**, Supplement 21, 99–101.

111. Sundqvist G (1976) Bacteriological studies of necrotic dental pulps. Thesis no. 7. Umeå, Sweden: Umeå University.

112. Sundqvist G (1994) Taxonomy, ecology, and pathogenicity of the root canal flora. *Oral Surgery, Oral Medicine, Oral Pathology* **78**, 522–530.

113. Sundqvist G, Figdor D, Persson S, Sjögren U (1998) Microbiologic analysis of teeth with failed endodontic treatment and the outcome of conservative re-treatment. *Oral Surgery, Oral Medicine, Oral Pathology, Oral Radiology, Endodontics* **85**, 86–93.

114. Taylor GN, Madonia JV, Wood NK, Heuer MA (1977) In vivo autoradiographic study of relative penetrating abilities of aqueous 2% parachlorophenol and camphorated 35% parachlorophenol. *Journal of Endodontics* **2**, 81–86.

115. Thompson KS, Seale NS, Nunn ME, Huff G (2001) Alternative method of hemorrhage control in full strength formocresol pulpotomy. *Pediatric Dentistry* **23**, 217–222.

116. Torabinejad M, Cymerman JJ, Frankson M, Lemon RR, Maggio JD, Schilder H (1994) Effectiveness of various medications on postoperative pain following complete instrumentation. *Journal of Endodontics* **20**, 345–354.

117. Tronstad L, Andreasen JO, Hasselgren G, Kristerson L, Riis I (1981) pH changes in dental tissues after root canal filling with calcium hydroxide. *Journal of Endodontics* **7**, 17–21.

118. Tronstad L, Kreshtool D, Barnett F (1990) Microbiological monitoring and results of treatment of extraradicular endodontic infection. *Endodontics and Dental Traumatology* **6**, 129–136.

119. Trope M (1990) Relationship of intracanal medicaments to endodontic flare-ups. *Endodontics and Dental Traumatology* **6**, 226–229.

120. Trope M (1995) Clinical management of the avulsed tooth. *Dental Clinics of North America* **39**, 93–112.

121. Trope M, Delano EO, Ørstavik D (1999) Endodontic treatment of teeth with apical periodontitis: single vs. multivisit treatment. *Journal of Endodontics* **25**, 345–350.

122. Vahdaty A, Pitt Ford TR, Wilson RF (1993) Efficacy of chlorhexidine in disinfecting dentinal tubules in vitro. *Endodontics and Dental Traumatology* **9**, 243–248.

123. Valderhaug J (1974) A histologic study of experimentally induced periapical inflammation in primary teeth in monkeys. *International Journal of Oral Surgery* **3**, 111–123.

124. Van Joost T, Dikland W, Stolz E, Prens E (1986) Sensitization to chloramphenicol; a persistent problem. *Contact Dermatitis* **14**, 176–178.

125. Wade WG, Moran J, Morgan JR, Newcombe R, Addy M (1992) The effects of antimicrobial acrylic strips on the subgingival microflora in chronic periodontitis. *Journal of Clinical Periodontology* **19**, 127–134.

126. Walkhoff O (1928) *Mein System der Medikamentösen Behandlung Schwerer Erkrankungen der Zahnpulpa und des Periodontiums*. Berlin, Germany: Hermann Meusser.

127. Waltimo TM, Ørstavik D, Siren EK, Haapasalo MP (1999) In vitro susceptibility of *Candida albicans* to four disinfectants and their combinations. *International Endodontic Journal* **32**, 421–429.

128. Waltimo TM, Siren EK, Ørstavik D, Haapasalo MP (1999) Susceptibility of oral Candida species to calcium hydroxide in vitro. *International Endodontic Journal* **32**, 94–98.

129. Waltimo TM, Siren EK, Torkko HL, Olsen I, Haapasalo MP (1997) Fungi in therapy-resistant apical periodontitis. *International Endodontic Journal* **30**, 96–101.

130. Weiss M (1966) Pulp capping in older patients. *New York State Dental Journal* **32**, 451–457.

131. Wennberg A (1980) Biological evaluation of root canal antiseptics using in vitro and in vivo methods. *Scandinavian Journal of Dental Research* **88**, 46–52.

132. Wesley DJ, Marshall FJ, Rosen S (1970) The quantitation of formocresol as a root canal medicament. *Oral Surgery, Oral Medicine, Oral Pathology* **29**, 603–612.

133. Yared GM, Dagher FE (1994) Influence of apical enlargement on bacterial infection during treatment of apical periodontitis. *Journal of Endodontics* **20**, 535–537.

# Root canal filling

## P. M. H. Dummer

Introduction 113

Canal anatomy 114

Access and canal preparation 114

Criteria for filling 114

Materials used to fill root canals 115

Sealers 115
   Functions of sealer 115

Smear layer 117

Gutta-percha 118
   Canal filling with gutta-percha 118
   Cold gutta-percha techniques 118
   Heat-softened gutta-percha techniques 125
   Solvent-softened gutta-percha 130

Apical dentine plug 132

Other methods of root canal filling 132
   Mineral trioxide aggregate 132
   Non-instrumentation technology 132
   Silver points 133
   Paste fillers 134

Restoration of the root filled tooth 135

Follow-up 135

Criteria of success 135

References 136

## INTRODUCTION

The entire root canal system should be filled following cleaning and shaping. The objectives of filling are:

1. To prevent microorganisms left in the canal system after preparation from proliferating and escaping into the periradicular tissues via the apical foramina and lateral and/or furcation canals.
2. To seal the pulp chamber and canal system from leakage via the crown in order to prevent passage of microorganisms and/or toxins along the root canal and into the periradicular tissues via the apical foramina and lateral and/or furcation canals.
3. To prevent percolation of periradicular exudate and possibly microorganisms into the pulp space via the apical foramina and/or lateral and furcation canals.
4. To prevent percolation of gingival exudate and microorganisms into the pulp space via lateral canals opening into the gingival sulcus or through exposed, patent dentinal tubules around the neck of the tooth.

The quality of canal filling depends on the complexity of the canal system, the efficacy of canal preparation, the materials and techniques used, and the skill and experience of the operator. Filling of the canal system is not the final stage in root canal treatment as restoration of the clinical crown to prevent leakage of fluids and oral microorganisms into the pulp space is critical to the long-term success of treatment [146]. Indeed, there is evidence to suggest that the quality of the final restoration has a significant impact on long-term success of root canal treatment [177] and may even be more important than the quality of canal filling [137].

Over the years a number of materials and techniques have been used to fill canals. At present, the material of choice is gutta-percha combined with a sealer, because it is versatile and can be used in a variety of techniques. It is essential that several filling techniques be mastered to undertake a range of cases. The aim of this chapter is to describe the fundamental principles of canal filling, to describe canal filling techniques using gutta-percha and to give a brief overview of alternative methods of canal filling.

## CANAL ANATOMY

Pulp anatomy is complex with a significant number of canals having apical deltas, lateral canals and other aberrations; posterior teeth are noted for accessory canals, fins, and anastomoses. These features, together with the results of pathological dentine deposition and procedural accidents during preparation, provide a challenge for even the most experienced clinician. Clearly, the anatomy of the canal system will have a major influence on the techniques used to obturate canals and on the quality of the final canal filling.

## ACCESS AND CANAL PREPARATION

The aims of preparation are to clean and shape the canal system. Although access and preparation have been discussed in Chapters 3 and 6, it is worth emphasizing that meticulous attention to the preparation stage will facilitate filling. The preparation stage should not only remove microorganisms and debris from within the canal system but also shape the canal to receive the root canal filling. Cleaning of the canal can often be achieved with irrigating fluids and minimal removal of dentine from canal walls; however, achieving the correct shape invariably requires additional effort to create the flowing flared preparation demanded by most methods of filling. Inappropriate access and canal preparation can leave microorganisms, pulpal remnants and dentine debris within the canal system. These will invariably prevent proper adaptation of the filling to the walls, and affect the physical properties of the sealer and thus the effectiveness of the seal produced. Furthermore, creation of an inappropriate shape will make it difficult to introduce material along the length of the canal, resulting in a

poorly condensed filling with voids. Thus, the ability to fill canals predictably is dependent to a large degree on the quality of access and canal preparation.

The method of canal filling will be dictated by the preparation technique and the shaping objectives determined by the operator. Thus, some operators prefer to create an apical stop at the dentine–cementum junction where they believe that a natural apical constriction occurs; in this way instrumentation does not extend beyond the apical foramen [193]. With this shape of canal, the filling technique of choice is cold lateral condensation of gutta-percha. Other operators create a continuously tapering canal shape where the smallest diameter is at the foramen [21]. With this shape one of the wide range of warm gutta-percha filling techniques is more appropriate as the lack of an apical stop will predispose to the master cone used in lateral condensation being stretched through the foramen when a cold spreader is introduced.

## CRITERIA FOR FILLING

Historically, canal filling was delayed for one or more visits after preparation to give time for medicaments sealed into the canal to reduce or eliminate the microbial population and for the patient's signs and symptoms to resolve [22,23]. Unfortunately, delaying filling can lead to other problems such as leakage of microorganisms or toxins along the interface of temporary filling and tooth, and even total loss of the temporary restoration. In addition, it is clear that most medicaments (other than calcium hydroxide) have a limited antibacterial action [23] and are effective for only a short period after placement [117]. The problems inherent in delaying canal filling and the fact that modern canal preparation is effective at eliminating microorganisms from the canal system has meant that many cases can be prepared and filled in one visit [120,163].

There is no doubt that the decision when to fill canals is controversial and has polarized endodontic practitioners into two groups. There are those who support the immediate filling of canals following preparation in the belief their regimen for eliminating microorganisms with continuously tapering canal shapes [21] and with extensive use of concentrated sodium hypochlorite and EDTA (or alternative) irrigation is effective. These practitioners argue that at the end of their cleaning and shaping procedures the canal system is likely to be sufficiently devoid of microorganism and substrate to allow filling to proceed [129]. On the other hand, it has been reported extensively that delaying filling and the use of a medicament will reduce the microbial population further [24] and enhance the long-term outcome when the canal system is infected, resulting in more rapid resolution of apical periodontitis and an improved prognosis [158,178]. To confuse the issue further, recent reports [184] have found no difference between the outcome of one-visit or two-visit treatment incorporating calcium hydroxide medication.

Although each case should be considered individually, it seems sensible to suggest that, in general, those teeth with non-infected pulps and no signs of apical periodontitis should be prepared and filled in one visit, whereas infected cases with apical periodontitis should be treated with more caution, and filling delayed until a further appointment by which time the medicament will have had an opportunity to reduce further the microbial population. Unfortunately, research in this critical area of clinical practice is difficult and time-consuming to carry out and has so far failed to provide a clear and definitive answer to the issue [183]. Whatever strategy is selected it is essential that the canal system is thoroughly dried at the filling stage to avoid compromising the physical properties of the sealer.

## MATERIALS USED TO FILL ROOT CANALS

A large number of materials have been used to fill canals, ranging from orangewood sticks through precious metals to dental cements. Requirements for a canal filling material have been described for many years [19,57]. Most materials have been shown to be inadequate and rejected as impractical or biologically unacceptable.

## SEALERS

A root canal sealer (cement) is used in combination with root canal filling materials, e.g. gutta-percha.

At one time it was thought that the sealer played a secondary role by simply cementing (binding, luting) the core filling material into the canal, however, it is now appreciated that the sealer has a primary role in sealing the canal by obliterating the irregularities between the canal wall and the core material. All modern filling techniques make use of sealer to enhance the seal of the root canal filling [42,73, 87,112]. However, assessment of sealing ability is not included in the requirements specified in the current International Standard covering sealers [3].

### Functions of sealer

Root canal sealers are used in conjunction with core filling materials for the following purposes:

- cementing (luting, binding) the core material into the canal;
- filling the discrepancies between the canal walls and core material;
- acting as a lubricant to enhance the positioning of the core filling material;
- acting as a bactericidal agent;
- acting as a marker for accessory canals, resorptive defects, root fractures and other spaces into which the main core material may not penetrate.

The requirements and characteristics of an ideal sealer are [59]:

- non-irritating to periapical tissues;
- insoluble in tissue fluids;
- dimensionally stable;
- hermetic sealing ability;
- radiopaque;
- bacteriostatic;
- sticky and good adhesion to canal wall when set;
- easily mixed;
- non-staining to dentine;
- good working time;
- readily removable if necessary.

Inevitably, no single material satisfies all the requirements but several do function adequately in clinical practice. The choice of canal sealer is not only dependent on its ability to create a sound seal, but it must also be well tolerated by the periradicular tissues and be relatively easy to manipulate so that its optimum physical properties can be achieved.

Sealers are toxic when freshly prepared [95,164]; however, their toxicity is reduced substantially after setting [125]. Thus, although sealers produce varying degrees of periradicular inflammation, it is normally only temporary and does not appear to prevent tissue healing [155].

Most sealers are absorbed to some extent when exposed to tissue fluid [123]. Thus, the volume of sealer must be kept to a minimum with the vast majority of the filling being made up by the core material. In essence, the core material should force the less viscous sealer into inaccessible areas such as canal anastomoses and apical deltas and into irregularities along the canal walls created during preparation. Excess sealer should ideally flow backwards out of the canal orifice, although a number of gutta-percha techniques tend to force sealer apically and laterally via the foramina and accessory canals [2,40,53]. Passage of sealer into the periradicular tissues is not encouraged; however, there is no evidence that it will reduce the success rate of treatment provided that canal preparation and filling have been carried out meticulously. Furthermore, clinical experience suggests that excess sealer forced into the periradicular region is absorbed with time.

Sealers in use today can be divided into four groups based on their constituents:

- zinc oxide–eugenol sealers;
- calcium hydroxide sealers;
- resin sealers;
- glass ionomer sealers.

### Zinc oxide–eugenol sealers

Most of the zinc oxide–eugenol sealers are based on Grossman's formula [58], which is itself a modification of the original Rickert's sealer [140]. Commercial products include Tubliseal (Kerr, Romulus, MI, USA), Pulp Canal Sealer (Kerr) and Roth Sealer (Roth, Chicago, IL, USA). A number of products are available with extended working times.

Once set, zinc oxide–eugenol sealers form relatively weak, porous materials that are susceptible to decomposition in tissue fluids [188], particularly when forced into the periradicular tissues [176]. All zinc oxide–eugenol cements are cytotoxic and the response may last longer than those produced by other materials [125]. The materials have the potential for sensitization [74] and have been shown to be mutagenic in extremely high doses [191]. However, these problems are not apparent when the materials are used clinically. They are probably used more often than all the other sealers combined and give satisfactory results. The various products have a range of setting times and flow characteristics so that for each case some thought should be given to the choice of sealer. For example, difficult canals that need some time to fill require a sealer with an extended working time. The influence of heat on the setting time of sealers should also be taken into account.

### Calcium hydroxide sealers

Calcium hydroxide-based sealers have been developed on the assumption that they preserve the vitality of the pulp stump and stimulate healing and hard tissue formation at the foramen. Commercial products include Sealapex (Kerr), a calcium hydroxide-containing polymeric resin, and Apexit (Ivoclar-Vivadent, Lichtenstein).

Laboratory research has demonstrated their sealing ability to be similar to zinc oxide–eugenol materials [82] although it remains to be seen whether during long-term exposure to tissue fluids the materials maintain their integrity since calcium hydroxide is soluble and may leach out and weaken the remaining cement [176].

### Resin sealers

Resin based materials have been available for many years [152] but remain less popular than zinc oxide–eugenol and calcium hydroxide sealers. The first resin sealer, AH26 (Dentsply, Konstanz, Germany), consisted of an epoxy resin base which set slowly when mixed with an activator. It had good sealing [99,119] and adhesive properties and antibacterial activity but gave an initial severe inflammatory reaction [125]. The initial reaction subsided after some weeks and the material was then tolerated well by the periradicular tissues [44,125]. The resin has a strong allergenic and mutagenic potential [153], and cases of contact allergy [78] and paraesthesia [7] have been reported. The material has also been shown to release formaldehyde [165]. AH26 has been superseded by AH Plus (Dentsply).

### Glass ionomer sealers

The ability of glass ionomer cement to adhere to dentine [187] would appear to provide a number of potential advantages over conventional sealers. Indeed, its endodontic potential was recognized not long after it became available commercially as a restorative material [131]. Initial evaluation of the material was confined to tests on cements designed for intracoronal restorations and it was many years before a product for specific endodontic use was formulated [136].

The physical, chemical and biocompatibility properties of glass ionomer cements have been reported extensively [182,187]. As with many other materials, unset glass ionomer cement has been found to be cytotoxic [35,88]. However, after setting, cytotoxic reactions and inflammatory responses are reduced with time [12,25,84].

The physical properties of the endodontic sealer Ketac Endo (Espe Gmbh, Seefeld, Germany) have been reported as superior to Grossman's sealer [136]. However, studies on the apical sealing properties of the material have been equivocal with some reports showing glass ionomers to be less effective than others [37,77,161], whilst others have shown no differences [18]. When using glass ionomer cements there would appear to be no differences in coronal leakage between techniques involving single points or lateral condensation [169], between presence or absence of smear layer [147], or between lateral condensation and filling with heat softened gutta-percha [147]. However, less coronal leakage has been demonstrated with glass ionomer cement than with a proprietary zinc oxide–eugenol sealer [145]. Pilot studies have also demonstrated that the shear bond strength of gutta-percha to glass ionomer cement was similar to that with zinc oxide–eugenol sealers and that fluoride leached out of the cement and was taken up by dentine [148]. Use of glass ionomer cement to fill the pulp chamber of molar teeth following root canal filling has been shown to reduce coronal leakage [26,144].

Of particular interest are the results of a clinical trial evaluating the performance of a glass ionomer sealer [48]. The results from this multicentre trial suggested that the outcome of root canal treatment with Ketac-Endo (ESPE) was similar to those reported in previous studies using traditional sealers.

## SMEAR LAYER

The smear layer is a layer of debris, comprising both organic and inorganic components, found on canal walls after endodontic instrumentation [106,114,156]. It is made up largely of particulate dentine debris removed by endodontic instruments during canal preparation but also contains pulpal remnants and microorganisms. With further instrumentation the material is forced against the canal walls forming a friable and loosely adherent layer. The smear layer is typically 1–2 μm thick, although it can also be found within the dentinal tubules for up to 40 μm [106].

The smear layer has received much attention [156], not only because it may harbour microorganisms already in the canal but also because it may create an avenue for leakage of microorganisms and act as a substrate for microbial proliferation [17,128]. It may also be broken down by bacterial action [33] to provide a pathway for leakage. The smear layer also has the potential to interfere with the adaptation of sealer against the canal walls and prevent tubular penetration, thereby increasing the likelihood of leakage [60,145,146]. Indeed, it has been shown that most leakage occurs between the root canal sealer and the wall of the root canal [79].

For these reasons removal of the smear layer prior to filling would appear to be desirable as it would eliminate microorganisms and allow for better adaptation of sealer. However, this procedure has been questioned since opening of the tubules might increase the diffusion of potentially irritant filling materials through the tubules to the root surface [49], allow microorganisms trapped in the tubules to escape [38] or to proliferate within the tubules [118], and even increase leakage [46]. Nevertheless, the present consensus is that removal of the smear layer is beneficial and thus desirable.

In laboratory studies a number of methods have been effective in removing the smear layer [156]. One involves the use of 17% EDTA as a chelating agent, along with sodium hypochlorite to dissolve the organic part [60]. Another involves use of 10–55% citric acid to dissolve the inorganic component, followed by rinsing with sodium hypochlorite [148]. Smear layer removal is easier in the coronal and middle parts of the canal compared with the apical part [148].

# GUTTA-PERCHA

Gutta-percha has been used to fill root canals for over 100 years [14] and is the most widely used and accepted filling material. Gutta-percha is a form of rubber obtained from a number of tropical trees. It is a *trans*-polyisoprene, which in its pure form is hard, brittle and less elastic than *cis*-polyisoprene, natural rubber. It is mixed with a variety of other materials to produce a blend that can be used effectively within the root canal. Thus, the points of gutta-percha available commercially contain gutta-percha (19–22%), zinc oxide (59–75%) and various waxes, colouring agents, antioxidants, and metal salts to provide radiopacity. The proportions of the constituents vary from brand to brand with the result that there is considerable variation in the stiffness, brittleness and tensile strength of commercially available gutta-percha points [47] and obturating products [31].

Gutta-percha points have many advantages as they are:

- inert;
- dimensionally stable;
- non-allergenic;
- antibacterial;
- non-staining to dentine;
- radiopaque;
- compactible;
- softened by heat;
- softened by organic solvents;
- removable from the root canal when necessary.

As with all materials gutta-percha points have some disadvantages as they:

- lack rigidity;
- do not adhere to dentine;
- can be stretched.

## Canal filling with gutta-percha

The objective of canal filling is to fill completely the canal system in an attempt to seal the canal from leakage in apical and coronal directions. Gutta-percha can be used in a variety of techniques because of its versatility; however, it must be emphasized that a sealer is always required to lute the material to the canal wall and to fill minor irregularities that cannot be filled by gutta-percha itself.

In recent years a large number of filling techniques have been described often accompanied by unsubstantiated claims of greater efficacy, reduced leakage or improved economics. Although it is essential to strive for improved filling techniques, the clinician must be aware that 'newer' does not necessarily mean 'better'. Indeed, there is little evidence from clinical trials to suggest that any differences exist between the techniques in terms of the ultimate success or failure of the procedure. In general terms, clinicians should be cautious in their approach to new filling techniques and await the outcome of laboratory and clinical studies before adopting a new regime.

Broadly speaking, techniques of filling canals with gutta-percha can be divided into three main groups:

- use of cold gutta-percha;
- use of heat-softened gutta-percha;
- use of solvent-softened gutta-percha.

## Cold gutta-percha techniques

Cold gutta-percha techniques are generally simple to master as they are not complicated by needing to soften the material with heat or solvents; neither do they require expensive and often complicated devices or equipment. However, it should be clear that cold gutta-percha cannot be compacted into irregularities within the canal system, with the result that this role must be fulfilled entirely by sealer.

Cold gutta-percha can be used in a number of ways but the lateral condensation technique is the most appropriate and popular; use of single cones with 0.02 taper is contraindicated.

## Lateral condensation

With the advent of the standardized preparation technique [80], the method of filling canals with a single full length gutta-percha point and sealer became popular. The theory behind the technique was simple and attractive; the canal was prepared to a round cross-sectional shape of standard size by use of reamers and then obturated by a gutta-percha point of matching diameter. However, it soon became apparent that a round canal shape was rarely achieved, especially in curved canals [72,86,151], and that single point filling was likely to be less than ideal as it would rely inevitably on substantial amounts of sealer to fill the gaps resulting in increased leakage [8,11]. It was also clear that discrepancies in size [71,90] and taper [66] between points and equivalent numbered instruments were prevalent. Unfortunately, although some clinicians appreciated these problems and adopted alternative filling techniques, a large number of clinicians were oblivious to the research findings and continued to use the technique (Fig. 8.1).

Current canal preparation techniques that are intended to flare canals to produce a flowing conical funnel shape cannot be filled adequately with a conventional 0.02 taper single point and therefore this should not be attempted. Recently, gutta-percha points with ISO standardized tip sizes but with 0.04 or 0.06 tapers have become available (Fig. 8.2). The manufacturers claim that these greater taper points can fill tapered canals more effectively as they are more likely to correspond to canal shapes created by instruments with similar degrees of taper. However, there are no laboratory or clinical reports to substantiate these claims and such evidence must be available before these new points can be recommended.

Lateral condensation of cold gutta-percha is taught and practised throughout the world [39,134] and is the technique of choice for many clinicians. It is simple and rapid to carry out, can be used in virtually all cases where canal preparation results in an apical stop, and is the standard against which many new techniques are compared (Fig. 8.3).

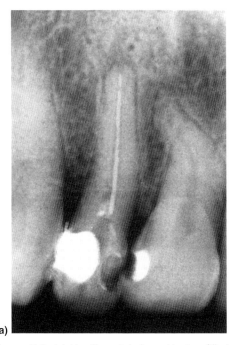
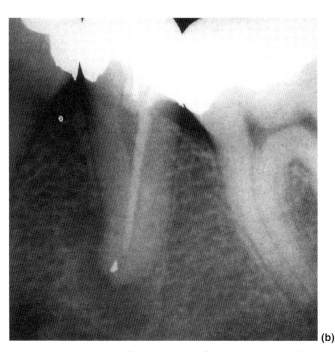

(a)　　　　　　　　　　　　　　　　　　　　　　　　　　　　(b)

**Figure 8.1** (**a**) Maxillary right lateral incisor filled with single gutta-percha point. (**b**) Mandibular left second premolar filled with single gutta-percha point. Note voids alongside fillings and periapical radiolucencies on both teeth.

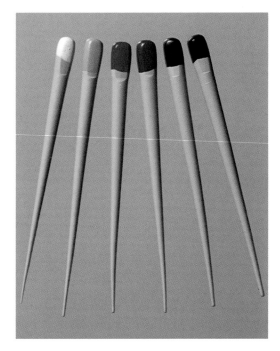

**Figure 8.2** Gutta-percha points with standardized 15–40 tip sizes but with 0.06 tapers.

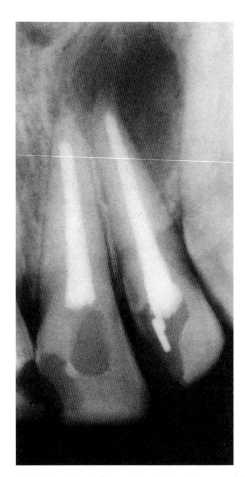

**Figure 8.3** Maxillary left central and lateral incisors filled with laterally condensed gutta-percha.

Lateral condensation involves the placement of a master (primary) point at the end-point of preparation followed by the insertion of additional (accessory) points alongside (Fig. 8.4). The use of a standardized master point provides the possibility of a predictable apical fit at the apical stop whereas the accessory points obturate the space produced as a result of the flared canal shape. The resultant filling consists of numerous points cemented together and to the canal wall by sealer; it does not result in a merging of the points into a homogeneous mass of gutta-percha. The technique is not recommended when the canal has no apical stop and files can pass through the foramen (e.g. when the canal has a continuous taper with the foramen being the narrowest).

A spreader is inserted alongside the master point to improve the adaptation of the master point at the end-point of preparation and to create the space for accessory points. When inserted to within 1 mm of the end-point of preparation the spreader compacts effectively the master point apically [195] and laterally, resulting in considerably less leakage than if the spreader had only entered part-way into the

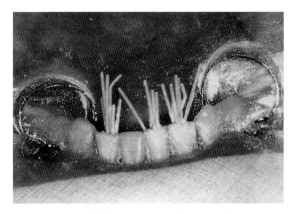

**Figure 8.4** Mandibular incisors with gutta-percha points protruding from access cavities after lateral condensation (reproduced courtesy of Dr DH Edmunds).

canal [5]. In fact, the necessity to advance the spreader well into the canal is one of the main reasons why canals are flared; a narrow, parallel canal shape would not allow a spreader to advance sufficiently to influence the adaptation of the apical region of the master point. Narrow preparations also predispose to the unwanted removal of the master point upon withdrawal of the spreader as it tends to pierce the master point rather than lie alongside it.

The requirements for successful lateral condensation are therefore:

- a flared canal preparation with an apical stop;
- a well-fitting master gutta-percha point of standard size and 0.02 taper; the new 0.04 and 0.06 taper points would tend to prevent deep spreader penetration;
- a series of spreaders of the appropriate size and shape;
- an assortment of accessory points which match the size and taper of spreaders;
- an appropriate sealer.

*Well-fitting master point.* The master point must fit to the full length of the preparation, be tight at the end-point of preparation (tug-back), and it must be impossible to force (stretch) it through the foramen.

The size of the master point is guided by the master apical file used in the final preparation of the apical stop. The selected point is held with tweezers at a length equivalent to the working distance and then inserted into the canal. Ideally, the point should:

- pass down to the full working distance so that the beaks of the tweezers touch the reference point;
- be impossible to push beyond this position, i.e. through the foramen;
- fit tightly at the end-point of preparation giving some resistance to withdrawal (tug-back).

The tweezers are squeezed slightly so as to notch the point and are then released leaving the point *in situ* (Fig. 8.5). A radiograph is then exposed to confirm its position in relation to the end-point of preparation and the radiographic apex. If the original estimate of the working distance was correct the point should be in the appropriate position and canal filling can proceed. Some clinicians condense the master point with a spreader prior to taking the

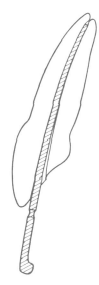

**Figure 8.5** Master gutta-percha point notched at working distance corresponding to the level of incisal edge reference point.

radiograph to ensure that it reaches the end-point of preparation.

However, a number of problems can occur, either as a result of technical difficulties during canal preparation or because of size discrepancies in the gutta-percha points and/or instruments. Most of these problems can be overcome with little effort but they require some thought to ensure that the exact problem is identified.

*Point reaches working distance but is loose.* This may occur for a number of reasons.

- *The gutta-percha point was smaller than expected.* During the manufacture of points a tolerance of ±0.05 mm is allowed at $d_1$ so that it is possible for the point with the correct nominal size to be smaller than the equivalent file size and prepared canal width. The solution is either to try-in a selection of other points of the same size in the hope that one of the correct size will be found, to remove 1 mm increments off the tip of the point with a sharp blade to increase the tip diameter, or to try-in a point of larger nominal diameter. If a point is reduced in length, care should be taken to ensure that the tip has not been flattened before it is reinserted into the canal.

- *The end-point of preparation was wider than expected.* Just as the size of points may vary so can the size of files. The tolerance of files can be ±0.02 mm at $d_1$ so that it is possible for the canal to be wider than anticipated. The solution is the same as described above.

  The canal can become wider than expected through inappropriate choice of instruments and/or preparation technique leading to the removal of excess tissue from the outer wall of the canal apically [6]. Should this problem be identified then either a selection of points can be tried-in until one is found to fit or an alternative filling method chosen.

*Point passes beyond working distance through foramen.* This can occur when the apical stop is inadequate or when the point is too small. If the stop is not sufficiently definite, then the point will pass more deeply into the canal and through the foramen. The solution is either to reprepare the canal with larger instruments until a distinct stop is created at the end-point of preparation or to remove 1 mm increments from the point until its diameter is sufficient to bind in the canal at the working distance. In general terms the creation of a definite apical stop is the solution of choice although care should be taken to avoid the creation of zips.

*Point does not reach working distance.* This is the most common problem that occurs with the positioning of the master point, and there are a number of reasons:

- *The point was larger than expected.* Just as points can be smaller than the nominal size and appear loose, they can also be larger and not seat fully. Thus, if a point is a short distance (< 2 mm) away from the end-point of preparation it may be possible to try a selection of points of the same nominal diameter with the intention of finding one that fits.
- *The canal was not widened sufficiently at the end-point or the canal taper was too narrow.* This is a common problem and occurs when the master apical file is either smaller than its nominal size or, more likely, that it was not used sufficiently to widen the canal fully. In this way, either the apical dimensions of the canal are too small or

the curved region of the canal is too narrow and causes the gutta-percha point to bind. It is essential that the master apical file be manipulated until it can pass down freely to the end-point of preparation without any undue force being applied. With insufficient preparation it may be possible to force the master apical file to the working distance; however, if the same technique is adopted with a gutta-percha point then it will bind and buckle short of the expected length. The solution to this problem is to select a new file and reinstrument the canal to the working length until the file is loose. Increasing the taper along the length of the canal may also be necessary.

- *Dentine debris is blocking the apical region of the canal.* This is another common problem that occurs as a result of insufficient irrigation. Prevention is better than cure as many blockages are difficult to eliminate. Thus, during canal preparation copious volumes of irrigant should be used and canal preparation should include frequent and effective recapitulation at the end-point of preparation.

  The solution to this problem is to irrigate the canal thoroughly and then to manipulate gently small files deep within the canal in an attempt to disrupt the compacted dentine and float out the debris in the irrigant. These small files can be rotated to improve their effectiveness but care should be exercised to prevent the files creating their own canal and perforating the canal wall. The use of large inflexible files with *sharp* tips must be avoided. Endosonic devices enhance debris removal and are more likely to clear canal blockages.

*Selection of spreaders and accessory gutta-percha points.* Once the master apical point has been selected, it is important to select and try-in the spreader to ensure that it can pass down the canal to within 1 mm of the end-point of preparation. Spreaders should be precurved in curved canals and a rubber stop used to identify the length of insertion. To eliminate the risk of root fracture excessive condensation pressures should be avoided by the use of finger spreaders [64].

The working part of spreaders can have a non-standardized taper or standardized ISO 0.02 taper, the same as most files. Non-standardised spreaders have relatively small diameters at the tip but a range of tapers from extra-fine through fine, medium to large; some manufacturers use letters rather than words to denote the degree of taper, e.g. A–D. Spreaders with a standardized taper are manufactured with ISO diameters such as size 20 up to size 40.

The choice of spreader design, that is, with non-standardized or standardized taper, is determined by operator preference and the type of accessory points to be used. When non-standardized spreaders are used the points should be non-standardized; however, standardized spreaders require standardized accessory gutta-percha points. In this way the point will fill the space created by the spreader. It is important to realise that space created by a standardized spreader cannot be filled adequately with a non-standardized point. It is sound clinical practice to use spreaders and points from the same manufacturer to ensure compatibility.

The size of spreader, and thus points, are determined by the size of the canal. Large canals with substantial taper are more efficiently filled with more tapered points, whilst smaller canals with narrower tapers should be filled by finer points. On most occasions an extra-fine or fine (A, B) spreader is required along with matching points.

## Completion of lateral condensation

The initial phases of lateral condensation have already been described. After these preliminary stages, the filling procedure is relatively straightforward:

1. The master point, spreader, accessory points and sealer should be arranged carefully to ensure they can be handled efficiently.
2. The canal should be dried thoroughly with paper points. Use of alcohol to promote effective drying is not recommended for inexperienced operators.
3. The sealer should be mixed, carried into the canal and smeared (buttered) onto the canal wall. Sealer application can be achieved using a hand file rotated anticlockwise, by coating a paper point and inserting into the canal, or by coating the master point itself. There is no need

to apply a large volume of sealer with a spiral filler.
4. The master point should be buttered lightly with sealer and then inserted immediately to the full distance so that the notch made by the tweezers lies at the reference point.
5. The spreader is then placed alongside the point and pushed apically with controlled force until it reaches the appropriate depth, 1 mm from the end-point of preparation. The direction of force should be apical with no lateral rocking of the spreader to prevent root fracture. Apical pressure should be applied in a constant manner for approximately 10 s to achieve the appropriate compaction of the gutta-percha in an apical and lateral direction. In curved canals the spreader should be precurved and applied either lateral to or on the outer aspect of the master point; it should not be applied along the inner aspect of the curve as the spreader could pierce the point and drag it out subsequently.
6. The first accessory point should be inserted into the space created by the spreader and seated fully.
7. The spreader is then cleaned and reinserted immediately into the canal as described above. On this occasion the spreader will not enter the canal to the same length.
8. The second accessory point is inserted into the space.
9. The sequence of spreader application and point insertion continues until the canal is full. The number of additional points required will vary from case to case. Where a post-retained restoration is planned lateral condensation need not continue along the whole length of the canal but can stop when the apical 5–6 mm have been filled.
10. If the final restoration is not post-retained the excess gutta-percha emerging from the canal should be removed with a hot instrument and condensed vertically at the orifice with a plugger that fits the canal tightly to ensure a satisfactory coronal seal. In anterior teeth the gutta-percha should be reduced to below the gingival level in order to maintain the translucency of the crown and to prevent the possibility of sealer staining the dentine [179]; in posterior teeth the gutta-percha should be

seared off at the canal orifice and condensed vertically.

When the final restoration is to be post-retained the gutta-percha can be removed immediately to the appropriate level within the canal, normally leaving approximately 4–5 mm of apical filling undisturbed [107,201]. Preparation of the post space at this stage is useful since the operator will be aware of the anatomy of the canal system and know what length of post is possible.

Lateral condensation is relatively simple to carry out, rapid, and has been used for many years with considerable success (Figs 8.6–8.9) [24,91]. However, since it is impossible for cold gutta-percha to flow into irregularities within the canal system, parts of the canal must either remain unfilled [192] or be filled only with sealer that has been forced into these regions by the pressure exerted through the insertion of spreaders and points. Recently, the importance of cleaning irregularities in oval canals has been emphasized otherwise they remain packed with debris and reduce the quality of the filling [192,194].

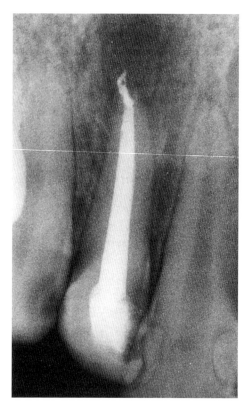

**Figure 8.7** Maxillary right lateral incisor filled with laterally condensed gutta-percha. A small amount of sealer has escaped into the periradicular region.

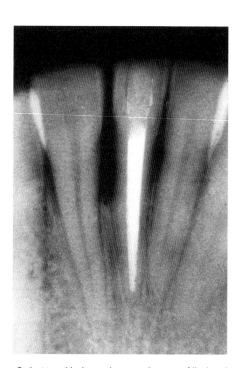

**Figure 8.6** Mandibular right central incisor filled with laterally condensed gutta-percha.

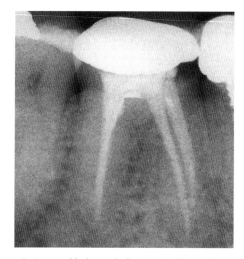

**Figure 8.8** Mandibular right first molar filled with laterally condensed gutta-percha prior to coronal restoration.

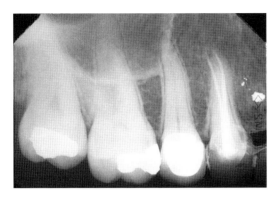

**Figure 8.9** Maxillary right first premolar filled with laterally condensed gutta-percha.

The perceived deficiency of lateral condensation has resulted in the development of techniques whereby gutta-percha is softened by heat or solvents with the intention that the core material can be condensed into irregularities [194]. Some of these techniques rely on the predictability of cold lateral condensation in the apical region and use heat simply to facilitate filling in the coronal two thirds whilst other techniques rely on heat to soften the gutta-percha throughout the whole length of the canal.

## Heat-softened gutta-percha techniques

For many years the only technique that used heat-softened gutta-percha was that of warm vertical condensation [150]. More recently a large number of innovative methods of warming and condensing gutta-percha have been described. Some techniques involve placing cold gutta-percha into the canal and then warming it *in situ*; these can be referred to as *intracanal heating techniques*, whilst others rely on warming gutta-percha outside the canal before its placement, the *extracanal heating techniques*.

For canals prepared with an apical stop lateral condensation of gutta-percha is the most appropriate and popular method of filling and the one recommended for most operators. In general, the heat-softened techniques are technically more difficult and should be used with caution by inexperienced and non-specialist operators. Prior to use in patients the techniques must be practised in simulated canals and extracted teeth to ensure competence.

### Intracanal heating techniques

These techniques include all those where cold gutta-percha is inserted into the canal and then heated within the canal so that it becomes softened and condensable. All the techniques are used in conjunction with sealer. Intracanal heating techniques are not new, but their popularity was limited until Schilder [150] elegantly described his method for filling canals in three dimensions using warm vertical condensation.

*Continuous wave of condensation technique.* In recent years the traditional warm vertical condensation technique has been simplified considerably through the use of electrically heated spreaders and pluggers (Touch 'n Heat and System B Heat Source, SybronEndo, CA, USA). As a result, there has been a resurgence of interest in vertical condensation techniques [20,141].

The continuous wave of condensation technique [20] uses the System B Heat Source. It consists of two stages, *down-packing* and *back-packing*. In down-packing a wave of heat is carried along the length of the master point starting coronally and ending in apical 'corkage'. The apical and lateral movement of thermosoftened gutta-percha is referred to as a *wave of condensation*. Back-packing involves filling the middle and coronal regions of the canal and can be accomplished using thermoplastic devices that can deposit increments of warm gutta-percha, e.g. injection delivery systems.

The System B controls the temperature at the tip of the plugger (set at maximum power, 200°C), to maintain the right temperature throughout down-packing. The technique is simpler and more rapid than other techniques because down-packing is completed in a single continuous vertical movement.

The continuous wave technique requires a continuously tapering canal shape with the smallest diameter at the foramen. A non-standardized point of similar taper is then selected and tried in to ensure it achieves the correct length and fits snuggly, with 'tugback'. This should allow the tip of the point to fit into, but not protrude through, the foramen. Good fit of the point at the foramen is essential to provide resistance during condensation and prevent the point being pushed into the periodontal ligament space. Thus, the matching taper of the point and canal preparation along with a snug fit at the foramen is meant to prevent overfilling. The tip of the point can be adjusted to provide a snug fit by removing increments with a scalpel until tugback is achieved (at length); radiographs should be exposed to confirm the position.

A Buchanan Plugger that matches the canal taper is attached to the System B and then tried in the canal so that it stops some 4–5 mm from the end-point of preparation, a position termed the 'binding point'. It is important that the taper of the plugger matches the taper produced in the canal during the preparation phase and that it does not contact the canal walls at this point. The pluggers can be pre-curved when appropriate.

Following sealer application, the pre-selected non-standardized point is positioned at length and the excess protruding out of the orifice removed with the heated plugger. Although not essential, a cold plugger can be used to condense the point in the orifice in order to provide a flat surface onto which the heated plugger can be placed. The plugger is then placed on the point, activated (maximum power, 200°C) and driven down (down-packed) through the gutta-percha to the level of the binding point (indicated by a rubber stop on the plugger). After 1 s, the activating button is released and the cooling plugger pushed vertically for some 10 s (sustained push) to counteract cooling shrinkage. Finally, the heat source is activated for a further second whilst apical pressure is maintained before the plugger is withdrawn. The withdrawal of the plugger removes most of the gutta-percha in the middle and coronal region but should leave the apical region and irregularities full. Back-filling can be completed using the System B, gutta-percha plugs and Buchanan Pluggers, or more effectively with heated delivery devices such as the Obtura II (Texceed Corporation, Fenton, MO, USA).

This technique appears to be simple but the skills necessary to achieve predictable results can be difficult to master, particularly in those teeth with confluent canal systems. Considerable practice on extracted teeth is essential to avoid unnecessary clinical problems. No evidence is available to confirm whether the technique has a greater clinical success rate but the radiological appearance of the final filling often demonstrates material forced into irregularities and lateral canals (Figs 8.10–8.12)

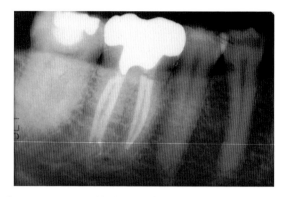

**Figure 8.10** Mandibular right first molar filled with System B and Obtura.

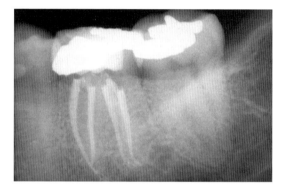

**Figure 8.11** Mandibular left first molar filled with System B and Obtura prior to coronal restoration.

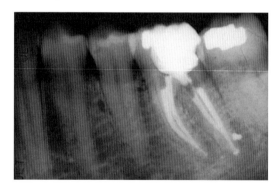

**Figure 8.12** Mandibular left first molar filled with System B and Obtura prior to coronal restoration.

implying that complete filling has been achieved. Unfortunately, the technique is also associated with material (probably sealer) passing beyond the foramen. Indeed, given that achieving patency is an essential step when preparing canals with a continuous taper, this is an inevitable outcome. The passage of sealer into the periradicular region is of concern as, although evidence exists that it will be absorbed [122], there is also evidence that suggests excess material may cause inflammation.

*Warm vertical condensation.* Vertical condensation of warm gutta-percha was suggested by Schilder [150], who modified the sectional gutta-percha technique of Coolidge [32]. The aim of this technique is to obliterate the canal with heat softened gutta-percha packed with sufficient vertical pressure to force it to flow into the entire root canal system, including accessory and lateral canals. The traditional technique requires a flared canal preparation with a definite apical stop. The flared nature of the canal is necessary to accommodate the pluggers used to condense the gutta-percha and facilitate the flow of the material apically. Excessive widening of the canal at the end-point is counterproductive and actually results in more apical leakage [196] and an increased incidence of over-extensions [197].

The traditional warm vertical condensation technique uses spreaders heated by a flame, but electrically heated spreaders (Touch 'n Heat, SybronEndo) provide a more convenient method. The technique produces homogeneous, compact fillings with gutta-percha flowing into irregularities, apical deltas and lateral canals [189]; signs of sealer and gutta-percha extrusion into the apical and lateral periodontal ligament are frequently observed. However, no substantial improvement in apical [46] or coronal seal [92] has been demonstrated over cold lateral condensation. Despite the use of very hot instruments the actual rise in temperature within the mass of gutta-percha is minimal [110] with no long-term effects that may endanger the integrity of the periodontium [68].

Intracanal heating of gutta-percha with endosonic devices has also been described. However, reports of their clinical efficacy are awaited.

*Rotating condenser.* The use of an engine-driven rotating compactor to soften and condense gutta-percha vertically and laterally was first described by McSpadden [116]. The technique was termed 'thermatic condensation' and relied upon a rotating stainless steel compactor generating sufficient frictional heat within the canal to plasticize the cold master point and then drive it apically. The original

instruments have been discontinued and only the Gutta-Condensor (Dentsply Maillefer, Ballaigues, Switzerland) is available.

The original technique demanded that the condenser be activated in the canal, alongside the master point, at approximately 12 000 rpm without apical pressure. After a matter of seconds the gutta-percha became softened and was driven apically by the controlled advance of the condenser to a point some 2 mm from the end-point of preparation. As the apical region filled with material the condenser tended to back-out of the canal whereupon the instrument was slowly withdrawn while still rotating at the optimum speed. In large canals a second point was condensed in order to fill deficiencies in the middle and coronal regions.

Following concerns about the unpredictable nature of the technique, the original method was modified [168]. The so-called 'hybrid technique' combined the predictability of lateral condensation in the apical region with the speed and efficacy of the rotating condenser in the middle and coronal areas. Thus, a master point was cemented and lateral condensation of accessory points completed in the apical 3–4 mm before undertaking thermal compaction.

In recent years the design and manufacture of condensers has been modified along with the technique of using them. Modern condensers are manufactured from nickel-titanium, not stainless steel, and used with gutta-percha that has already been softened out of the mouth. These techniques are described next.

### Extracanal heating techniques

These rely on gutta-percha being warmed and softened out of the mouth prior to its insertion within the canal. All the techniques are used with sealer.

*Precoated carriers.* An innovative approach to filling canals using a carrier to introduce thermally softened gutta-percha to the tooth was described many years ago [83]. The efficacy of the technique was based on the flow characteristics of the gutta-percha and the ability of the carrier to transport and condense the material.

The technique was subsequently modified and made available commercially using a series of carriers made from plastic (Thermafil Endodontic Obturators, Dentsply Maillefer). Special gutta-percha coats the shaft of the carriers making the warmed material sticky and adhesive but with excellent flow characteristics. The system includes an oven to warm the obturators in a controlled and reproducible manner. In addition, a series of verifiers are provided to check the diameter of the end-point of preparation and to simplify the selection of the appropriately sized obturator. Within the last few years a variety of similarly precoated carriers made by other companies have been marketed.

The technique for using precoated carriers is simple but it is important to appreciate that the taper of the carriers is at least 0.04 and so canal shaping procedures must take this into account. Following preparation and drying of the canal, an uncoated carrier (or a verifier) of the estimated size is inserted to the full working distance; a radiograph can confirm the position. If it passes down to the end-point of preparation without using force, the equivalent size of obturator is selected and the working distance marked with the silicone stop. The canal is dried, then coated with a small amount of sealer placed at the entrance to the orifice. The obturator is then placed in the heating chamber of the oven for the appropriate time. The obturator is removed from the oven and immediately seated into the canal; it should not be inserted so that the tip of the carrier reaches the apical extent of preparation, rather the aim is to ensure the tip of the carrier is some 0.5 mm from this point leaving the apical region filled only with gutta-percha and sealer. Thus, the canal length must be measured accurately and the rubber stop on the Obturator moved to the appropriate position.

The excess gutta-percha in the chamber is removed and the remainder condensed vertically to enhance the coronal seal; additional gutta-percha can be introduced in oval or C-shaped canals if required. After the gutta-percha has cooled the shaft is severed with a bur and the handle discarded.

A clear disadvantage of these devices, particularly when a post-retained restoration is planned, is the fact that the shaft of the carrier remains within the bulk of gutta-percha. However, although some studies have shown that this does not affect the apical seal [142,149], one has reported substantially more leakage after immediate post preparation [138].

The results of most laboratory studies on precoated carriers suggest the technique is significantly quicker than lateral condensation [40,41,62], produces fillings of similar radiographic quality [40,41] and an equivalent or better apical seal with both the original metal [10,41,98,115] and plastic carriers [29,36,40,63]. A minority of studies have reported that lateral condensation produced a better apical seal [28,65,97,135]. In laboratory studies the use of precoated carriers has been associated with an increased incidence of sealer and gutta-percha extrusion [29,41,98,154]. Although no clinical reports have been published to confirm whether this phenomenon occurs in vivo, it is clearly a common occurrence (Figs 8.13 and 8.14). Recently, a technique of backfilling with Thermafil Obturators has been described following the initial placement of a cold master gutta-percha point. Laboratory

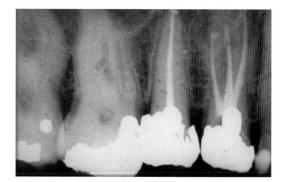

**Figure 8.13** Maxillary right first and second premolars filled with Thermafil Obturators (reproduced courtesy of Mr SJ Hayes).

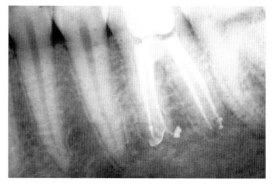

**Figure 8.14** Mandibular left first molar filled with Thermafil Obturators.

studies have shown the extrusion of sealer and gutta-percha has been eliminated when this technique is adopted [34].

Studies have also reported that the carriers are often in direct contact with the canal wall and not embedded entirely within gutta-percha [29,85,97]. Concerns have also been expressed about the problems of removing carriers should retreatment be necessary [67,185,186]. No clinical study has been carried out to determine whether the use of precoated carriers results in a higher success rate compared with more conventional filling techniques.

The development of coated carriers is continuing and a new series of obturators matching the GT rotary instruments is now available (Dentsply Maillefer). In this system there are 0.04, 0.06, 0.08 and 0.10 taper GT instruments in sizes 20, 30 and 40 and obturators of similar dimensions. However, it must be emphasized that no evidence is available to confirm their efficacy.

Although precoated carriers are convenient they are relatively expensive and cannot be customized easily for specific canals. A number of techniques were developed where the operator could coat the carrier with gutta-percha at the chairside prior to insertion. The SuccessFil technique (Hygenic, Akron, OH, USA) and the AlphaSeal technique (NT Company, Chattanooga, TN, USA) provided syringes of gutta-percha, which were heated and then applied to a carrier. There is no data on the efficacy of these carriers and many have been discontinued.

*Thermoplastic delivery systems.* The technique involves heating gutta-percha to a molten state and then forcing it under mechanical pressure (injection) into a relatively cool mould (the root canal) [198]. On dissipation of the heat, the material solidifies and retains the shape determined by the internal outline of the mould. The techniques used in endodontics for injecting softened gutta-percha are not true injection-moulding systems as the pressure applied to the gutta-percha by the delivery systems is sufficient only to deposit the material into the canal; vertical condensation is then required to ensure adaptation of the gutta-percha to the canal wall and three-dimensional filling of the canal system.

Injection of gutta-percha produces a seal comparable to lateral condensation [198], although extrusion of material may occur. The adaptation of gutta-

percha to the canal walls has been confirmed [173]. In a commercially available delivery system [75], the gutta-percha was heated to 160°C and delivered through the needle tip at approximately 60°C [55]. The original device has been superseded by the Obtura II system (Obtura Corporation) with improved temperature control.

The high-temperature Obtura device has been shown to produce clinically acceptable results (Fig. 8.15) [109,111,162], whilst a number of laboratory studies have demonstrated an apical seal as good as lateral condensation [42,46,73,159]. Warm injected gutta-percha can also penetrate dentinal tubules [60]. On the other hand, some studies have reported the apical seal to be less effective [15,94] and the incidence of gutta-percha under or over-extension to be high [42,108].

Clinical experience and the results of various laboratory studies have emphasized the need to limit enlargement of the foramen [139] and for the prepared canal to include a definite stop at the endpoint of preparation [50,52,61]. The use of a sectional injection technique whereby the gutta-percha is deposited and condensed in several increments rather than in one has also been found to improve the apical seal as it allows better condensation of the material deposited apically [180,181]. Improvement of the apical seal has also been found when a conventional master gutta-percha point is cemented before injection of the heated gutta-percha [121].

Injection delivery systems are more popular now for back-filling the middle and coronal regions following vertical condensation [20,141] or lateral condensation [30].

*Operator-coated carrier-condenser.* The original technique of thermatic condensation of gutta-percha used conventional gutta-percha points and a rotating condenser to generate heat [116]. Concerns about instrument fracture, inability to be used effectively in curved canals, heat generation and lack of predictability led to the development of a new generation of nickel-titanium condensers and a technique in which the condenser is coated with heat softened gutta-percha prior to insertion into the canal (AlphaSeal, NT Company). The special gutta-percha was available in two formulations, one relatively viscous and the other more fluid.

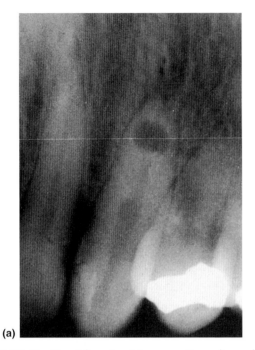 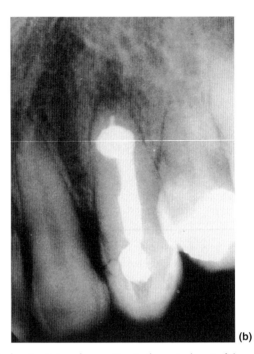

(a)  (b)

**Figure 8.15** Maxillary left canine: (**a**) preoperative radiograph showing internal resorption in the apical part of the root canal. (**b**) Root canal and resorptive defect filled with warm gutta-percha using an injection delivery system (reproduced courtesy of Mr N Claydon).

A number of methods could be used to obturate canals; one involved sealing a conventional master point into the canal followed by the immediate use of a condenser coated with heat-softened material [54]. Alternatively, the compactor can first be coated with the more viscous material and then with an additional layer of the more fluid material. Few reports have so far been published on the use of this technique [53].

The AlphaSeal system has been superseded recently by the MicroSeal system (SybronEndo, CA, USA). The concept of the new system remains as before, but it has been enhanced by provision of master cones having a different gutta-percha formulation to the one that is warmed and injected onto the condenser. The manufacturer recommends the fitting of a cold master cone prior to the introduction of the warmed gutta-percha on the condenser [54].

## Solvent-softened gutta-percha

Chloroform-softened gutta-percha has a long tradition in endodontics, and associated filling techniques are still taught in many institutions and practised widely. The forerunner of the current methods was the Johnston–Callahan method of root canal filling. Following extensive drying of the canal with alcohol, it was filled with a solution of rosin (colophony) in chloroform into which was seated a gutta-percha master point. The chloroform softened the surface of the gutta-percha and made it swell, and the rosin acted as a glue to make the mass stick to the canal walls. This method is still taught with only minor modification in Sweden, as the rosin–chloroform filling method.

The high degree of evaporation and the fluid nature of the rosin solution led to the development of chloro-percha. Primarily a thick suspension of fine carvings of gutta-percha in chloroform, chloro-percha was soon modified by the addition of zinc oxide and metal salts to act as much as a conventional sealer as merely softening the points. The Kloroperka of Nygaard-Östby, which has some 50% zinc oxide and 20% metal salts in addition to gutta-percha, Canada balsam and waxes is the best known formulation.

Chloroform is also used to aid in the production of custom-formed master points. This has been popularized as the chloroform dip technique [9,89]. In this method the apical 2–5 mm of the master gutta-percha point is dipped in chloroform for a few seconds (Fig. 8.16) and inserted into the canal to the end-point of preparation. The point is then withdrawn and allowed to dry (Fig. 8.17). The chloroform softens the outer layer of the gutta-percha so that when it is seated fully it takes up the shape of the apical portion of the canal. Because the volume of solvent is small and the thickness of gutta-percha affected is minimal there is little shrinkage following solvent evaporation [96,190]. The customized point is then cemented in place with a conventional sealer and the remainder of the canal filled with laterally condensed gutta-percha. The apical seal obtained with this technique has been shown to be comparable with traditional cold lateral condensation [160].

Chloroform is a potent organic solvent with potentially undesirable biological effects. There are limits for the concentration in the working environment, and if chloroform is used injudiciously in the dental surgery these may be exceeded. Other solvents with less potentially harmful side-effects have been tested as alternatives, some of which have found practical application.

Oil of eucalyptus has long been used as an alternative to chloroform in endodontics. It has a strong smell that may be less agreeable, and its ability to soften gutta-percha is much less than that of chloroform. Xylene and rectified turpentine also have substantially less dissolving ability compared with chloroform. Halothane, which is an inhalation anaesthetic agent, is bioacceptable and softens gutta-percha, even if not to the same extent as chloroform. Citrus extracts also have ability to soften

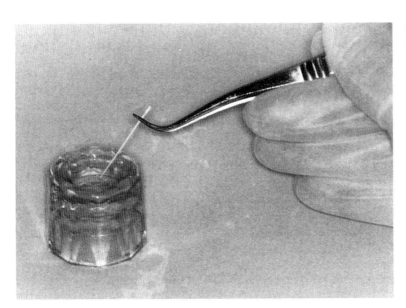

**Figure 8.16** Apical 2 mm of gutta-percha point immersed in chloroform for 1–2 seconds to soften the surface.

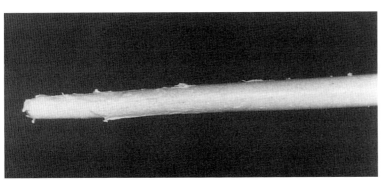

**Figure 8.17** Apical portion of gutta-percha cone, following chloroform softening and insertion into the canal, showing canal wall irregularities.

gutta-percha. Common to most, if not all, alternatives to chloroform is that, because of their lower vapour pressure, it takes longer for them to evaporate, and therefore their tissue-irritating properties last for longer.

Set specimens of Kloroperka or rosin–chloroform-softened gutta-percha are among the least irritating or cytotoxic endodontic materials. Further, histological examination of periapical tissues of teeth root filled with Kloroperka has shown a favourable response. These materials have performed consistently poorly in leakage studies where dyes were used; this is because of the shrinkage caused by the evaporation of chloroform (or other solvent). Chloroform does not actually dissolve gutta-percha: its main effect is to cause a swelling of the resin structure. Even if massive shrinkage is prevented because the bulk of the gutta-percha point is unaffected, the 5–7% linear shrinkage at the interface of sealer and dentine may be sufficient to allow dye penetration. The clinical significance of this is unknown, and so far solvent-based filling methods have not been tested by bacterial leakage. These root canal fillings are dominant in Scandinavian studies on clinical performance of root canal treatment [24,56,167], and they appear successful.

## APICAL DENTINE PLUG

Problems with the biocompatibility of root canal filling materials and the potential for their extrusion through the foramen into the surrounding periradicular tissues led to the intentional use of an apical dentine plug during canal filling. The apical dentine plug is built up from clean dentine filings packed into the apical foramen of the canal prior to filling with conventional techniques. The rationale for this procedure is that dentine filings (shavings), when impinged on the vital apical pulp stump or periradicular tissue, act as a nidus for the deposition of cementum or intermediate-type hard tissue, while the plug acts as a barrier between the root canal-filling material and connective tissue [113,130]. Studies in experimental animals revealed that packing uninfected shavings in the foramina stimulated the formation of cementum and bone at the apex [132,175]. On the other hand, use of infected dentine

chips has a negative effect on healing [76,174]. Unfortunately, the results of investigations into the efficacy of apical dentine plugs have been contradictory. Some studies have reported more rapid healing [127] and that an effective barrier could be created [43], particularly when heat softened gutta-percha techniques are used [154], whilst other studies have reported greater leakage [81] and the technique to be of dubious value [199].

## OTHER METHODS OF ROOT CANAL FILLING

### Mineral trioxide aggregate

Mineral trioxide aggregate (MTA) is a powder that consists of hydrophilic particles that sets in the presence of moisture [172]. Hydration of the powder results in a colloidal gel with a pH of 12.5 that solidifies to a hard structure. This material has been investigated as a potential compound to seal off the pathways of communication between the root canal system and the external surface of the tooth [171]. Several in vitro and in vivo studies have shown that MTA prevents microleakage, is biocompatible, and promotes regeneration of the original tissues when placed in contact with the dental pulp or periradicular tissues [171].

To date, the clinical applications suggested for MTA include capping of pulps with reversible pulpitis, apexification, surgical and non-surgical repair of root perforations and fractures, as well as a root-end filling material. However, MTA has a potential use as a conventional root filling material if problems of placement within the canal can be overcome. If not used to fill the entire canal system, it can be used as a base material in canal orifices and pulp chambers to create a coronal barrier to leakage.

The use of MTA as an apical plug in cases of teeth with immature, open apices has been described [171]. The MTA can create a hard tissue barrier [157,170] and prevent extrusion of conventional filling material (Figs 8.18 and 8.19).

### Non-instrumentation technology

A new method for root canal treatment has been described that allows the cleaning, disinfection and

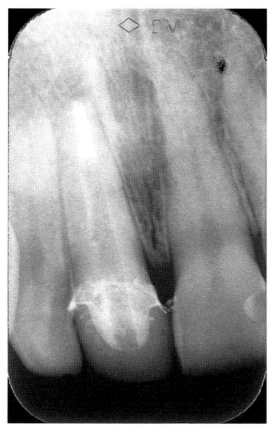

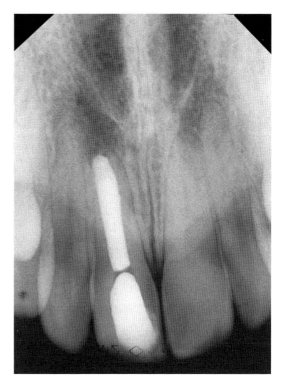

**Figure 8.19** Maxillary right central incisor with open apex filled with MTA and Obtura (reproduced courtesy of Mr SJ Hayes).

**Figure 8.18** Maxillary right central incisor with open apex filled with MTA (reproduced courtesy of Mr SJ Hayes).

filling of the root canal system without the use of traditional instruments [101,102,104]. The canals are cleansed by irrigation with sodium hypochlorite under alternating pressure generated by a vacuum pump; the canals are not enlarged. Filling of the canal system is performed using a vacuum pump that produces a negative pressure. When this is achieved, a valve is opened to a reservoir containing freshly mixed sealer and the material is sucked into the canal system. Laboratory studies of the technique are promising and demonstrate good filling of the canal system and sealing comparable to lateral condensation [133,103]; clinical studies are limited but show promise [105].

## Silver points

Silver points were introduced in the 1930s as a method for filling fine tortuous canals. With the

instruments and preparation techniques available at the time, such canals were difficult to enlarge adequately in order to accept gutta-percha points. The rigidity of silver points made it easier and quicker to complete the filling procedure since apical pressure on the points forced them down narrow canals to the end-point of preparation. Resultant radiographs invariably revealed a dense radiopaque filling which appeared to obturate the entire length of the canal (Fig. 8.20). Unfortunately, because silver points could be forced down canals many clinicians spent little time cleaning and shaping the canal system with the result that pulpal debris and microorganisms were often left in situ. This abuse of silver points led to frequent failure as leakage of microorganisms and toxins into the periradicular tissues occurred over time.

Use of silver points is contraindicated as they have a number of other inherent disadvantages. Silver points are round in cross-section and perform best when filling canals that have been prepared to

133

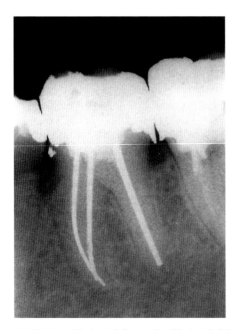

**Figure 8.20** Mandibular left first molar filled with full length silver points.

a round cross-section of matching diameter. Unfortunately, a number of studies have shown that few canals are round or can be made round, particularly in more coronal regions [151]. Consequently, the seal in such circumstances relies heavily on relatively large volumes of sealer. Silver points are also prone to corrosion when exposed to tissue fluids [16]. The corrosion products can leak into the periradicular tissues and compound the problems caused by simple sealer dissolution. Finally, full length silver points cannot be used in teeth where post-retained restorations are planned as the coronal portion of the point occupies the space required by the post.

## Paste fillers

Paste fillers were introduced to simplify and speed up root canal treatment [143], just as silver points were introduced to facilitate filling of difficult canals. The paste fillers should not be confused with sealers or cements designed to lute solid or semi-solid materials into the canal. Rather, the paste fillers contain strong disinfectants (paraformaldehyde) and anti-inflammatory agents (corticosteroids) and were introduced in the belief that their use could bypass the accepted principles of canal preparation, disinfection and filling. The proponents of paste fillers argued that the medicaments would allow canals to be treated without the need for thorough cleaning and shaping since the powerful disinfectants would eliminate microorganisms and because the anti-inflammatory agents would reduce the host response.

Unfortunately, the attraction of a rapid and simple method for root canal treatment found favour with many practitioners and numerous teeth were root filled using paste fillers (Fig. 8.21). Not surprisingly, this concept resulted in repeated problems and some patients suffered permanent injury as a result of toxic materials being passed into the periradicular tissues and beyond [1,4]. Clearly, there is no place for these materials in modern practice and their use is contraindicated.

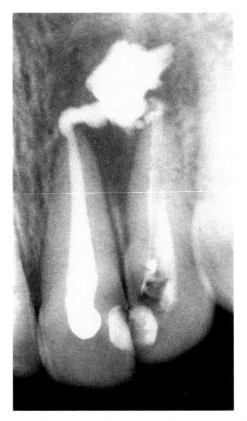

**Figure 8.21** Maxillary left central and lateral incisors filled with paste. A substantial amount of paste has been extruded into the periradicular region. The filling in the lateral incisor is poorly condensed and contains numerous voids.

## Paraformaldehyde

Most of the paste fillers (Endomethasone, Septodont, St Maur des Fosses, France; N2, Indrag Agsa, Locarno, Switzerland; SPAD, Quetigny, France) contain paraformaldehyde. If deposited in the periradicular tissues this may give rise to severe inflammatory reactions and long-lasting or permanent injury, particularly if nerve bundles are affected [4,126].

The application of paraformaldehyde to vital tissue will result in traces of the material or its components being spread throughout the body [13,176]. This is undesirable since not only can individuals show a hypersensitivity response [74,100] but the material may have both mutagenic and carcinogenic potency [124].

## Corticosteroids

Corticosteroid preparations severely affect the defence responses of the periradicular tissues by suppressing phagocytosis, providing the opportunity for microorganisms to multiply. Their use may possibly cause unwanted systemic side-effects [70,166].

## RESTORATION OF THE ROOT FILLED TOOTH

The completion of the root canal filling does not mean that treatment has been completed. Considerable evidence now exists to support the concept of coronal leakage [146] and the necessity to restore the tooth with a good quality coronal restoration [93,137,177]. Thus, following root canal filling the crown of the tooth must be restored permanently as soon as practicable to prevent the ingress of saliva and microorganisms into the chamber and along the root canal to the apical foramina.

## FOLLOW-UP

Immediately following root canal preparation and filling, teeth may be tender and it advisable to warn patients that this may occur [27,51]. Fortunately, the incidence of severe pain following root canal filling is low [69,200]. In most cases the pain is mild and transient and no active intervention is required. However, if an episode of severe pain occurs over an extended period then further investigation is necessary and a diagnosis should be established. In particular, the quality of treatment should be reviewed so that it can be established whether poor technique and/or procedural accidents have contributed to the problem. Once the cause has been identified then the correct treatment can be instituted; this may be root canal retreatment or surgical intervention.

Follow-up of root-filled teeth is important. The patient should be recalled and the tooth examined clinically and radiologically over an extended period. Because each case is different it is impossible to give firm guidelines for when recall should take place and when clinical examination should be supplemented by radiography. However, it is essential that a radiograph should be taken straight after root canal filling to record the immediate postoperative condition. A further radiological check after one year is advisable [45]. The strategy for further radiographic screening will depend on the case.

## CRITERIA OF SUCCESS

Success of root canal treatment should be judged using a combination of clinical and radiological criteria:

- The tooth should be functional with no signs of swelling or sinus tract.
- The patient should be free from symptoms.
- The radiological appearance of the periradicular tissues should either remain normal (if there was no evidence of bone involvement at the commencement of treatment) or return to normality as a result of the complete healing of any periradicular bone loss.

Success or failure cannot be judged immediately after treatment. For example, large areas of periradicular bone loss may take months and sometimes years to heal completely, whilst it can take many months for loss of bone in failing cases to become obvious radiologically.

## REFERENCES

1. Alantar A, Tarragano H, Lefevre B (1994) Extrusion of endodontic filling material into the insertions of the mylohyoid muscle. A case report. *Oral Surgery, Oral Medicine, Oral Pathology* **78**, 646–649.

2. Al-Dewani N, Hayes SJ, Dummer PMH (2000) Comparison of laterally condensed and low temperature thermoplasticized gutta-percha root fillings. *Journal of Endodontics* **26**, 733–738.

3. AliGhamdi A, Wennberg A (1994) Testing of sealing ability of endodontic filling materials. *Endodontics and Dental Traumatology* **10**, 249–255.

4. Allard KUB (1986) Paraesthesia – a consequence of a controversial root-filling material? A case report. *International Endodontic Journal* **19**, 205–208.

5. Allison DA, Weber CR, Walton RE (1979) The influence of the method of canal preparation on the quality of apical and coronal obturation. *Journal of Endodontics* **5**, 298–304.

6. Alodeh M, Doller R, Dummer PMH (1989) Shaping of simulated root canals in resin blocks using the step-back technique with K-files manipulated in a simple in/out filing motion. *International Endodontic Journal* **22**, 107–117.

7. Barkhordar RA, Ngyuyen NT (1985) Paraesthesia of the mental nerve after overextension with AH26 and gutta-percha: report of a case. *Journal of the American Dental Association* **110**, 202–203.

8. Beatty RG (1987) The effect of standard or serial preparation on single cone obturation. *International Endodontic Journal* **20**, 276–281.

9. Beatty RG, Zakariasen KL (1984) Apical leakage associated with three obturation techniques in large and small root canals. *International Endodontic Journal* **17**, 67–72.

10. Beatty RG, Baker PS, Haddix J, Hart F (1989) The efficacy of four root canal obturation techniques in preventing apical dye penetration. *Journal of the American Dental Association* **119**, 633–637.

11. Beer R, Gängler P, Beer M (1986) In-vitro-Untersuchungen unterschiedlicher Wurzelkanalfülltechniken und-materialien. *Zahn-, Mund-, und Kieferheilkunde mit Zentralblatt* **74**, 800–806.

12. Blackman R, Gross M, Seltzer S (1988) An evaluation of the biocompatibility of a glass ionomer-silver cement in rat connective tissue. *Journal of Endodontics* **15**, 76–79.

13. Block RM, Lewis RD, Hirsch J, Coffey J, Langeland K (1983) Systemic distribution of [$^{14}$C]-labeled paraformaldehyde incorporated within formocresol following pulpotomies in dogs. *Journal of Endodontics* **9**, 176–189.

14. Bowman GA (1876) Root filling. *Missouri Dental Journal* **8**, 372–376.

15. Bradshaw GB, Hall A, Edmunds DH (1989) The sealing ability of injection-moulded thermoplasticized gutta-percha. *International Endodontic Journal* **22**, 17–20.

16. Brady JM, del Rio CE (1975) Corrosion of endodontic silver cones in humans: a scanning electron microscope and X-ray microprobe study. *Journal of Endodontics* **1**, 205–210.

17. Brännström M (1984) Smear layer: pathological and treatment considerations. *Operative Dentistry* Supplement **3**, 35–42.

18. Brown RC, Jackson CR, Skidmore AE (1994) An evaluation of apical leakage of a glass ionomer root canal sealer. *Journal of Endodontics* **20**, 288–291.

19. Brownlee WA (1900) Filling of root canals in recently devitalized teeth. *Dominion Dental Journal* **12**, 254–256.

20. Buchanan LS (1994) The Buchanan continuous wave of condensation technique. A convergence of conceptual and procedural advances in obturation. *Dentistry Today* **October**, 80–85.

21. Buchanan LS (2000) The standardized-taper root canal preparation – Part 1. Concepts for variably tapered shaping instruments. *International Endodontic Journal* **33**, 516–529.

22. Byström A, Sundqvist G (1981) Bacteriologic evaluation of the efficacy of mechanical root canal instrumentation in endodontic therapy. *Scandinavian Journal of Dental Research* **89**, 321–328.

23. Byström A, Claesson R, Sundqvist G (1985) The antibacterial effect of camphorated paramonochlorophenol, camphorated phenol and calcium hydroxide in the treatment of infected root canals. *Endodontics and Dental Traumatology* **1**, 170–175.

24. Byström A, Happonen RP, Sjögren U, Sundqvist G (1987) Healing of periapical lesions of pulpless teeth after endodontic treatment with controlled asepsis. *Endodontics and Dental Traumatology* **3**, 58–63.

25. Callis PD, Santini A (1987) Tissue response to retrograde root fillings in the ferret canine: a comparison of a glass ionomer cement and gutta-percha with sealer. *Oral Surgery, Oral Medicine, Oral Pathology* **64**, 475–479.

26. Carman JE, Wallace JA (1994) An in vitro comparison of microleakage of restorative materials in the pulp chambers of human molar teeth. *Journal of Endodontics* **20**, 571–575.

27. Chapman CR (1984) New directions in the understanding and management of pain. *Social Science and Medicine* **19**, 1261–1277.

28. Chohayeb AA (1992) Comparison of conventional root canal obturation techniques with Thermafil obturators. *Journal of Endodontics* **18**, 10–12.

29. Clark DS, ElDeeb ME (1993) Apical sealing ability of metal versus plastic carrier Thermafil obturators. *Journal of Endodontics* **19**, 4–9.

30. Coletti P, Beatty R, Campbell J (1988) Effect of combined lateral condensation-injected warm gutta-percha obturations. *Journal of Dental Research* **67**, 219 (Abstract 848).

31. Combe EC, Cohen BD, Cummings K (2001) Alpha- and beta-forms of gutta-percha in products for root canal filling. *International Endodontic Journal* **34**, 447–451.

32. Coolidge ED (1950) *Endodontia*. Philadelphia, USA: Lea and Febiger, pp. 190–207.

33. Czonstkowsky M, Wilson EG, Holstein FA (1990) The smear layer in endodontics. *Dental Clinics of North America* **34**, 13–25.

34. Da Silva D, Endal U, Reynaud A, Portenier I, Ørstavik D, Haapasalo M (2002) An in vitro study of a Thermafil backfilling technique. *International Endodontic Journal* **35**, 88.

35. Dahl BL, Tronstad L (1976) Biological tests on an experimental glass ionomer (silicopolyacrylate) cement. *Journal of Oral Rehabilitation* **3**, 19–24.

36. Dalat DM, Spångberg LSW (1994) Comparison of apical leakage in root canals obturated with various gutta-percha techniques using a dye vacuum tracing method. *Journal of Endodontics* **20**, 315–319.

37. de Gee AJ, Wu MK, Wesselink PR (1994) Sealing properties of Ketac-Endo glass ionomer cement and AH26 root canal sealers. *International Endodontic Journal* **27**, 239–244.

38. Drake DR, Wiemann AH, Rivera EM, Walton RE (1994) Bacterial retention in canal walls in vitro: effect of smear layer. *Journal of Endodontics* **20**, 78–82.

39. Dummer PMH (1991) Comparison of undergraduate endodontic teaching programmes in the United Kingdom and in some dental schools in Europe and the United States. *International Endodontic Journal* **24**, 169–177.

40. Dummer PMH, Lyle L, Rawle J, Kennedy JK (1994) A laboratory study of root fillings in teeth obturated by lateral condensation of gutta-percha or Thermafil obturators. *International Endodontic Journal* **27**, 32–38.

41. Dummer PMH, Kelly T, Meghji A, Sheikh I, Vanitchai JT (1993) An in vitro study of the quality of root fillings in teeth obturated by lateral condensation of gutta-percha or Thermafil obturators. *International Endodontic Journal* **26**, 99–105.

42. ElDeeb ME (1985) The sealing ability of injection-molded thermoplasticized gutta-percha. *Journal of Endodontics* **11**, 84–86.

43. ElDeeb ME, Nguyen TTQ, Jensen JR (1983) The dentinal plug: its effects on confining substances to the canal and on the apical seal. *Journal of Endodontics* **9**, 355–359.

44. Erausquin J, Muruzabal M (1968) Tissue reaction to root canal cements in the rat molar. *Oral Surgery, Oral Medicine, Oral Pathology* **26**, 360–373.

45. European Society of Endodontology (1994) Consensus report of the European Society of Endodontology on quality guidelines for endodontic treatment. *International Endodontic Journal* **27**, 115–124.

46. Evans JT, Simon JH (1986) Evaluation of the apical seal produced by injected thermoplasticized gutta-percha in the absence of smear layer and root canal sealer. *Journal of Endodontics* **12**, 100–107.

47. Friedman CE, Sandrik JL, Heuer MA, Rapp GW (1977) Composition and physical properties of gutta-percha endodontic filling materials. *Journal of Endodontics* **3**, 304–308.

48. Friedman S, Löst C, Zarrabian M, Trope M (1995) Evaluation of success and failure after endodontic therapy using a glass ionomer cement sealer. *Journal of Endodontics* **21**, 384–390.

49. Galvan DA, Ciarlone AE, Pashley DH, Kulild JC, Primack PD, Simpson MD (1994) Effect of smear layer removal on the diffusion permeability of human roots. *Journal of Endodontics* **20**, 83–86.

50. Gatot A, Peist M, Mozes M (1989) Endodontic overextension produced by injected thermoplasticized gutta-percha. *Journal of Endodontics* **15**, 273–274.

51. George JM, Scott DS (1982) The effects of psychological factors on recovery from surgery. *Journal of the American Dental Association* **105**, 251–258.

52. George JW, Michanowicz AE, Michanowicz JP (1987) A method of canal preparation to control apical extrusion of low-temperature thermoplasticized gutta-percha. *Journal of Endodontics* **13**, 18–23.

53. Gilhooly RMP, Hayes SJ, Bryant ST, Dummer PMH (2000) Comparison of cold lateral condensation and a warm multiphase gutta-percha technique for obturating curved root canals. *International Endodontic Journal* **33**, 415–420.

54. Gilhooly RMP, Hayes SJ, Bryant ST, Dummer PMH (2001) Comparison of lateral condensation and thermomechanically compacted warm alpha-phase gutta-percha with a single cone for obturating curved root canals. *Oral Surgery, Oral Medicine, Oral Pathology, Oral Radiology, Endodontics* **91**, 89–94.

55. Glickman GN, Gutmann JL (1992) Contemporary perspectives on canal obturation. *Dental Clinics of North America* **36**, 327–341.

56. Grahnen H, Hansson L (1961) The prognosis of pulp and root canal therapy. A clinical and radiographic follow-up examination. *Odontologisk Revy* **12**, 146–165.

57. Grossman LI (1940) *Root Canal Therapy*. Philadelphia, PA, USA: Lea and Febiger.

58. Grossman LI (1958) An improved root canal cement. *Journal of the American Dental Association* **56**, 381–385.

59. Grossman LI, Oliet S, del Rio CE (1988) *Endodontic Practice*. 11th edn. Philadelphia, PA, USA: Lea and Febiger, pp. 242–270.

60. Gutmann JL (1993) Adaptation of injected thermoplasticized gutta-percha in the absence of the dentinal smear layer. *International Endodontic Journal* **26**, 87–92.

61. Gutmann JL, Rakusin H (1987) Perspectives on root canal obturation with thermoplasticized injectable gutta-percha. *International Endodontic Journal* **20**, 261–270.

62. Gutmann JL, Saunders WP, Saunders EM, Nguyen L (1993) An assessment of the plastic Thermafil obturation technique. Part 1. Radiographic evaluation of adaptation and placement. *International Endodontic Journal* **26**, 173–178.

63. Gutmann JL, Saunders WP, Saunders EM, Nguyen L (1993) An assessment of the plastic Thermafil obturation technique. Part 2. Material adaptation and sealability. *International Endodontic Journal* **26**, 179–183.

64. Haddix JE, Oguntebi BR (1989) Endodontic obturation with gutta-percha: an update. *Florida Dental Journal* **60**, 18–26.

65. Haddix JE, Jarrell M, Mattison GD, Pink FE (1991) An in vitro investigation of the apical seal produced by a new thermoplasticized gutta-percha obturation technique. *Quintessence International* **22**, 159–163.

66. Haga CS (1968) Microscopic measurements of root canal preparations following instrumentation. *Journal of the British Endodontic Society* **2**, 41–46.

67. Hamburg L (1992) Current developments in the filling of root canals. *Ontario Dentist* **69**, 13–15.

68. Hand RE, Huget EF, Tsaknis PJ (1976) Effects of a warm gutta-percha technique on the lateral periodontium. *Oral Surgery, Oral Medicine, Oral Pathology* **42**, 395–401.

69. Harrison JW, Baumgartner JC, Svec TA (1983) Incidence of pain associated with clinical factors during and after root canal therapy. Part 2. Postobturation pain. *Journal of Endodontics* **9**, 434–438.

70. Hartmann F (1981) Clinical applications of corticoids. *International Dental Journal* **31**, 273–285.

71. Harty FJ, Sondoozi AE (1972) The status of standardised endodontic instruments. *Journal of the British Endodontic Society* **6**, 57–62.

72. Harty FJ, Stock CJR (1974) The giromatic system compared with hand instrumentation in endodontics. *British Dental Journal* **137**, 239–244.

73. Hata G, Kawazoe S, Toda T, Weine FS (1995) Sealing ability of thermoplasticized gutta-percha fill techniques as assessed by a new method of determining apical leakage. *Journal of Endodontics* **21**, 167–172.

74. Hensten-Pettersen A, Ørstavik D, Wennberg A (1985) Allergenic potential of root canal sealers. *Endodontics and Dental Traumatology* **1**, 61–65.

75. Herschowitz SB, Marlin J, Stiglitz MR (1981) US Patent No. 831714.

76. Holland R, de Souza V, Nery MJ, de Mello W, Bernabé PFE, Otoboni Filho JA (1980) Tissue reactions following apical plugging of the root canal with infected dentin chips. *Oral Surgery, Oral Medicine, Oral Pathology* **49**, 366–369.

77. Horning TG, Kessler JR (1995) A comparison of three different root canal sealers when used to obturate a moisture-contaminated root canal system. *Journal of Endodontics* **21**, 354–357.

78. Hørsted P, Søholm B (1976) Overfølsomhed over for rodfyldnings materialet AH26. *Tandlaegebladet* **80**, 194–197.

79. Hovland EJ, Dumsha TC (1985) Leakage evaluation in vitro of the root canal sealer cement Sealapex. *International Endodontic Journal* **18**, 179–182.

80. Ingle JI (1961) A standardized endodontic technique utilizing newly designed instruments and filling materials. *Oral Surgery, Oral Medicine, Oral Pathology* **14**, 83–91.

81. Jacobsen EL, Bery PF, BeGole EA (1985) The effectiveness of apical dentine plugs in sealing endodontically treated teeth. *Journal of Endodontics* **11**, 289–293.

82. Jacobsen EL, BeGole EA, Vitkus DD, Daniel JC (1987) An evaluation of two newly formulated calcium hydroxide cements: a leakage study. *Journal of Endodontics* **13**, 164–169.

83. Johnson WB (1978) A new gutta-percha filling technique. *Journal of Endodontics* **4**, 184–188.

84. Jonck LM, Grobbelaar CJ, Strating H (1989) Biological evaluation of glass-ionomer cement (Ketac-O) as an interface material in total joint replacement. A screening test. *Clinical Materials* **4**, 201–224.

85. Juhlin JJ, Walton RE, Dovgan JS (1993) Adaptation of Thermafil components to canal walls. *Journal of Endodontics* **19**, 130–135.

86. Jungmann CL, Uchin RA, Bucher JF (1975) Effect of instrumentation on the shape of the root canal. *Journal of Endodontics* **1**, 66–68.

87. Kapsimalis P, Evans R (1966) Sealing properties of endodontic filling materials using radioactive polar and nonpolar isotopes. *Oral Surgery, Oral Medicine, Oral Pathology* **22**, 386–393.

88. Kawahara H, Imanishi Y, Oshima H (1979) Biological evaluation of glass ionomer cement. *Journal of Dental Research* **58**, 1080–1086.

89. Keane KM, Harrington GW (1984) The use of chloroform-softened gutta-percha master cone and its effect on the apical seal. *Journal of Endodontics* **10**, 57–63.

90. Kerekes K (1979) Evaluation of standardized root canal instruments and obturating points. *Journal of Endodontics* **5**, 145–150.

91. Kerekes K, Tronstad L (1979) Long-term results of endodontic treatment performed with a standardized technique. *Journal of Endodontics* **5**, 83–90.

92. Khayat A, Lee SJ, Torabinejad M (1993) Human saliva penetration of coronally unsealed obturated root canals. *Journal of Endodontics* **19**, 458–461.

93. Kirkevang L-L, Ørstavik D, Hörsted-Bindslev P, Wenzel A (2000) Periapical status and quality of root fillings and coronal restorations in a Danish population. *International Endodontic Journal* **33**, 509–515.

94. LaCombe JS, Campbell AD, Hicks ML, Pelleu GB (1988) A comparison of the apical seal produced by two thermoplasticized injectable gutta-percha techniques. *Journal of Endodontics* **14**, 445–450.

95. Langeland K (1974) Root canal sealants and pastes. *Dental Clinics of North America* **18**, 309–327.

96. Larder TC, Prescott AJ, Brayton SM (1976) Gutta-percha: a comparative study of three methods of obturation. *Journal of Endodontics* **2**, 289–294.

97. Lares C, ElDeeb ME (1990) The sealing ability of the Thermafil obturation technique. *Journal of Endodontics* **16**, 474–479.

98. Leung SF, Gulabivala K (1994) An in vitro evaluation of the influence of canal curvature on the sealing ability of Thermafil. *International Endodontic Journal* **27**, 190–196.

99. Limkangwalmongkol S, Abbott PV, Sandler AB (1992) Apical dye penetration with four root canal sealers and gutta-percha using longitudinal sectioning. *Journal of Endodontics* **18**, 535–539.

100. Longwill DG, Marshall FJ, Creamer RH (1982) Reactivity of human lymphocytes to pulp antigens. *Journal of Endodontics* **8**, 27–32.

101. Lussi A, Nussbächer U, Grosrey J (1993) A novel noninstrumented technique for cleansing the root canal system. *Journal of Endodontics* **19**, 549–553.

102. Lussi A, Messerli L, Hotz P, Grosrey J (1995) A new non-instrumental technique for cleaning and filling root canals. *International Endodontic Journal* **28**, 1–6.

103. Lussi A, Imwinkelried S, Hotz P, Grosrey J (2000) Long-term obturation quality using noninstrumentation technology. *Journal of Endodontics* **26**, 491–493.

104. Lussi A, Portmann P, Nussbächer U, Imwinkelried S, Grosrey J (1999) Comparison of two devices for root canal cleansing by the noninstrumentation technology. *Journal of Endodontics* **25**, 9–13.

105. Lussi A, Suter B, Fritzsche A, Gygax M, Portmann P (2002) In vivo performance of the new non-instrumentation technology (NIT) for root canal obturation. *International Endodontic Journal* **35**, 352–358.

106. Mader CL, Baumgartner JC, Peters DD (1984) Scanning electron microscopic investigation of the smeared layer on root canal walls. *Journal of Endodontics* **10**, 477–483.

107. Madison S, Zakariasen KL (1984) Linear and volumetric analysis of apical leakage in teeth prepared for posts. *Journal of Endodontics* **10**, 422–427.

108. Mann SR, McWalter GM (1987) Evaluation of apical seal and placement control in straight and curved canals obturated by laterally condensed and thermoplasticised gutta-percha. *Journal of Endodontics* **13**, 10–17.

109. Marlin J (1986) Injectable standard gutta-percha as a method of filling the root canal system. *Journal of Endodontics* **12**, 354–358.

110. Marlin J, Schilder H (1973) Physical properties of gutta-percha when subjected to heat and vertical condensation. *Oral Surgery, Oral Medicine, Oral Pathology* **36**, 872–879.

111. Marlin J, Krakow AA, Desilets RP, Gron P (1981) Clinical use of injection-molded thermoplasticized gutta-percha for obturation of the root canal system: a preliminary report. *Journal of Endodontics* **7**, 277–281.

112. Marshall FJ, Massler M (1961) Sealing of pulpless teeth evaluated with radioisotopes. *Journal of Dental Medicine* **16**, 172–184.

113. Mayer A, Ketterl W (1958) Dauererfolge bei der Pulpitisbehandlung. *Deutsche Zahnärztliche Zeitung* **13**, 883–898.

114. McComb D, Smith D (1975) A preliminary scanning electron microscopic study of root canals after endodontic procedures. *Journal of Endodontics* **1**, 238–242.

115. McMurtrey LG, Krell KV, Wilcox LR (1992) A comparison between Thermafil and lateral condensation in highly curved canals. *Journal of Endodontics* **18**, 68–71.

116. McSpadden J (1980) *Self-study course for the thermatic condensation of gutta-percha.* York, PA, USA: Dentsply.

117. Messer HH, Chen RS (1984) The duration of effectiveness of root canal medicaments. *Journal of Endodontics* **10**, 240–245.

118. Michelich VJ, Shuster GS, Pashley DH (1980) Bacterial penetration of human dentin in vitro. *Journal of Dental Research* **59**, 1398–1403.

119. Oguntebi BR, Shen C (1992) Effect of different sealers on thermoplasticized gutta-percha root canal obturations. *Journal of Endodontics* **18**, 363–366.

120. Oliet S (1983) Single-visit endodontics: a clinical study. *Journal of Endodontics* **9**, 147–152.

121. Olson AK, Hartwell GR, Weller RN (1989) Evaluation of the controlled placement of injected thermoplasticized gutta-percha. *Journal of Endodontics* **15**, 306–309.

122. Olsson B, Sliwkowski A, Langeland K (1981) Subcutaneous implantation for the biological evaluation of endodontic materials. *Journal of Endodontics* **7**, 355–367.

123. Ørstavik D (1983) Weight loss of endodontic sealers, cements and pastes in water. *Scandinavian Journal of Dental Research* **91**, 316–319.

124. Ørstavik D, Hongslo JK (1985) Mutagenicity of endodontic sealers. *Biomaterials* **6**, 129–132.

125. Ørstavik D, Mjör IA (1988) Histopathology and X-ray microanalysis of the subcutaneous tissue response to endodontic sealers. *Journal of Endodontics* **14**, 13–23.

126. Ørstavik D, Brodin P, Aas E (1983) Paraesthesia following endodontic treatment: survey of the literature and report of a case. *International Endodontic Journal* **16**, 167–172.

127. Oswald RJ, Friedman CE (1980) Periapical response to dentin fillings. *Oral Surgery, Oral Medicine, Oral Pathology* **49**, 344–355.

128. Pashley DH (1984) Smear layer: physiological considerations. *Operative Dentistry* **Supplement 3**, 13–29.

129. Peters LB, Wesselink PR, Moorer WR (1995) The fate and the role of bacteria left in root canal tubules. *International Endodontic Journal* **28**, 95–99.

130. Petersson K, Hasselgren G, Petersson A, Tronstad L (1982) Clinical experience with the use of dentine chips in pulpectomies. *International Endodontic Journal* **15**, 161–167.

131. Pitt Ford TR (1979) The leakage of root fillings using glass ionomer cement and other materials. *British Dental Journal* **146**, 273–278.

132. Pitts DL, Jones JE, Oswald RJ (1984) A histological comparison of calcium hydroxide plugs and dentin plugs used for the control of gutta-percha root canal filling material. *Journal of Endodontics* **10**, 283–293.

133. Portmann P, Lussi A (1994) A comparison between a new vacuum obturation technique and lateral condensation: an in vitro study. *Journal of Endodontics* **20**, 292–295.

134. Qualtrough AJ, Whitworth JM, Dummer PMH (1999) Preclinical endodontology: an international comparison. *International Endodontic Journal* **32**, 406–414.

135. Ravanshad S, Torabinejad M (1992) Coronal dye penetration of the apical filling materials after post space preparation. *Oral Surgery, Oral Medicine, Oral Pathology* **74**, 644–647.

136. Ray H, Seltzer S (1991) A new glass ionomer root canal sealer. *Journal of Endodontics* **17**, 598–603.

137. Ray HA, Trope M (1995) Periapical status of endodontically treated teeth in relation to the technical quality of the root filling and the coronal restoration. *International Endodontic Journal* **28**, 12–18.

138. Ricci ER, Kessler JR (1994) Apical seal of teeth obturated by the laterally condensed gutta-percha, the Thermafil plastic and Thermafil metal obturator techniques after post space preparation. *Journal of Endodontics* **20**, 123–126.

139. Richie GM, Anderson DM, Sakumura JS (1988) Apical extrusion of thermoplasticized gutta-percha used as a root canal filling. *Journal of Endodontics* **14**, 128–132.

140. Rickert UG, Dixon CM (1931) The controlling of root surgery. *Proceedings of Eighth International Dental Congress,* Paris, France. **IIIa**, 15–22.

141. Ruddle CJ (1994) Three dimensional obturation: the rationale and application of warm gutta-percha with vertical condensation. In: Cohen S, Burns RC (eds) *Pathways of the Pulp,* 6th edn. St Louis, MO, USA: Mosby-Year Book, pp. 243–247.

142. Rybicki R, Zillich R (1994) Apical sealing ability of Thermafil following immediate and delayed post space preparations. *Journal of Endodontics* **20**, 64–66.

143. Sargenti A, Richter SL (1965) *Rationalized Root Canal Treatment.* New York, NY, USA: AGSA.

144. Saunders WP, Saunders EM (1990) Assessment of leakage in the restored pulp chamber of endodontically treated multirooted teeth. *International Endodontic Journal* **23**, 28–33.

145. Saunders WP, Saunders EM (1992) The effect of smear layer upon the coronal leakage of gutta-percha root fillings and a glass ionomer sealer. *International Endodontic Journal* **25**, 245–249.

146. Saunders WP, Saunders EM (1994) Coronal leakage as a cause of failure in root canal therapy: a review. *Endodontics and Dental Traumatology* **10**, 105–108.

147. Saunders WP, Saunders EM (1994) Influence of smear layer on the coronal leakage of Thermafil and laterally condensed gutta-percha root fillings with a glass ionomer sealer. *Journal of Endodontics* **20**, 155–158.

148. Saunders WP, Saunders EM, Herd D, Stephens E (1992) The use of glass ionomer as a root canal sealer – a pilot study. *International Endodontic Journal* **25**, 238–244.

149. Saunders WP, Saunder EM, Gutmann JL, Gutmann ML (1993) An assessment of the plastic Thermafil obturation technique. Part 3. The effect of post space preparation on the apical seal. *International Endodontic Journal* **26**, 184–189.

150. Schilder H (1967) Filling root canals in three dimensions. *Dental Clinics of North America* **11**, 723–744.

151. Schneider SW (1971) A comparison of canal preparations in straight and curved root canals. *Oral Surgery, Oral Medicine, Oral Pathology* **32**, 271–275.

152. Schroeder A (1954) Mitteilungen über die Abschlussdichtigkeit von Wurzelfüllmaterialen und erster Hinweis auf ein neuartiges Wurzelfüllmittel. *Schweizer Monatschrift Zahnärztliche* **64**, 921–931.

153. Schweikl H, Schmalz G, Stimmelmayr H, Bey B (1995) Mutagenicity of AH26 in an in vitro mammalian cell mutation assay. *Journal of Endodontics* **21**, 407–410.

154. Scott AC, Vire DE (1992) An evaluation of the ability of a dentin plug to control extrusion of thermoplasticized gutta-percha. *Journal of Endodontics* **18**, 52–57.

155. Seltzer S, Soltanoff W, Smith J (1973) Biologic aspects of endodontics. V. Periapical tissue reactions to root canal instrumentation beyond the apex and root canal fillings short of and beyond the apex. *Oral Surgery, Oral Medicine, Oral Pathology* **36**, 725–737.

156. Sen BH, Wesselink PR, Türkün M (1995) The smear layer: a phenomenon in root canal therapy. *International Endodontic Journal* **28**, 141–148.

157. Shabahang S, Torabinejad M, Boyne P, Abedi H, McMillan P (1999) A comparative study of root-end induction using osteogenic protein-1, calcium hydroxide, and mineral trioxide aggregate in dogs. *Journal of Endodontics* **25**, 1–5.

158. Sjögren U, Figdor D, Persson S, Sundqvist G (1997) Influence of infection at the time of root filling on the outcome of endodontic treatment of teeth with apical periodontitis. *International Endodontic Journal* **30**, 297–306.

159. Skinner RL, Himel VT (1987) The sealing ability of injection-molded thermoplasticized gutta-percha with and without the use of sealers. *Journal of Endodontics* **13**, 315–317.

160. Smith JJ, Montgomery S (1992) A comparison of apical seal: chloroform versus halothane-dipped gutta-percha cones. *Journal of Endodontics* **18**, 156–160.

161. Smith MA, Steiman, HR (1994) An in vitro evaluation of microleakage of two new and two old root canal sealers. *Journal of Endodontics* **20**, 18–21.

162. Sobarzo-Navarro V (1991) Clinical experience in root canal obturation by an injection thermoplasticized gutta-percha technique. *Journal of Endodontics* **17**, 389–391.

163. Soltanoff W (1978) A comparative study of the single-visit and multiple-visit endodontic procedure. *Journal of Endodontics* **4**, 278–281.

164. Spångberg LSW, Langeland K (1973) Biologic effects of dental materials. 1. Toxicity of root canal filling materials on Hela cells in vitro. *Oral Surgery, Oral Medicine, Oral Pathology* **35**, 402–414.

165. Spångberg LSW, Barbosa SV, Lavigne GD (1993) AH26 releases formaldehyde. *Journal of Endodontics* **19**, 596–598.

166. Spector RG (1981) Pharmacological properties of the glucocorticoids. *International Dental Journal* **31**, 152–155.

167. Strindberg LZ (1956) The dependence of the results of pulp therapy on certain factors. An analytic study based on radiographic and clinical follow-up examinations. *Acta Odontologica Scandinavica* **14**, Supplement 21, 1–175.

168. Tagger M, Tamse A, Katz A, Korzen BH (1984) Evaluation of apical seal produced by a hybrid root canal filling method combining lateral condensation and thermatic compaction. *Journal of Endodontics* **10**, 299–303.

169. Tidswell HE, Saunders EM, Saunders WP (1994) Assessment of coronal leakage in teeth root filled with gutta-percha and a glass ionomer root canal sealer. *International Endodontic Journal* **27**, 208–212.

170. Tittle K, Farley J, Linkhardt T, Torabinejad M (1996) Apical closure induction using bone growth factors and mineral trioxide aggregate. *Journal of Endodontics* **22**, 198.

171. Torabinejad M, Chivian N (1999) Clinical applications of mineral trioxide aggregate. *Journal of Endodontics* **25**, 197–205.

172. Torabinejad M, Hong CU, McDonald F, Pitt Ford TR (1995) Physical and chemical properties of a new root end filling material. *Journal of Endodontics* **21**, 349–353.

173. Torabinejad M, Skobe Z, Trombly PL, Krakow AA, Grøn P, Marlin J (1978) Scanning electron microscopic study of root canal obturation using thermoplasticized gutta-percha. *Journal of Endodontics* **4**, 245–250.

174. Torneck CD, Smith JS, Grindall P (1973) Biologic effects of procedures on developing incisor teeth. II. Effect of pulp injury and oral contamination. *Oral Surgery, Oral Medicine, Oral Pathology* **35**, 378–388.

175. Tronstad L (1978) Tissue reactions following apical plugging of the root canal with dentin chips in monkey teeth subject to pulpectomy. *Oral Surgery, Oral Medicine, Oral Pathology* **45**, 297–304.

176. Tronstad L, Barnett F, Flax M (1988) Solubility and biocompatibility of calcium hydroxide-containing root canal sealers. *Endodontics and Dental Traumatology* **4**, 152–159.

177. Tronstad L, Asbjørnsen K, Døving L, Pedersen I, Eriksen HM (2000) Influence of coronal restorations on the periapical health of endodontically treated teeth. *Endodontics and Dental Traumatology* **16**, 218–221.

178. Trope M, Delano EO, Ørstavik D (1999) Endodontic treatment of teeth with apical periodontitis: single visit vs. multivisit treatment. *Journal of Endodontics* **25**, 345–350.

179. Van der Burgt TP, Eronat C, Plasschaert AJM (1986) Staining patterns in teeth discolored by endodontic sealers. *Journal of Endodontics* **12**, 187–191.

180. Veis A, Beltes P, Liolios E (1989) Sealing ability of thermoplasticized gutta-percha in root canal obturation using a sectional vs a single-phase technique. *Endodontics and Dental Traumatology* **5**, 87–91.

181. Veis A, Lambrianidis T, Molyvdas I, Zervas P (1992) Sealing ability of sectional injection thermoplasticized gutta-percha technique with varying distances between needle tip and apical foramen. *Endodontics and Dental Traumatology* **8**, 63–66.

182. Walls AWG (1986) Glass polyalkenoate (glass-ionomer) cements: a review. *Journal of Dentistry* **14**, 231–246.

183. Weiger R, Axmann-Krcmar D, Löst C (1998) Prognosis of conventional root canal treatment reconsidered. *Endodontics and Dental Traumatology* **14**, 1–9.

184. Weiger R, Rosendahl R, Löst C (2000) Influence of calcium hydroxide intracanal dressings on the prognosis of teeth with endodontically induced periapical lesions. *International Endodontic Journal* **33**, 219–226.

185. Wilcox LR (1993) Thermafil retreatment with and without chloroform solvent. *Journal of Endodontics* **19**, 563–566.

186. Wilcox LR, Juhlin JJ (1994) Endodontic retreatment of Thermafil versus laterally condensed gutta-percha. *Journal of Endodontics* **20**, 115–117.

187. Wilson AD, Kent BE (1971) The glass-ionomer cement: a new translucent dental filling material. *Journal of Applied Chemistry and Biotechnology* **21**, 313–318.

188. Wilson AD, Clinton DJ, Miller RP (1973) Zinc oxide–eugenol cements: IV. Microstructure and hydrolysis. *Journal of Dental Research* **52**, 253–260.

189. Wong M, Peters DD, Lorton L (1981) Comparison of gutta-percha filling techniques, compaction (mechanical), vertical (warm), and lateral condensation techniques, part 1. *Journal of Endodontics* **7**, 551–558.

190. Wong M, Peters DD, Lorton L, Bernier WE (1982) Comparison of gutta-percha filling techniques: three chloroform-gutta-percha filling techniques, part 2. *Journal of Endodontics* **8**, 4–9.

191. Woolverton CJ, Fotos PG, Mokas J, Mermigas ME (1986) Evaluation of eugenol for mutagenicity by the mouse micronucleus test. *Journal of Oral Pathology* **15**, 450–453.

192. Wu MK, Wesselink PR (2001) A primary observation on the preparation and obturation of oval canals. *International Endodontic Journal* **34**, 137–141.

193. Wu MK, Wesselink PR, Walton RE (2000) Apical terminus location of root canal treatment procedures. *Oral Surgery, Oral Medicine, Oral Pathology, Oral Radiology, Endodontics* **89**, 99–103.

194. Wu MK, Kast'áková A, Wesselink PR (2001) Quality of cold and warm gutta-percha fillings in oval canals in mandibular premolars. *International Endodontic Journal* **34**, 485–491.

195. Yared GM, Bou Dagher FE (1993) Elongation and movement of the gutta-percha master cone during initial lateral condensation. *Journal of Endodontics* **19**, 395–397.

196. Yared GM, Bou Dagher FE (1994) Apical enlargement: influence on the sealing ability of the vertical compaction technique. *Journal of Endodontics* **20**, 313–314.

197. Yared GM, Bou Dagher FE (1994) Apical enlargement: influence on overextensions during in vitro vertical compaction. *Journal of Endodontics* **20**, 269–271.

198. Yee FS, Marlin J, Krakow AA, Gron P (1977) Three-dimensional obturation of the root canal using injection-molded, thermoplasticized dental gutta-percha. *Journal of Endodontics* **3**, 168–174.

199. Yee RDJ, Newton CW, Patterson SS, Swartz ML (1984) The effect of canal preparation on the formation and leakage characteristics of the apical dentin plug. *Journal of Endodontics* **10**, 308–317.

200. Yesiloy C, Koren LZ, Morse DR, Rankow H, Bolanus OR, Furst ML (1988) Post-endodontic obturation pain: a comparative evaluation. *Quintessence International* **19**, 431–438.

201. Zmener O (1980) Effect of dowel preparation on the apical seal of endodontically treated teeth. *Journal of Endodontics* **6**, 687–690.

# Surgical endodontics

J. L. Gutmann and J. D. Regan

Introduction  143

Indications for periradicular surgery  143

Preoperative assessment  144

Surgical kit  145

Surgical technique  146
  Tissue anaesthesia and haemostasis  146
  Soft tissue incision and reflection  147
  Osseous entry and root identification  151
  Removal of diseased soft tissue (periradicular
    curettage)  152
  Root-end resection  153
  Root-end cavity preparation  157
  Root-end cavity filling  159
  Root-end filling materials  162
  Treatment of the root face  164
  Closure of the surgical site  164
  Postoperative radiological assessment  167
  Postoperative patient instructions  167
  Postoperative examination and review  168

Periradicular surgery of particular teeth  168
  Maxillary anterior teeth  168
  Maxillary premolars  168
  Maxillary molars  168
  Mandibular anterior teeth  169
  Mandibular premolars  169
  Mandibular molars  169
  General anatomical considerations  169

Repair of perforation  170

Replantation/transplantation  171

Regenerative procedures  172
  Clinical techniques in regenerative procedures  173

Success and failure – aetiology and evaluation  173

Retreatment of surgical procedures  174

References  175

## INTRODUCTION

A high degree of success is normally achievable with root canal treatment. Occasionally, however, surgery may be indicated to achieve what was not possible with root canal treatment or to secure a biopsy. In recent years the terminology used in endodontic surgery has been clarified [7]. Likewise, research in endodontic surgery has helped to improve clinical practice based on scientific concepts.

The most common endodontic surgical procedure (periradicular surgery) consists of periradicular curettage, root-end resection, root-end preparation and root-end filling. Other procedures include perforation repair, root and tooth resection, crown-lengthening, intentional replantation, regenerative techniques, incision and drainage, and cortical trephination. This chapter will focus primarily on the essentials of periradicular surgery.

## INDICATIONS FOR PERIRADICULAR SURGERY

Historically, most texts on endodontic surgery list multiple, 'cook-book' type indications for surgical intervention [11,72]. These often include instrument separation, apical fracture, inadequate root canal filling, and presence of a cyst. Advances in the understanding of apical periodontitis and in clinical techniques have eliminated most of these indications for surgery. Studies on the success and failure of root canal treatment versus surgical treatment have clearly shown a higher success rate with high quality root canal treatment. Unfortunately however, in a recent report most of the teeth referred by dental practitioners for surgical endodontic treatment would more appropriately have been treated non-surgically (44). Periradicular tissues usually heal following removal of infection from the root canal system, and the prevention of further contamination [94, 150]. Additionally, the main cause of failure following surgical treatment is inadequate cleaning, shaping and filling of the root canal system [145]. Therefore the routine selection of surgery without full case assessment, in particular the status of the root canal system, is unwarranted as is selection for the convenience of the clinician.

Few true indications exist for surgery. These indications must always be in the best interest of the patient and within the realm of the clinician's understanding and expertise [61]. First, if failure has resulted from root canal treatment, and retreatment is impossible or would not achieve a better result, surgery may be indicated, e.g. non-negotiable canal, perforation or ledge with signs and/or symptoms. Secondly, if there is a strong possibility of failure with root canal treatment, surgery may be indicated, e.g. calcified canal with concomitant patient signs and/or symptoms. Thirdly, if a biopsy is necessary at or near the root apex, surgery will be indicated.

Contraindications to surgery are very few and are usually limited to patient (psychological and systemic), clinician (experience and expertise), and anatomical (extremely unusual bony or root configurations and/or complete lack of surgical access). Few cases, however, will not be amenable to surgical intervention.

## PREOPERATIVE ASSESSMENT

The prognosis following surgery is dependent on careful patient assessment, evidence-based diagnosis and long-term treatment planning [16]. Contraindications involving the patient's psychological or systemic condition can be identified, as well as patient acceptance of and cooperation with the anticipated surgical procedure. Procedures to minimize stress for patients who are particularly susceptible to pain and anxiety may be required [64].

**Table 9.1** General medical conditions

| | |
|---|---|
| Hypertension | Coronary atherosclerotic disease |
| Stable angina | Myocardial infarction |
| Infective endocarditis | Chronic obstructive pulmonary disease |
| Asthma | Cerebrovascular accident |
| Epilepsy | Diabetes |
| Adrenal insufficiency | Steroid therapy |
| Organ transplant | Impaired hepatic or renal function |

General patient systemic factors, which usually require medical consultation, are listed in Table 9.1. As a general rule, no special precautions need to be taken when surgery is planned other than those that normally apply to routine dental procedures [64].

Local patient factors focus on the management of both soft and hard tissues. These factors include the possible need to remove previous dental restorations that are failing and the need to retreat the tooth as part of overall management. More favourable results have been obtained when root canal systems are retreated prior to surgical management [51,82,105,106]. The tooth must also be assessed for restorability, and its place in the overall treatment plan determined.

Radiological examination is essential, including prior radiographs if available [16]. Radiographs from different angles should be taken, identifying the number, curvature and angle of the roots requiring surgery and the position of the apices relative to adjacent structures. Anatomical structures that may impair surgical or visual access to the surgical site must be identified. These include the mental foramen, zygomatic process, anterior nasal spine and external oblique ridge. The following factors are particularly important in a radiological assessment:

- relation of the apices to the inferior dental canal, mental foramen, the maxillary sinus or adjacent roots;
- number of roots;
- approximate length of the roots; this may sometimes be ascertained from the patient's records if non-surgical treatment had been performed;
- approximate extent of any visible lesion.

Communication with the patient concerning the need for surgery, outline of the procedure, anticipated difficulties and problems, the prognosis, pre-operative medication or mouth rinses, post-operative care and long-term assessment is essential [64]. Provision of written information and instructions is beneficial and can help to allay some of the patient's fears.

The following pretreatment regimens are recommended:

- A periodontal examination must be performed prior to surgery to assess for periodontal pockets and/or sinus tracts. Scaling and/or root planing may be required. The patient's oral hygiene practices should be assessed and reinforced.
- Patients should be placed on 0.12% chlorhexidine rinses in an attempt to reduce the oral microorganisms. These rinses should be performed one day prior to surgery, immediately before surgery and should continue for at least 2–3 days afterwards.
- Patients can begin taking non-steroidal anti-inflammatory medication one day prior to surgery, or at the latest one hour before treatment.
- Patients should be advised to refrain from smoking.
- If sedation is to be used, the patient must bring an accompanying person, who will be responsible for escorting the patient home and for compliance with postoperative instructions.

## SURGICAL KIT

A plethora of instruments are available for endodontic surgical procedures. Particular instruments should be chosen that facilitate the procedure according to the individual operator's requirements. Instruments must be sterile, sharp, undamaged and enable the surgeon to maintain total control of the surgical site. A basic kit should contain the most commonly used instruments and should be readily supplemented with any other instrument considered necessary. Key instruments and their general use are listed in Table 9.2 and illustrated in Figure 9.1.

Instruments that have been designed in recent years for use in endodontic surgical procedures

**Table 9.2** Surgical kit

*Presurgical assessment*
Mirror and curved explorer
Straight and curved periodontal probes

*Soft tissue incision, elevation & reflection*
Sharp scalpels – numbers 15, 15c, 11, and 12
Micro scalpels
Broad-based periosteal elevator
Broad-based periosteal retractor
Tissue forceps
Surgical aspirator
Irrigating syringes and needles

*Periradicular curettage*
Straight and angled bone curettes
Small endodontic spoon curette
Periodontal curettes
Fine, curved mosquito forceps
Small, curved surgical scissors

*Bone removal and root-end resection*
Surgical length round and tapered fissure burs
Straight and angled bone curettes
Rear-venting high speed handpiece
Contra-angled slow speed handpiece

*Root-end preparation/placement of root-end filling/finish of resected root end*
Ultrasonic or sonic unit with appropriate root-end preparation tips
Root-end filling material
Haemostatic agent (avoid bone wax)
Miniature material carriers and condensers
Small ball burnisher
Paper points or fine aspirator tip
Small, fine explorer

*Suturing and soft tissue closure*
Surgical scissors
Haemostat or fine needle holders
Various suture types and sizes (3-0 to 6-0)
Sterile gauze for soft tissue compression

*Miscellaneous (or readily available)*
Adequate aspiration equipment
Additional light source – magnification
Root canal filling materials
Anaesthetic syringes and anaesthetic

include miniature surgical blades and mirrors, rear-venting surgical handpieces, ultrasonically energized root-end preparation tips and root-end pluggers. Visual aids such as loupes and the operating microscope provide the operator with excellent lighting and magnification, and facilitate the surgical procedures.

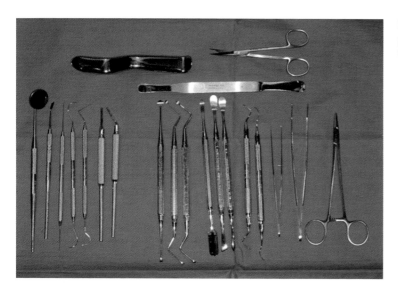

**Figure 9.1** Basic instruments for periradicular surgery (see Table 9.2 for details).

## SURGICAL TECHNIQUE

### Tissue anaesthesia and haemostasis

The ability to achieve profound anaesthesia and tissue haemostasis in the surgical site is essential to successful surgery. Profound anaesthesia will minimize or eliminate patient discomfort during the procedure and for a significant period thereafter, whilst good haemostasis will improve vision in the surgical site, improve root-end cavity preparation and filling, minimize surgical time, and reduce surgical blood loss, postsurgical haemorrhage and postsurgical swelling [64]. An anaesthetic solution containing a vasoconstrictor is indicated to achieve these objectives [73].

The choice of the anaesthetic-vasoconstrictor combination is dependent on the health status of the patient and surgical needs. Lidocaine (lignocaine) with adrenaline (epinephrine) has long been recognized as an excellent anaesthetic agent for periradicular surgery because of its clinical success in producing profound and prolonged analgesia [36,96]. Although several studies support the efficacy of 2% lidocaine with 1:200 000 to 1:100 000 concentrations of adrenaline for profound anaesthesia [55,80,85], clinical evidence suggests that a 1:50 000 concentration provides better haemostasis [25,36].

Assessment of the patient's systemic status is essential prior to the use of 2% lidocaine with 1:50 000 adrenaline. This is important because lidocaine with adrenaline can elevate systemic plasma levels of the vasoconstrictor [173], although the haemodynamic response to this increase is still controversial [68,86]. This potential rise in adrenaline concentration suggests that high-risk patients should be carefully monitored. Great care should be taken during injection to prevent intravascular placement of the solution [73]. When an anaesthetic with 1:50 000 adrenaline is unavailable, 1:80 000 is clinically acceptable. While 2% lidocaine with 1:100 000 is recommended for regional nerve blocks prior to endodontic surgery, this level of vasoconstrictor does not suffice for local haemostasis at the surgical site. Haemostasis must also be established at the surgical site [18] by additional injections supraperiosteally using 2% lidocaine with 1:50 000 [62]. In healthy patients a dose of 2–4 ml is recommended. In the maxilla achievement of both anaesthesia and haemostasis can be accomplished simultaneously. This requires multiple injections, depositing the solution throughout the entire submucosa superficial to the periosteum at the level of the root apices in the surgical site. The needle, with the bevel toward the bone, is advanced to the target site and, following aspiration, 0.5 ml of solution is deposited slowly (Fig. 9.2). The needle may be moved peripherally and similar small amounts of solution deposited. Additional injections can be made to ensure that the entire surgical field has been covered. Slow, peripheral supraperiosteal

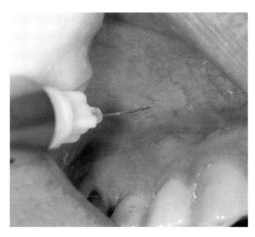

**Figure 9.2** Placement of anaesthetic solution around the root apex of the tooth to be treated surgically.

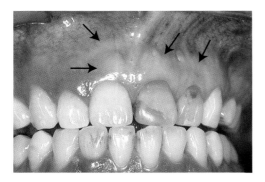

**Figure 9.3** Slow and careful infiltration of the anaesthetic solution provides widespread and effective tissue haemostasis (delineated by arrows) for treatment of left maxillary central incisor.

infiltration into the submucosa promotes maximum diffusion (Fig. 9.3). In the mandible the anaesthetic–vasoconstrictor solution is injected slowly adjacent to the root apices, in addition to the block injection of the inferior alveolar nerve. Incisions that are made in alignment with the long axis of the supporting supraperiosteal vasculature, and tissues that are carefully elevated and reflected, will minimize haemorrhage at the surgical site [64].

The amount of anaesthetic solution containing 1:50 000 adrenaline that is necessary to achieve anaesthesia and haemostasis is dependent on the surgical site, but 2.0 to 3.0 ml will generally suffice. The rate of injection can also influence the degree of haemostasis and anaesthesia obtained, with a rate of 1 to 2 ml/min recommended [141]. Injecting at

higher rates results in the localized pooling of solution, delayed and limited diffusion into the adjacent tissues, and less than optimal anaesthesia and haemostasis. Predictable anaesthesia and haemostasis is most likely to be achieved prior to any incisions. Later attempts during surgery are less successful. Following administration of the local anaesthetic sufficient time must elapse prior to the initial incision (5–10 min), to allow for proper vascular constriction throughout the surgical site.

## Soft tissue incision and reflection

Good surgical access requires the incision and elevation of the soft tissue from the underlying bone. The design of this tissue flap is crucial not only to surgical entry and management of the root structure, but also to healing of the surgical wound. The design of soft tissue flaps has received wide and varied attention. For years the semilunar flap (Partsch incision) in the apical loose alveolar mucosa was recommended but this has now been largely superseded. Various flap designs have been advocated based on a biological approach to tissue management and wound healing. Table 9.3 outlines the range of contemporary surgical flap designs [64]. There are strong biological reasons to consider the use of full mucoperiosteal tissue flaps whenever possible (Table 9.3). Figures 9.4–9.9 detail diagram-

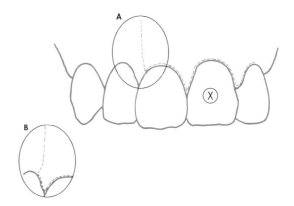

**Figure 9.4** Triangular tissue flap design with single vertical releasing incision. The vertical releasing incision can be performed in different ways. Either (**A**) the incision leaves the interdental papilla intact or (**B**; insert) the incision includes the interdental papilla. In either case the incision line should meet the tooth at 90°.

147

**Table 9.3** Periradicular surgical soft-tissue flap designs

| Type of flap | Advantages/disadvantages |
|---|---|
| *Full mucoperiosteal tissue flaps* | |
| Triangular | Maintains intact vertical blood supply |
| Rectangular | Minimizes haemorrhage |
| Trapezoidal | Primary wound closure and rapid healing |
| Horizontal (envelope) | Allows survey of bone and root structure |
| | Excellent surgical orientation |
| | Minimal postoperative sequelae |
| | May have loss of tissue attachment |
| | May have loss of crestal bone height |
| | Possibility of tissue flap dislodgement |
| | Possible loss of interdental papilla integrity |
| *Limited mucoperiosteal flaps* | |
| Submarginal curved (semilunar) | Marginal and interdental papilla intact |
| Submarginal rectangular (Luebke–Ochsenbein) | Unaltered soft tissue attachment |
| | Adequate surgical access – may be compromised in posterior cases or cases with lateral defects |
| | Good healing potential |
| | Disruption of blood supply |
| | Possibility of tissue shrinkage |
| | Delayed secondary healing/scarring |
| | Limited orientation to apical region |
| | Very limited in posterior surgery |
| Papilla-base incision | Unproven technique |
| | May interrupt blood supply leading to delayed healing |
| | Difficult to perform |
| | Good healing potential |

matically each design whilst the subsequent text gives a brief description of their application.

## Full mucoperiosteal tissue flap

The horizontal incision begins in the gingival sulcus, extending through the gingival fibres to the crestal bone. The scalpel blade is held in a near

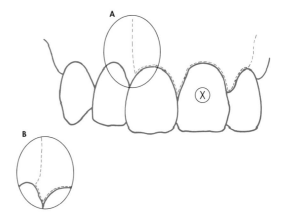

**Figure 9.5** Rectangular tissue flap design with double vertical releasing incisions. As with the triangular flap design, variations can be used with the vertical incisions (**A** and **B**); a description has been included in Figure 9.4.

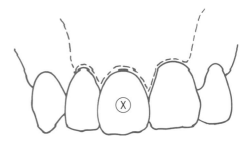

**Figure 9.6** Trapezoidal tissue flap design. Note vertical releasing incisions are angled towards the base of the flap.

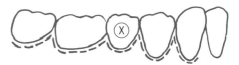

**Figure 9.7** Horizontal tissue flap design. No vertical releasing incisions are used initially but they can be added later to enhance surgical access if necessary.

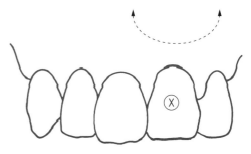

**Figure 9.8** Semilunar tissue flap design. Note that the scope of this flap limits extension if necessary.

vertical position (Fig. 9.10). In the interdental region, the incision should pass through the mid-col area, separating the buccal and lingual papillae, and severing the gingival fibres to the depth of the interdental crestal bone (Fig. 9.11). This is critical to

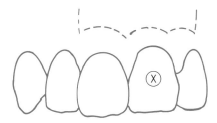

**Figure 9.9** Luebke–Ochsenbein (submarginal) tissue flap design. This flap may have one or two vertical releasing incisions, or may be limited to a horizontal incision, only if sufficient surgical and visual access can be obtained.

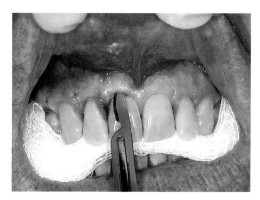

**Figure 9.10** Intrasulcular incision with a no. 15 scalpel blade. Note the vertical position of the scalpel as it cuts through and releases the crestal fibres.

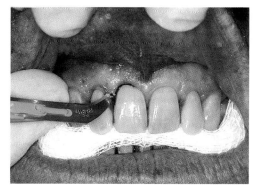

**Figure 9.11** Use of a no. 12 scalpel blade to release the fibres of the interdental papilla. Note the depth and angulation of the blade.

prevent sloughing of the papillae due to a compromised blood supply. Because of the shape of the embrasure space it may be necessary to use a curved scalpel blade or a miniature surgical blade to follow the interproximal tooth contours (Fig. 9.11).

Vertical (releasing) incisions are used in the triangular and rectangular flap designs (Figs 9.4 and 9.5), and are vertically oriented passing between the roots of adjacent teeth and coursing parallel to the long axes of the roots. The incision should be over intact bone and to the depth of the bone. Vertical incisions should terminate at the mesial or distal line angles of teeth, and never in papillae or in the mid-root area. Incisions should be positioned to ensure that at closure the re-apposed soft tissue will overlie solid bone.

The trapezoidal flap design (Fig. 9.6) incorporates angled releasing incisions and is not considered biologically acceptable for periradicular surgery because it cuts across the vertically positioned supra-periosteal vasculature and tissue-supportive collagen fibres. The horizontal or envelope flap design (Fig. 9.7) is often used for maxillary or mandibular molars, or palatal flaps. However, some type of releasing incision is generally incorporated, albeit not as long as that used with triangular or rectangular flaps.

Tissue reflection always begins in the attached gingiva of the vertical incision. The periosteal elevator is positioned to apply reflective forces in a lateral direction against the cortical bone while elevating the tougher fibrous-based tissue of the gingiva (Fig. 9.12). This also elevates the periosteum and its superficial tissues from the cortical plate. Subsequently, the elevator is directed coronally (Fig. 9.13) to elevate the marginal and interdental gingiva with minimal traumatic force (Fig. 9.14). All reflective forces should be applied to the bone and

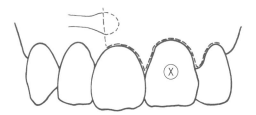

**Figure 9.12** The periosteum is initially elevated by applying force against the cortical bone in the region of the attached tissues.

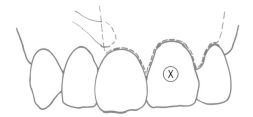

**Figure 9.13** The periosteal elevator is subsequently moved coronally to elevate the marginal tissues.

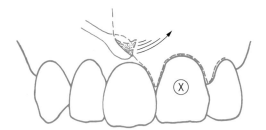

**Figure 9.14** The entire tissue flap is elevated with minimal force being directed on the marginal and interdental gingival tissues.

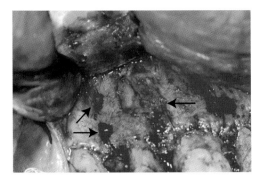

**Figure 9.15** Tissue tags remain on the cortical bone after flap elevation (arrowed).

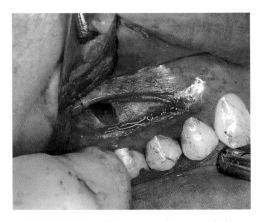

**Figure 9.16** Pinching of the mucosal tissue with the periosteal retractor should be avoided during surgery.

periosteum, with minimal forces on the gingival elements; this is referred to as undermining elevation [64]. After tissue reflection, bleeding tissue tags are often seen on the cortical surface in the crestal region and between root eminences (Fig. 9.15). Because these tissue tags play an important role in healing they should not be removed during surgery.

Adequate retraction of the tissue flap is necessary for surgical access to the periradicular tissues. The retractor must always rest on sound bone with light but firm pressure. Pinching of the soft tissue flap with the retractor must be avoided to minimize tissue damage and untoward postsurgical sequelae (Fig. 9.16). If this is not possible the reflected tissue must be elevated further or the tissue flap extended to release its attachment from the bone.

### Limited mucoperiosteal tissue flap

These tissue flaps do not include the marginal and interdental gingiva. The horizontal incision of these flaps should be in the attached gingiva with the vertical incisions involving both the attached gingiva and alveolar mucosa. An absolute minimum of 2 mm of attached gingiva from the depth of the

gingival sulcus must be present before this flap design is chosen. However, there is a very narrow limit for safe incision between the sulcular depth and the mucogingival junction in most patients, especially in the mandible [2].

The rectangular submarginal flap design (Luebke–Ochsenbein flap) is formed by a scalloped horizontal incision in the attached gingiva and two vertical releasing incisions (Fig. 9.9). Scalloping reflects the contour of the marginal gingivae and provides an adequate distance from the depths of the gingival sulci. Here also, the vasculature and collagen fibres are severed. It may be used in maxillary anterior or posterior teeth in which reflection of marginal and interdental gingival is contraindicated because of tissue inflammation or aesthetic concerns with extensive fixed prostheses. Often, anatomical factors negate the use of a limited mucoperiosteal flap design.

## Osseous entry and root identification

Prior to root-end resection and removal of diseased soft tissue that may surround the root, bone may need to be removed to gain visual access to the surgical site. Removal is usually accomplished with a large round bur (ISO size 018 or 024), using a low- or high-speed handpiece. The bone is removed in a brush-stroke fashion [163] with copious irrigation, creating a window over the root apex. Adherence to this technique will reduce the heat produced during the osteotomy procedure thereby minimizing the potential for damage to the living bone tissue. In many cases the approach may need to be from a coronal position on the bone, moving apically once the root structure has been identified. Care should be taken not to remove cementum from the root surface to prevent later resorption. Entry as close to the apex, however, is recommended, with the angle of entry facilitating visibility and surgical access. Measuring the approximate length of the root on the bone, as estimated from the preoperative radiological assessment, facilitates location of the root apex (Fig. 9.17).

The apex may also be identified during osseous palpation after soft tissue reflection. Where the bone is thin, or the root apex is prominent, a straight bone curette can be used in a rotating motion to penetrate the cortical plate and identify the root structure (Fig. 9.18). In cases with large periradicular lesions, the loss of the cortical plate of bone may directly expose the root apex. Once exposed, the bur can be used to create a greater window to outline the root apex. In those cases where the bone is thick and location of the apex is difficult, the same type of initial osseous penetration can be made and a sterile radiopaque object placed in the small hole. A radiograph will provide additional information on the location of the root apex.

Root structure can be identified from bone by texture (smooth and hard), lack of bleeding upon

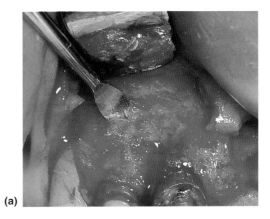

(a)

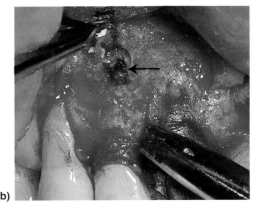

(b)

**Figure 9.18** (a) Use of a straight curette to peel away the surface cortical bone. (b) Penetration through the bone with a curette alone to expose the root (arrowed). Note bone chips on curette.

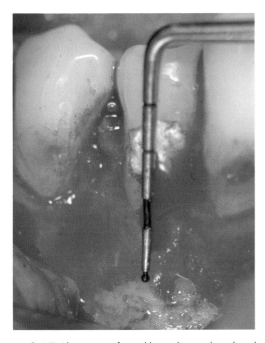

**Figure 9.17** Placement of a calibrated periodontal probe to determine the approximate position of the root apex.

probing, outline (presence of periodontal ligament, PDL), and colour (yellowish) [13]. The perimeter of the root and its periodontal ligament (PDL) may also be identified by painting 1% methylene blue on the surface [29].

## Removal of diseased soft tissue (periradicular curettage)

This procedure can often be performed prior to or in conjunction with root-end resection. The purpose is to remove the reactive tissue [157]. Failure to remove every remnant of this soft reactive tissue will not lead to failure, as the tissue elements in the periphery of these lesions usually contain fibroblasts, vascular buds, new collagen and bone matrix. In those cases in which the soft tissue mass is exposed upon flap reflection or initial bone removal, curettage can proceed prior to root-end resection. In other cases resection is necessary to gain access to most of the tissue.

Curettage is accomplished with straight or angled surgical bone curettes and periodontal curettes (Fig. 9.19). Initially the bone curettes are used to peel the soft tissue from the lateral borders of the bony crypt. This is performed with the concave surface of the curette facing the bony wall, applying pressure only against the bone (Fig. 9.20) [13,59]. It is desirable to avoid penetration of the soft tissue as this may sever the vascular network, and increase local haemorrhage. Once the tissue is freed along the lateral margins, the bone curettes can be turned and used in scraping fashion along

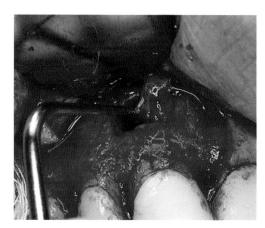

**Figure 9.20** Use of the bone curette to peel the soft-tissue lesion from the bone cavity.

the deep walls of the crypt. This will detach the soft tissue from its lingual or palatal base. Once loosened, tissue forceps are used to grasp the tissue gently as it is teased from its position with a bone curette. The tissue sample is placed directly into a bottle of neutral buffered formalin or transport medium for biopsy. In those cases that require root-end resection prior to curettage, the root structure must be sufficiently exposed to minimize shredding of the soft tissues during resection. Despite profound anaesthesia in the surgical site as a whole, it is often found that the centre of the periradicular lesion remains sensitive. This is explained by the proliferation of neural endings stimulated by inflammatory mediators [26]. Infiltration of local anaesthetic into the reactive tissue will invariably eliminate any residual sensation.

In the presence of large lesions, care must be exercised during curettage of the lateral surfaces of the bony crypt to avoid damage to adjacent roots and their pulpal vasculature. Presurgical radiographs should reveal this possibility, and tissue in these areas may need to be left in position. Caution is necessary to prevent damage to vital structures when operating close to the maxillary antrum, mental foramen, or mandibular canal. When soft tissue is adherent either lingually to the root, or in the furcation region, periodontal curettes facilitate its removal.

Periradicular curettage is normally performed in conjunction with resection of the root-end [63].

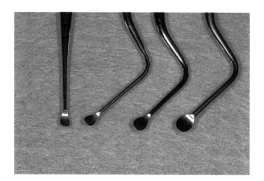

**Figure 9.19** Straight and angled bone curettes are useful to manage the wide variety of challenges encountered in bone and soft tissue removal.

## Root-end resection

The term root-end resection refers specifically to the removal of the apical portion of the root. There are many indications for resection of the root end during periradicular surgery, each designed to eliminate aetiological factors.

Historically, the technique of root-end resection involved the creation of a bevel on the root face, to improve surgical access and visibility [29,63,93,107, 144]. The angle of resection and its use were determined by the root inclination and curvature, number of roots, thickness of bone and position of the root in the bone. Current evidence indicates that reducing the angle of the bevel will reduce dentinal tubule exposure [164]. Based on the number of dentinal tubules communicating between the root canal and the resected root face, the angle of the bevel should be kept to a minimum [164]. A significant increase in leakage from the root canal system has been demonstrated as the bevel increased [56]. Ultrasonic instruments have been developed that greatly facilitate preparation along the long axis of the root and therefore eliminate the need for extensive bevelling of the root face.

The root end can be resected in one of two ways. First, after the root end has been exposed, the bur (narrow straight fissure) in a handpiece is positioned at the desired angle and the root is shaved away, beginning from the apex, cutting coronally (Fig. 9.21a). The bur is moved from mesial to distal, shaving the root smooth and flat, and exposing the entire canal system and root outline. This approach allows for continual observation of the root end during cutting. The second technique of resection is to predetermine the amount of root end to be resected. The bur and handpiece are positioned, and the apex is resected by cutting through the root from mesial to distal (Fig. 9.21). Once the apex is removed, the root face is gently shaved with the bur to smooth the surface and ensure complete resection and visibility of the root face. This technique works well when an apical biopsy is desired or to gain access to significant amounts of soft tissue located lingual to the root. It is also the technique of choice in cases where the root end is located in close proximity to structures such as the mental foramen or the inferior alveolar canal. The disadvantage however is that this approach may remove more root structure than is absolutely necessary.

The appearance of the root face following root-end resection will vary depending on the type of bur used, the external root anatomy, the anatomy of the canal system exposed at the particular angle of resection, and the nature and density of the root canal filling material. Various types of burs have been recommended for root-end resection [64]; each will leave a characteristic imprint on the root face, from rough-grooved and gouged to smooth [108]. To date, no study has determined the advantages of one type of bur over another, although for years clinical practice has favoured a smooth flat root surface [60,106,156,171].

The level to which the root end should be resected will be dictated by the following factors [64]:

- access and visibility to the surgical site;
- position and anatomy of the root within the alveolar bone;
- presence and position of additional roots, e.g. an additional palatal or lingual root;
- anatomy of the cut root surface relative to the number of canals and their configuration;
- need to place a root-end filling;
- presence and location of a perforation;
- presence of an intra-alveolar root fracture;
- anatomical considerations, e.g. proximity of adjacent teeth, mental foramen or inferior dental canal, level of remaining crestal bone;
- presence of significant accessory canals, which may dictate a more extensive resection.

Regardless of the rationale for the extent of root-end removal, there is no reason to resect the root to the base of a large periradicular lesion as was previously advised. Likewise, resection to the point where little (< 1 mm) or no crestal bone remains covering the buccal aspect of the root may very well doom the tooth to failure (Fig. 9.22). On the other hand, omitting to remove sufficient root structure to be able to inspect the resected root surface and place a root-end filling may also contribute to failure. Root canals or anastomoses may be missed, or may be improperly managed in confined spaces.

The complete root face must be identified and examined after resection. This is done with a fine sharp probe guided around the periphery of the root and the root canal. The external root anatomy

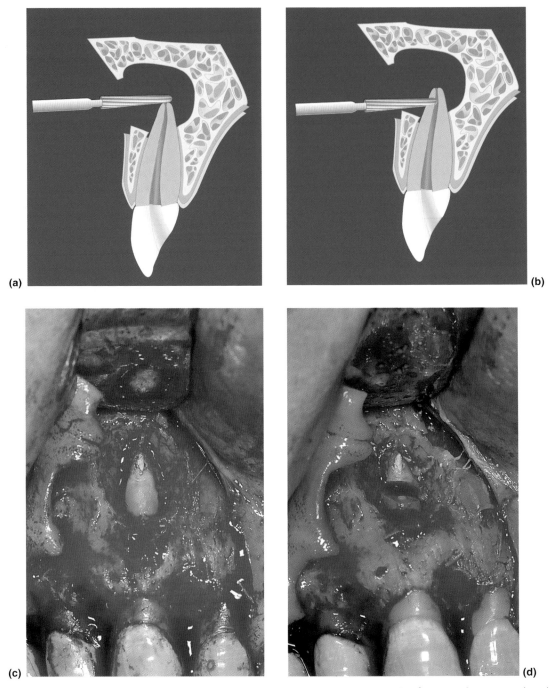

**Figure 9.21** Diagrammatic representation of (**a**) root-end resection from the apex coronally; (**b**) root-end resection when the amount of root to be resected has been determined. (**c**) Clinical case of root-end resection in which the amount of the root to be resected has been predetermined. (**d**) Resection of the root apex.

will determine the ultimate shape of the cut root end, as oval, round, dumb-bell shaped, kidney-bean shaped, or tear-drop shaped (Fig. 9.23). The outline of the resected root end will vary depending on the tooth, angle of any bevel and position of the cut on

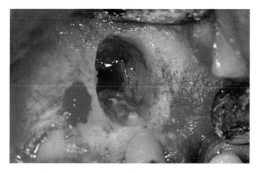

**Figure 9.22** Severely angled resections, often coupled with large periradicular lesions, compromise the amount of remaining crestal bone.

the root. However the entire surface must be visible. If visibility is impaired, or the root has an unusual cross-section, 1% methylene blue dye can be placed on the root surface for 5–10 s using a sterile sponge applicator to identify the periodontal ligament [29]. Subsequently the area is flushed with sterile water or saline. The dye will stain the periodontal ligament dark blue, highlighting the root outline. Cotton pellets should not be used as remnants of cotton fibres left in the surgical site have been shown to induce a foreign-body reaction in healing tissues [64]. The shape of the exposed canal system will vary depending on the angle of the bevel and the canal anatomy at that level. Canal systems will generally assume a more elongated and accentuated shape with increasing angles of bevel (Fig. 9.24).

Also visible on most resected root ends is the presence of root canal filling material. Variations in

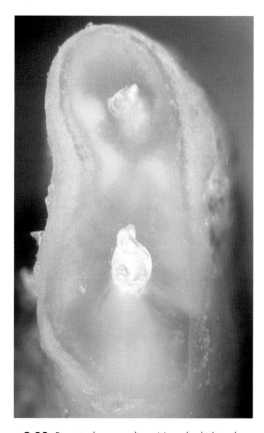

**Figure 9.23** Resected root outline. Note the kidney bean shape along with position of the canals. No canal anastomosis is visible.

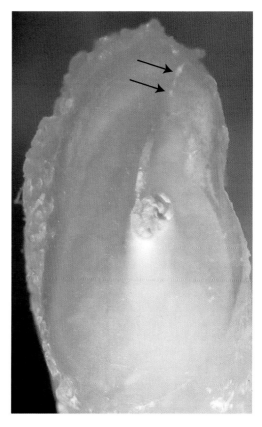

**Figure 9.24** Angled resection reveals an extended canal space. Removal of additional root palatally will be necessary to manage the uppermost part of the canal system (arrowed).

quality of the filling will be seen in both the type of filling material and the nature of the filling technique (Fig. 9.25). Furthermore, the different burs used for resection will create discrepancies in the surface of the filling material and adaptation to the canal walls. For example, coarse diamond burs will tend to rip and tear at the gutta-percha root canal filling, spreading the gutta-percha over the edge of the canal aperture and onto the resected root face (Fig. 9.26). Surface finishing with an ultra-fine diamond is recommended (Fig. 9.27) (Ultrafine no. 862-012 diamond bur, Brasseler, Savannah, GA, USA).

The presence of additional canals, anastomoses between them, fracture lines, and the quality of the apical adaptation of the root canal filling must be checked on the resected root surface (Fig. 9.28). If

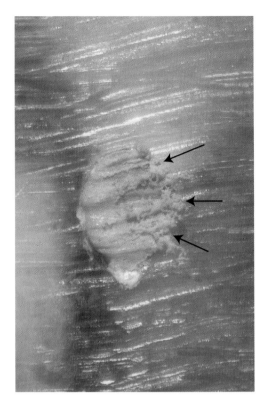

**Figure 9.26** Rough surface of resected root after being cut with a coarse diamond. Note the gutta-percha has been dragged across the surface of the root (arrowed).

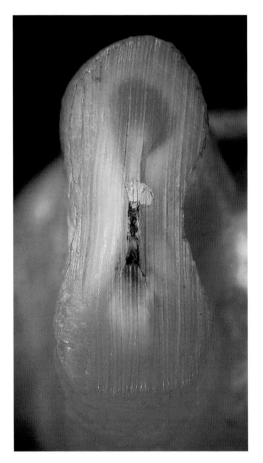

**Figure 9.25** Root-end resection reveals a poorly compacted gutta-percha filling. Voids filled with sealer are present between the gutta-percha cones, and an anastomosis is present that is filled with tissue remnants (bluish colour).

methylene blue has been used, it will also stain the periphery of the canal system and highlight fracture lines. A fibre-optic light can be aimed at or behind the root end to enhance visibility [11]. Sometimes it may be necessary to remove additional root structure to identify the canal system or, in the case of a fracture line, to observe its direction and extent.

A major area of concern following root-end resection and dentinal tubule exposure is the possibility that these tubules may serve as a direct source of contamination from uncleaned root canals into the periradicular tissues. Root ends resected from 45° to 60° have as many as 28 000 tubules/mm² immediately adjacent to the canal [164]. At the dentino–cemental junction, areas that may communicate with the root canal even in the presence of a root-end filling 13 000 tubules/mm² are found. Likewise, due to angular changes in the tubules at the apex, there could be patent communication with the main canal if the depth of the root-end

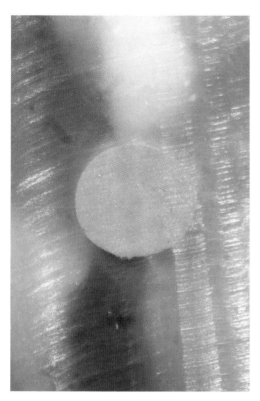

**Figure 9.27** Smooth surface of resected root and root filling created with an ultrafine diamond and waterspray. Note the adaptation of the filling material to the outline of the canal.

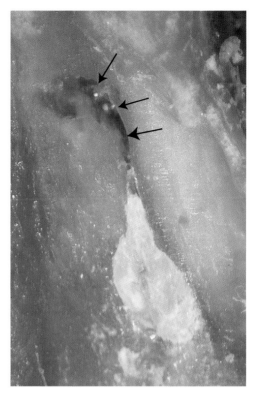

**Figure 9.28** Resected root end. The main canal has been obturated but the canal extension contains necrotic debris (arrowed). A root-end preparation and filling must be performed.

preparation in the buccal aspect of the cavity is insufficient [15,174]. Root-end resections in older teeth have shown less leakage than that seen in teeth from younger patients [71]; this corroborates with the findings of sclerosis and reduced patency in apical dentinal tubules [32].

Another concern following root-end resection is the formation of a contaminated smear layer over the resected root end (Fig. 9.29). This may serve as a source of irritation to the periradicular tissues, primarily preventing the intimate layering of cementum against the resected tubules. A thicker smear layer is usually created when cutting without waterspray [120], or when using coarse diamond burs rather than tungsten carbide burs [24]. Therefore it is recommended that root-end resection be performed under constant irrigation, which minimizes the dentinal smear layer. If diamond burs are used to resect the root, a medium grit is preferred, followed by a fine or ultrafine grit diamond.

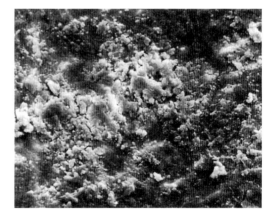

**Figure 9.29** Smear layer on the resected root end.

## Root-end cavity preparation

In order to seal the potential avenues of communication from the resected root end to the canal system adequately, a root-end preparation should be made into the root to the coronal extent of the resected apical tubules [56,174]. A depth of 2–4 mm is generally sufficient [14,144] depending on the angle of the resection. Increasing the depth of the root-end filling significantly decreases apical leakage [56]. The optimum depths for a root-end cavity, measured from the buccal aspect of the cavity, are 1.0, 2.1 and 2.5 mm for a 90°, 30° and 45° angle of resection, respectively [56]. Ideally this preparation is made in the long axis of the root, is parallel to the anatomical outline of the root, possesses adequate retention form, and encompasses all exposed orifices of the root canal system. If this is the case, then the depths indicated will be sufficient in all aspects of the preparation.

The final outline of the preparation will depend mainly on the anatomy of the exposed canal space, and in some cases, the nature of the root outline. For example in maxillary central incisors the shape of the root-end preparation will generally be round to oval in shape. In premolars or molars it may be very elongated and narrow in conjunction with oval or round shapes.

Root-end preparations are best created with specially designed, ultrasonically energized instruments (Fig. 9.30). These ultrasonic tips eliminate many of the difficulties associated with root-end preparation with burs. The small, angled tips allow for ultrasonic shaping of apical preparations parallel to the long axis of the root after minimal root-end resection and minimal bevelling of the root face (Fig. 9.31). They are effective in the debridement and enlargement of canal anastomoses and irregularities commonly found in molar roots (Fig. 9.32) [31]; the ability of this technique to achieve better-shaped and cleaner root-end preparations as opposed to bur preparations has been highlighted [66,159,160]. The creation of clean, good quality root-end preparations has also been achieved with the use of sonic tips [50,91,92] and clinical experience would support the routine use of either of these newer techniques. However, a note of caution has been sounded by some authors [1,151], who have demonstrated cracks in the root surface following use of ultrasonic root-end preparation instruments.

After root-end preparation the cavity should be irrigated with sterile saline or water. Small suction tips, made from 20- or 18-gauge needles that can be bent and adapted to a high-speed suction device,

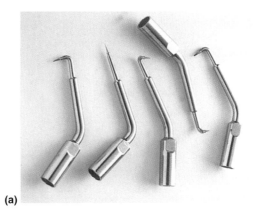

(a)

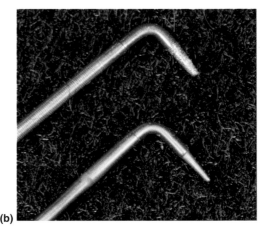

(b)

**Figure 9.30** (a) Variously shaped and angled ultrasonic tips for preparing a root-end cavity. (b) Top, Berutti ultrasonic tip; bottom, EMS RE-2 tip.

are used to remove fluid and debris from the cavity. Some clinicians prefer using paper points to dry the preparation. The Stropko irrigator/drier device (Ultradent Co) is a simple and effective means of drying the root-end preparation (Fig. 9.33a). Although rinsing the cavity with citric acid has been recommended to remove the smear layer [31], recent studies have indicated that this may actually enhance the amount of leakage after root-end filling [124,151]. Despite creating cleaner root-end cavity walls and assisting in debris removal, the routine use of citric acid is questionable. Following drying the cavity must be inspected to ensure that it is clean and that it encompasses all of the canal extensions. Small mirrors have been designed specifically for this purpose (Fig. 9.33b).

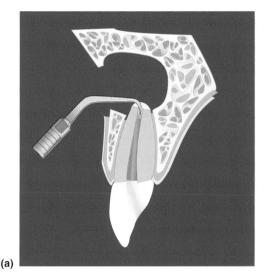
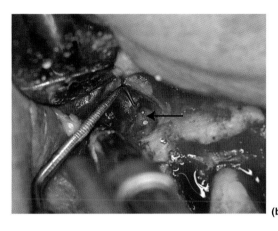

(a)

(b)

**Figure 9.31** (a) Diagrammatic representation of root-end cavity preparation along the root axis using an ultrasonic tip. (b) An ultrasonic tip near the resected root end. Note good access and two canals (identified by gutta-percha) united by a thin white line – anastomosis (arrowed). Preparation of the anastomosis is essential.

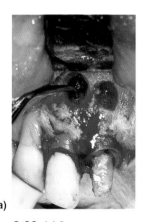
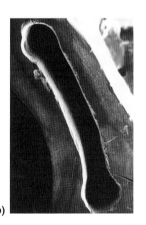
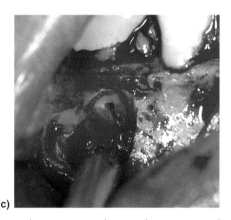

(a)

(b)

(c)

**Figure 9.32** (a) Preparing a root-end cavity with an ultrasonic tip. (b) Root-end cavity prepared in a molar root uniting the two mesial canals through the anastomosis (SEM). (c) Ultrasonic root-end preparation in the mesial root of a mandibular molar.

## Root-end cavity filling

Irrespective of whether a root-end filling is placed or not, it is important that the canal system is cleaned and sealed as well as possible. In many cases this necessitates that old root canal fillings should be redone prior to surgery. Under these circumstances many cases may be successful without the use of a root-end filling.

In some cases in which time is a factor or cases in which there are persistent exacerbations between visits, root canal retreatment can be done at the time of surgery. The elevated tissue is reflected, the root apex exposed and resected. The canal preparation is performed with the file tips protruding through the resected root end (Fig. 9.34a). Small aspirators can be placed next to the apical opening to prevent root canal irrigant entering the bony cavity. After adequate preparation, the canal is dried with paper points. Filling should follow with a suitable material, and excess removed (Fig. 9.34b). An ultra-fine diamond bur or composite finishing bur can be

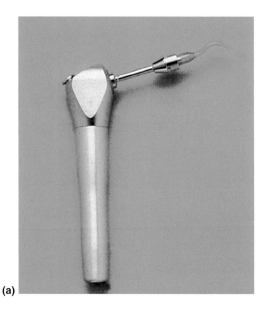

(a)

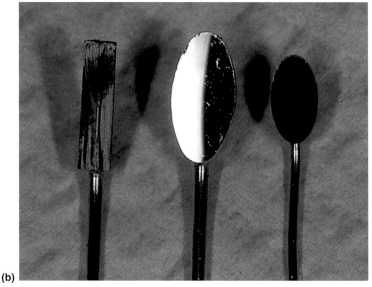

(b)

**Figure 9.33** (a) Stropko irrigator. (b) Miniature mirrors.

run over the root surface with a sterile water or saline spray (Fig. 9.34c). If the canal is filled properly, the result will be a very smooth, well-adapted root canal filling.

Prior to filling, the root-end cavity must be isolated to ensure moisture control. The appropriate use of vasoconstrictors will greatly reduce the blood flow in the surgical site but other supplementary agents are frequently used. Historically, bone wax was widely used, however studies have shown that any wax particles retained in the surgical site will provoke a prolonged inflammatory reaction. In recent years more biocompatible and biodegradable products have been developed; these include collagen-based products such as CollaPlug, Colla-Cote, Avitene or Superstat that can remain in the osseous cavity or be removed prior to closure (Fig. 9.35) [64]. Non-collagen products include Surgicel,

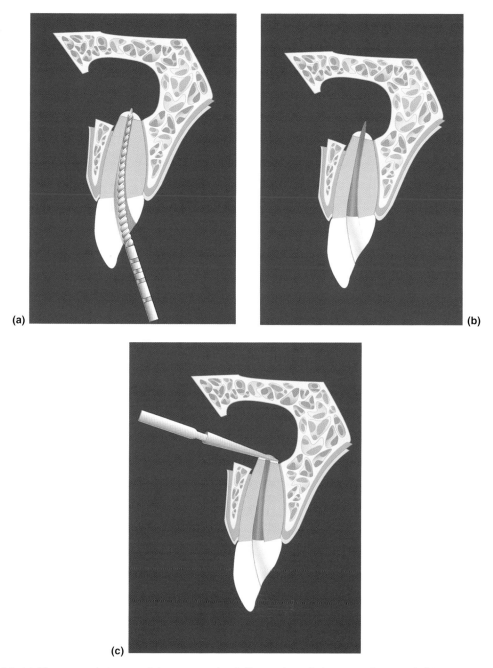

(a)

(b)

(c)

**Figure 9.34** (a) Cleaning and shaping of the root canal with file tips through the resected root end. (b) Compaction of the gutta-percha filling with the tip through the root-end. (c) Removal of excess filling material and finishing of the root surface with an ultrafine diamond bur.

Oxycel and Gelfoam. These products can exert their influence on haemostasis by stimulating the intrinsic clotting pathway and physically by introducing a tamponing effect when packed into the crypt. Other less biocompatible products include Astrigedent, Cut-Trol, and ViscoStat; these are solutions of ferric sulphate which must be removed as much as possible from the bone cavity prior to tissue closure

161

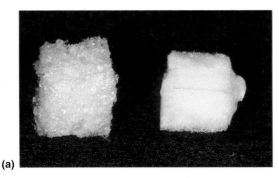

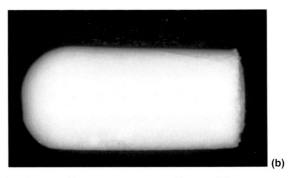

**(a)**                                                                 **(b)**

**Figure 9.35** Collagen sponge materials for haemorrhage control in the apical bony cavity: (**a**) Hemofibrine – left; Hemocollagene – right. (**b**) Collaplug.

[74,89]. Haemostasis in periradicular surgery has been reviewed thoroughly [181].

## Root-end filling materials

The purpose of the root-end filling is to seal the canal system apically and prevent the egress of bacteria and bacterial products into the periradicular tissues. Presently there are no commercially available materials that provide a perfect seal, therefore the materials that are used must be prepared and placed carefully to ensure the best possible adaptation to the cavity walls. When using modern materials as root-end fillings, adherence to manufacturers' recommendations in preparation, manipulation and placement is important. Table 9.4 lists current materials that are recommended for root-end filling. Amalgam has previously been the most widely used root-end filling material and has been associated with a reasonable level of success. However problems have existed with corrosion and tissue argyria, persistence of apical inflammation, and its long-term success [52]. Coupled with concerns over the mercury component, it is recommended that more biocompatible materials be used and several

**Table 9.4** Current root-end filling materials

Super EBA
Intermediate restorative material (IRM)
Glass ionomer
Diaket
Composite resin (dentine-bonded)
Mineral trioxide aggregate (MTA) – ProRoot

clinical studies support the use of alternative materials [45,75,136,167–170,184,185].

### Super-EBA

This material is modified zinc oxide–eugenol cement that has high compressive and tensile strengths, neutral pH, and low solubility. It adheres to the walls of the root-end preparation even in the presence of moisture. The in vitro short-term seal obtained with super EBA has been shown to be affected minimally by blood contamination [166], whilst its in vivo sealing ability as a root-end filling material to microorganisms has been shown to be better than that of amalgam [128]. There is evidence of osseous tissue repair following its use as a bone implant [115] and periradicular tissue repair when used as a root-end filling material [118]. A clinically high success rate (95%) has been reported over a long period of evaluation [45]. When used in bur- or ultrasonically prepared root-end cavities in which the smear layer had either been retained or removed, leakage was observed [114,151]. In spite of some of the variables seen with this material its widespread use as a root-end filling material has been advocated.

### Intermediate restorative material (IRM)

IRM is a resin reinforced zinc oxide–eugenol cement that has been shown to provide a better seal than amalgam, especially against the passage of microorganisms [127]. Healing of the periradicular tissues in the presence of IRM root-end fillings has been quite favourable [76,127]. Likewise, clinical studies have shown enhanced success with IRM root-end fillings (91%) compared with amalgam (75%) over long periods [45]. When using this material as a root-end filling a high powder-to-liquid ratio has been recommended to enhance placement, decrease setting time, reduce toxicity and reduce dissolution in tissue fluids [40]. Therefore the use of IRM as a root-end filling material is recommended when mixed at a high powder-to-liquid ratio.

*Glass ionomer cement*

Developed in the 1970s, the main components of these materials, aluminofluorosilicate glass, polyacids and water undergo an acid-base reaction to form the restorative material. Glass ionomer cements bond physicochemically to dentine. The biocompatibility is enhanced with setting, and marginal adaptation and adhesion to dentine have been shown to be improved with the use of acid conditioners [131,132]. The sealing ability of glass ionomer cements has been demonstrated in recent studies of their use for root-end filling [3,4,34,119]. Antibacterial activity is acceptable [33] and sealing ability is better than that of amalgam, heat-sealed gutta-percha or zinc polycarboxylate cement [33,116]. Bone healing adjacent to glass ionomers used as root-end fillings or implants has been clearly demonstrated [28,43, 129,185]. In addition, clinical studies support the use of glass ionomer cement for root-end filling [69,75, 83,184,185]. The occasional blood contamination does not appear to affect healing adversely with these materials used as root-end fillings over a 5-year period [75]. The careful use of glass ionomer cements as root-end fillings can be recommended.

*Dentine-bonded composite resin*

There has been limited use but promising results with dentine-bonded composite resin root-end fillings. Key to their success appears to be a combination of minimal toxicity of the dentine-bonding agent, placement in a moisture-free environment, and good adhesion to the underlying dentine with minimal polymerization contraction [148]. A clinical and radiological evaluation of 388 teeth over a one-year period showed healing with dentine-bonded composite resin root-end fillings to be much better than with amalgam [147]. Histological and scanning electron microscopic assessment of this technique have indicated reformation of the periodontium adjacent to the composite resin, including reformation of a lamina dura, insertion of Sharpey's fibres, and cementum deposited in intimate contact with the composite resin [9,10]. These findings would suggest that ideal healing can be achieved with this material; further long-term studies are warranted before widespread use can be recommended.

*Diaket*

Primarily a root canal sealer, this polyvinyl resin has been used as a root-end filling material for a number of years with a high level of empirical success. Diaket has excellent sealing ability [77,180] with a highly favourable tissue response in bone and periradicular tissues [109,136,180]. Histologically there is a suggestion that cementum can form immediately adjacent to or in intimate contact with Diaket, or with Diaket–tricalcium phosphate paste [136,180]. It is imperative that this material is mixed at a higher powder-to-liquid ratio than that for a root canal sealer [109,163]; a suggested ratio is at least 2 parts powder to 1 portion liquid [180]. This can be done on a glass slab 20–30 min prior to use, without risk of the material setting. It is carried to the apical cavity with a small carrier, such as a Messing carrier or the MAP System (Produits Dentaires, Vevey, Switzerland) (Fig. 9.36), compacted and burnished in a similar way to amalgam.

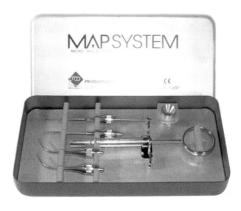

**Figure 9.36** Miniature carriers, such as the MAP System are used to carry small increments of root-end filling material.

*Mineral trioxide aggregate (MTA)*

MTA is a new material developed by Torabinejad and co-workers [165]. A series of studies have illustrated the useful properties of MTA as a root-end filling material including its biocompatibility, sealing properties and ability to promote regeneration [165–169]. Recent studies have demonstrated the superior sealing properties of MTA over other root-end filling materials using either dye leakage or electrochemical testing [166] or endotoxin [161]. The properties of this material have been shown to be relatively unaffected by blood contamination [166]. Complete regeneration of the periodontal apparatus has been demonstrated in some cases but not in all cases examined in a recent study [136]. In addition, in another recent study, the success rate associated with the use of MTA as a root-end filling material was not significantly greater than that with IRM [35]. Overall it would appear that MTA holds great promise for the future as a root-end filling material; however, in its current form it is not easy to manipulate in clinical situations.

## Treatment of the root face

Removal of the smear layer and exposure of the apical collagen fibres is recommended after root-end resection, primarily to remove potentially contaminated debris and to enhance the healing environment for cemental deposition. Various agents have been recommended and include phosphoric acid [57,120], EDTA [22], hydrochloric acid [137,149], and citric acid [21,39,138]. The optimal exposure of collagen and demineralization occurs with a burnishing application of citric acid (pH 1.0) for three minutes [37]. Longer applications result in collagen denaturation. The peak activity pH of citric acid is 1.42 [158]. Demineralization of resected root ends with a two-minute burnishing of 50% citric acid at pH 1.0 resulted in a rapid and predictable layering of a cementoid type of material on the resected surface of dogs' teeth after 45 days [38]. No direct application to human teeth under similar circumstances has been studied, although the omission of an acid cleaner does not preclude the formation of a viable cementum layer [101].

Recent studies have identified the use of the ferric ion, as an aqueous solution of 10% citric acid and

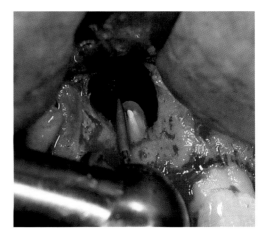

**Figure 9.37** Smoothing of the resected root end with an ultrafine diamond.

3% ferric chloride (10:3), to stabilize dentine collagen during the demineralization process [104,179]; however, applications were < 30 s, as longer exposure increased demineralization and denaturation of the collagen. This approach has enhanced the bonding that occurs with restorative materials, and may also stimulate adhesion of the exposed, intact collagen with fibrin and fibronectin [130] and the splicing of collagen with newly formed collagen fibrils [140] during the wound healing process. Further work on the resected root end is warranted.

The following treatment regimen is indicated for the resected root face after placement of a root-end filling, or root-end resection in which a well-condensed gutta-percha root filling is in place:

1. Finish the surface with an ultra-fine diamond or 30-flute tungsten-carbide composite-resin finishing-bur [31,65] (Fig. 9.37).
2. Burnish the surface gently with a weak acid cleaner (10%) for a short period (30 s) [65].

These procedures achieve the desired result of a smooth root face devoid of smear layer, regardless of the root or canal configuration type (Fig. 9.38). Such treatment of the root face is inappropriate if MTA is used as the root-end filling.

## Closure of the surgical site

Prior to repositioning the tissue flap, the underside of the reflected tissue, the surrounding bone, and

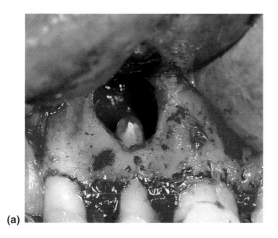

(a)

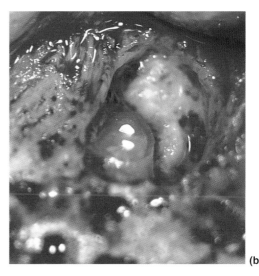

(b)

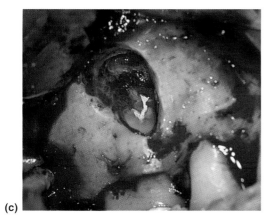

(c)

**Figure 9.38** Finished root ends prior to tissue closure. Note the smooth and varied appearance of the root and root-end filling material depending on the cross-section of the root canal anatomy in an (**a**) anterior tooth, (**b**) premolar tooth, and (**c**) molar tooth.

the periradicular bone cavity should be inspected for debris. The surgical site is carefully flushed with saline, except where MTA has been used as the root-end filling. A radiograph is taken to ensure that all debris including resected root-ends has been removed and that the goals of the surgical procedure have been accomplished. Final irrigation with saline is often warranted followed by tissue repositioning to the wound edges to ensure primary closure.

When surgery has been performed and there is a stable buccal cortical plate of bone to protect the root structure and no evidence of marginal perio-dontitis, tissue closure is straightforward. Intimate approximation of the healthy soft tissues and bone with sutures will suffice, and healing will occur uneventfully. Ideally, detection of bony dehiscences or large fenestrations should be made prior to surgery so that adjunct procedures such as guided-tissue regeneration can be planned (Fig. 9.39) [81,122,126]. When there has been loss of the cortical

bone, especially in the crestal region, or the presence of marginal periodontitis, the chances for long-term success are highly guarded [70,155].

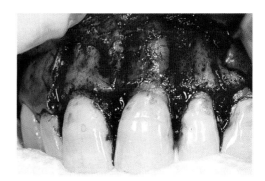

**Figure 9.39** Loss of buccal cortical bone over the root of a left maxillary central incisor with a periradicular lesion. Correct treatment planning should be able to determine, or at least anticipate the presence of this defect prior to surgical entry.

165

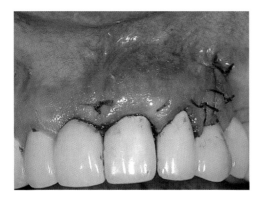

**Figure 9.40** Close tissue flap approximation with minimal suturing and tissue damage.

**Table 9.5** Suture materials

| Material | Advantages/disadvantages |
|---|---|
| Black silk | Non-resorbable<br>Historically the most commonly used<br>Good handling characteristics<br>Braided; wicking delays healing |
| Surgical gut (Collagen)<br>Chromic acid treated surgical gut | Absorbable; manufacturing process determines longevity of catgut sutures<br>Treatment with chromic acid prolongs retention in tissues<br>Difficult to handle |
| Nylon | Non-absorbable<br>Monofilament |
| Polyglycolic acid (PGA) | Absorbable<br>May be braided or monofilament |
| Expanded polytetrafluoroethylene (PTFE) (GORE-TEX) | Single filament; smooth, strong<br>Non-porous surface<br>Provokes little tissue reaction |
| Polyester | Non-absorbable |
| Coated polyester (Tecdek) | Usually braided |
| Polyamide | Non-absorbable<br>Strong<br>Smooth, non-porous |

Persistent periradicular inflammation following root-end surgery has been associated with marginal periodontitis at the time of surgery [145].

Many clinicians will also apply gentle pressure to the repositioned tissue at this time to remove residual blood and to begin the intimate reattachment process. Suturing will be necessary in most cases. A variety of suturing techniques are frequently used and include interrupted, mattress, continuous or sling sutures. The suture is first placed in the flap and is then carried into the attached tissues. Whilst there is no one formula for the number of sutures and their position, the clinician must exercise judgement in their placement to ensure adequate and stable positioning, especially in the crestal region. Vertical incisions may require several depending on the length and nature of the tissue (Fig. 9.40).

A variety of suture materials are available each demonstrating advantages and disadvantages. Suture materials are either absorbable or non-absorbable. They can also be either monofilament or braided; the latter have a tendency to facilitate the movement of saliva and bacteria along the suture into the tissues. This property called 'wicking' contributes to irritation of the tissues and may delay healing. A list of suitable suture materials is shown in Table 9.5.

For years silk sutures have been most widely used; their main disadvantage is bacterial colonization, which will delay healing. However, with proper suture placement, adequate cleaning of the surgical site by the patient, and timely suture removal in 48–72 h, this problem can be minimized. Gut sutures can also be used, but their handling characteristics can be a challenge. A number of new synthetic suture materials are now available and may have relegated the silk suture to history. Materials such as Polyglactin, Polypropylene, Polyethylene and Teflon (PTFE) cause minimal tissue reaction. With these newer monofilament synthetic materials, the preferred suture size for wound closure in periradicular surgery is either 5-0 or 6-0. Different needle sizes and shapes are often necessary due to osseous contours and tissue thickness. No single needle shape or radius is ideal for every situation. Thin tissue is often found along the vertical releasing incision and requires a small radius needle. Larger radius needles are generally used in the horizontal incision.

Suture knots should always be placed away from the incision line to minimize microbial colonization in that area (Fig. 9.41). Sutured tissue should be cleaned routinely by the patient with chlorhexidine or warm saline rinses. Immediately following suturing, the tissue must be compressed with firm finger pressure for 3–5 min to ensure correct tissue

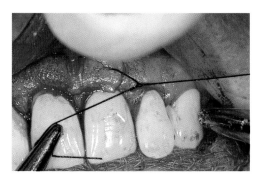

**Figure 9.41** Suture knots must be kept away from the incision line to minimize infection of the wound.

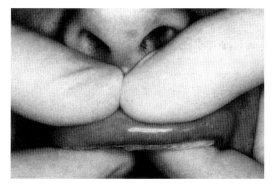

**Figure 9.42** Compression of the tissue flap with gauze and light pressure is essential to minimize blood clot between tissue and cortical bone.

position with a minimal blood clot between the bone and tissue flap (Fig. 9.42). During this time, the patient can be given postoperative instructions. All sutures should be removed in 48–72 h.

## Postoperative radiological assessment

As previously indicated, a postoperative radiograph should be taken prior to closure of the surgical site; mistakes can be rectified easily at this point. In some cases, especially posterior teeth, angled radiographs should be considered. Radiographs taken with a film-holding device are preferred. When review examination radiographs are taken with the same device, healing can be assessed more accurately. Some points for the clinician to consider are:

- Is there any remaining unresected root structure, or have the wrong roots been inadvertently damaged?

- Has any resected root tissue been left in the surgical site?
- Are the correct root ends surgically filled?
- Do the root-end fillings appear adequate in depth and adaptation and appear well compacted?
- Is there scattered radiopaque material within the surgical site?
- Has root-end filling material been pushed into the maxillary sinus or mandibular canal?
- Is there a fracture that was not seen clinically?

## Postoperative patient instructions

When the soft tissues are managed properly and surgical time is minimized, healing is generally uneventful. Careful attention to postoperative instructions, however, is essential for patient comfort and tissue healing during the next few days. The following postoperative instructions should be given verbally and supported in writing for the patient's reference.

- Strenuous activity should be avoided, along with drinking alcohol and smoking.
- An adequate diet consisting of fruit juices, soups, soft foods and liquid food supplements should be consumed after the effects of the local anaesthesia have worn off. Avoid hard, sticky or chewy foods.
- Do not pull on, or unnecessarily lift the facial tissues.
- Oozing of blood from the surgical site is normal for the first 24 h. Bleeding can be managed by applying a gauze pack to the site. Slight and transient facial swelling and bruising may be experienced.
- Postsurgical discomfort is minimal but the surgical site will be tender and sore. The use of analgesics for 24–48 h will help to alleviate this occurrence. Normally, continue with the analgesics given presurgically.
- For the first day place ice packs with firm pressure directly on the face over the surgical site for 20 min and remove for 20 min. Repeat until retiring that evening.
- Chlorhexidine rinses should be used twice daily. On the day following surgery and for the next 3–4 days, warm hypertonic salt water rinses can be used every 1–2 h if possible (half a teaspoon of salt in a glass of water).

- Sutures will be removed in 48–72 h.
- Brushing of the surgical site is not recommended until the sutures are removed. Prior to that the surgical area can be cleaned using a large cotton puff or ball saturated with warm salt solution.
- Telephone numbers are provided for your convenience should complications arise.

## Postoperative examination and review

Re-examination of the patient, both clinically and radiologically, is normally scheduled at one year. In most cases osseous repair is virtually complete at this time; evidence of this as well as clinical healing has been considered as a valid criterion for continued success. Therefore, no additional follow-up may be necessary [67,75,146]. Failure to observe complete repair or delayed healing should warrant additional evaluation for as long as four years [139], until repair is evident, or signs and symptoms indicate failure.

Radiological interpretation is highly variable and can easily be influenced by the quality and angulation of the film and processing irregularities. Therefore, the clinician should use a film-holding device for all follow-up radiographs. Likewise, familiarity with radiological classifications of healing (success–failure) is essential [64,104,145]. This will enable case outcomes to be based on a sound, logical and consistent decision-making process [61].

## PERIRADICULAR SURGERY OF PARTICULAR TEETH

### Maxillary anterior teeth

Surgical access to maxillary anterior teeth is relatively straightforward due to root position in relation to the labial cortical bone. The lateral incisor may pose more of a challenge due to its common disto-palatal root inclination and curvature. Deep osseous penetration is often necessary and the root apex may impinge on the palatal cortical plate of bone. Common also in this region is the excessively long canine that requires extensive soft tissue elevation for access to the root end. Anatomical cross-sections after root-end resection usually reveal a round, oval or slightly oblong root outline with canals placed centrally on the root surface. Because the lateral incisor is commonly positioned to the palatal, both the buccal and palatal cortical plates of bone may be destroyed from advancing periradicular disease or surgical intervention. This usually leads to a greater frequency of scar tissue (incomplete healing) as opposed to complete bony repair.

### Maxillary premolars

Surgical access to single-rooted premolars is also straightforward, with a minimal thickness of cortical plate covering the root apex. Complications generally occur when multiple roots are present, widely divergent in a buccopalatal dimension, and/or the position of the maxillary sinus is such that penetration into the sinus cannot be avoided. Often, these teeth have buccal apices that have fenestrated the buccal cortex and access is relatively simple.

Single-rooted maxillary premolar resected root outlines are oval, oblong, dumb-bell shaped or round. In multi-rooted premolars, canals are centrally placed and generally oval or circular on the resected root surface. In a two-canal, single-rooted premolar, two oval or round canals can be expected with a joining anastomosis. In this situation, the root-end cavity must encompass not only the canal openings but also the anastomosis, for which ultrasonic or sonic root-end preparation is indicated.

### Maxillary molars

When buccal fenestrations exist, surgical access to the buccal roots of maxillary molars is relatively easy. Depending on the position of the inferior border of the zygomatic process, extensive removal of bone may be necessary. Root outlines, after resection, are usually oval or circular for the disto-buccal root and oblong, teardrop shaped, figure-of-eight shaped, or narrow and curved for the mesio-buccal root. This root has a high incidence of two canals with a joining anastomosis, and therefore all orifices on the resected root face must be identified.

In palatal root surgery, soft tissue management is more difficult during reflection and retraction due to the thickness of the palatal flap and an irregular surface of the cortical plate. Palatal roots have a tendency to curve to the buccal and the root has seldom fenestrated the bone at the apex. This often implies that large amounts of bone must be removed in a site that has restricted access and visibility. Penetration into the sinus is not uncommon. The greater palatine nerve and vessels will invariably be encountered with the palatal root of a second molar. Resected root outlines are generally oval, round or oblong, with the canal placed centrally on the root surface.

## Mandibular anterior teeth

Surgical access to the root apices of mandibular anterior teeth is often difficult because of lingual tooth inclination, wide buccolingual roots, thick cortical bone apically with increased amounts of cancellous bone between the cortex and root, and root dehiscences in the coronal half of the root. It is common for the root apices of mandibular incisors to be in close proximity to each other, which may pose problems in root-end management. Resected root outlines are narrow, oblong, or figure-of-eight-shaped, with canal space on the resected root usually narrow mesiodistally and wide buccolingually. The incidence of two canals or joining canals on the root surface is high after root-end resection.

## Mandibular premolars

Surgical access to mandibular premolars is usually direct, except for the occasional presence of significant muscle attachments in the soft tissues and the mental foramen in the bone. Surgical entry is often from a superior direction to avoid the foramen, which is most commonly close to the second premolar. The thickness of the cortical bone overlying the root apices is variable depending on tooth inclination in the arch. Root outlines are generally oval to oblong in a buccolingual dimension, with a small incidence of multiple canals exiting on the resected root surface; preoperative radiographs should reveal warnings of this possibility.

## Mandibular molars

Surgical entry through the cortical plate to mandibular molars can be straightforward, but is more often complicated by limited access, shallow vestibule, thick cortical plate, external oblique ridge, root length, position and inclination. Although the apices of molar roots are inclined buccally [11], the roots are often housed within a thick cortical plate of bone. Additionally, individual root variations and curvatures often place the apices in positions difficult to reach. Therefore, these anatomical problems must be considered during treatment planning. Radiological assessment is essential; the location of the mandibular canal must be identified through the use of angled films in a superior or inferior direction. Likewise, proximally angled films will provide information about the number and curvature of roots.

Root outlines after resection are oval, dumb-bell-shaped, oblong, and wide in a buccolingual dimension. Canals often have joining anastomoses in both mesial and distal roots. The use of staining is strongly advised. Root-end cavities, by necessity, are oblong encompassing the entire canal system as it exits on the resected root surface (Fig. 9.32).

## General anatomical considerations

It is uncommon to penetrate the maxillary sinus during periradicular surgery. If this occurs, however, the opening must be protected to prevent debris entering the sinus during the management of the root end (Fig. 9.43). This can be done with collagen-based haemostatic agents as previously mentioned. Bone wax should not be used because it can be pushed into the sinus and evoke a significant foreign-body giant cell reaction along with delayed healing [48]. The postsurgical need for antibiotics or antihistamines has not been established [64]. Since primary closure can be achieved with soft tissue repositioning and suturing, an effective seal is obtained, avoiding the need for drug therapy.

The mental foramen also poses a challenge for many clinicians. Discussion with the patient in the treatment planning stage is essential to disclose the nature of the problem, the methods used to manage it, and the potential for untoward postoperative sequelae. The best way to manage this entity is to:

- identify its position;
- plan surgical entry away from it;
- use the periosteal retractor to protect the foramen and its contents during surgery;
- avoid pinching the soft tissues with the retractor.

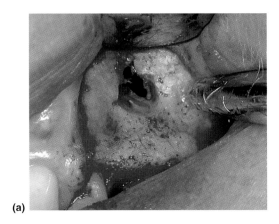
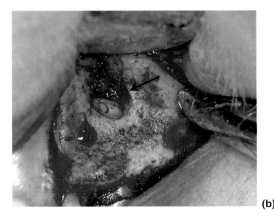

**(a)**
**(b)**

**Figure 9.43** (**a**) Penetration into the maxillary sinus apical and distal to a premolar. (**b**) Blocking of the sinus perforation with a collagen sponge (arrowed). Note root-end preparation has been made with good haemorrhage control around the resected apex. Collagen was left in place to serve as a matrix for closure of the sinus perforation.

An additional concern with all periradicular surgery is the presence of fenestrations and dehiscences, along with large penetrating periradicular lesions which have destroyed buccal and lingual cortical plates of bone [81,122,126]. Previous studies have identified less than favourable results when the surrounding bone has been compromised [70,146, 155]. Management of these osseous defects often requires a guided tissue/bone regenerative procedure, which is becoming more widespread. These situations should be diagnosed and treatment planned carefully; when appropriate, consider help from experienced specialists.

## REPAIR OF PERFORATION

Non-surgical repair of root perforations is reasonably successful [17,19,172,177], but when it fails or is impractical, surgery is necessary. The surgical repair of root perforations is generally more difficult than root-end procedures. Perforations pose greater radiological difficulties in identification, diagnosis and post-surgical assessment [53]. Surgical management of perforated roots depends on access to the defect and the relationship of the perforation to crestal bone and the epithelial attachment. Perforations have been classified according to their relationship to the epithelial attachment and the crestal bone – the 'critical crestal zone' [54,135].

Perforations occurring in the apical third pose the least problem in surgical management and are generally amenable to root-end resection [111,117, 154]. Mid-root perforations present a different set of challenges. Typically they are not in line with the coronal aspect of the canal, and may be identified by radiographs taken from different angles. Once identified surgically, they can be managed like any root end (Figs 9.44 and 9.45). Access to the defect margins, however, is more difficult when the perforation is located on the proximal surface of the root, and it is necessary to ensure complete marginal adaptation of the filling material while preventing its placement into the surrounding bone (Fig. 9.45). Access to lingual perforations is almost impossible on most teeth and other courses of treatment must be considered.

A common cause of perforation is due to post space preparation and placement [135]. Often the post must be removed prior to root repair and a shorter post placed. In some cases the post may be ground down so that it lies inside the root and a filling material is placed to seal the perforation.

The prognosis for surgically repaired root perforations is based on a number of factors, similar to those for non-surgical repair of root perforations. Success is highly dependent on the following factors:

- Proximity of the perforation to the critical crestal zone. The prognosis for furcation

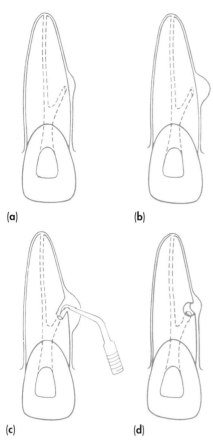

(a)  (b)

(c)  (d)

**Figure 9.44** Access to a midroot proximal perforation.
(a) Perforation; (b) access improved by careful removal of
overlying bone; (c) creation of a cavity with an ultrasonic tip;
(d) if necessary additional bone can be removed to enhance
access to the defect.

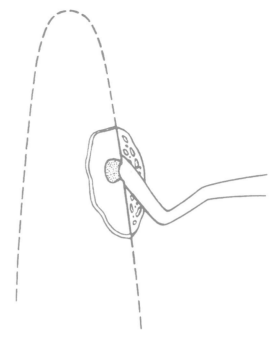

**Figure 9.45** Repair of perforation. A flat plastic instrument
or the convex side of a small curette may be used to apply
the filling material to the prepared cavity; it may also serve
as a matrix, against which the filling material is compacted
with pluggers.

- Sealing of the defect with minimal to no excess
  material in the surgical site that may cause
  persistent inflammation and possibly stimulate
  root resorption.
- Maintenance of optimal oral hygiene in the area
  of any perforation repair.

## REPLANTATION/TRANSPLANTATION

Replantation is defined as replacing a tooth in its
socket following deliberate or traumatic avulsion.
In the case of surgical or deliberate removal of a
tooth and its replacement, it is defined as intentional replantation [7]. Transplantion involves the
transfer of a tooth from one alveolar socket to
another either in the same or another person [7].

Few true indications exist for choosing intentional
replantation as a primary method of treatment [64].
The presence of calcified canals, separated instruments, non-negotiable root canals, perforations, or

perforations is very poor due to the potential
for microbial contamination.
- Microbial contamination of the perforation.
- Timely management of the perforation; the
  shorter the time interval between creation of the
  perforation and repair, the better the prognosis.
- Use of a biocompatible repair material. Any
  material that is cytotoxic will significantly
  reduce the prognosis. For example, the
  placement of phenolic compounds in the root
  canal after a perforation has occurred and
  before surgical repair will cause irreparable
  damage to the periodontium at the perforation
  site. Likewise the use of a cytotoxic material to
  seal the perforation will cause tissue damage.

anatomical closeness of, e.g. the mandibular canal, are not valid indications for choosing intentional replantation. The patient's symptoms and signs, the strategic value of the tooth, and the overall dental condition, including arch continuity, occlusion, function, tooth restorability and periodontal status must be considered along with the patient's understanding and cooperation. Finally, awareness of the potential for adverse sequelae such as bone loss, tooth resorption and tooth fractures during extraction must be considered. When viewed from this perspective the only true indication for intentional replantation is when there is absolutely no other treatment available to maintain a strategic tooth [47,152,179]. Even then it is essential that all phases of this planned procedure be communicated to the patient, providing a realistic appraisal of the treatment plan, sequelae, prognosis and alternatives.

Once a decision has been reached to perform intentional replantation, all efforts should be taken to ensure removal of all tissue debris within the tooth. Root canals must be as clean as possible, canals filled as far as possible, and the access opening closed with a permanent restoration. Occlusal adjustments and teeth cleaning should also be performed.

Ideally, a two-person team should perform the procedure, one to remove the tooth and the other to assess and fulfil the endodontic needs of the tooth. The surrounding tissue is disinfected with an antiseptic solution. Elevators should be carefully used to loosen the tooth, minimizing injuries to the soft tissue, bone and root. If necessary the extraction forceps can be wrapped with gauze to minimize damage to the root. Once removed the crown of the tooth is grasped with gauze sponges soaked in sterile saline. The socket is gently curetted to remove foreign debris. Care is exercised to avoid damage to the socket-retained periodontal fibres; gauze or cotton products should not be placed into the socket.

The extracted tooth is examined for fractures, extra roots or foramina, or any unusual anatomical configurations. Root ends are easily resected with a high-speed fine diamond bur under sterile saline spray. The nature of the canal system and its orifices are examined and if necessary, apically prepared with ultrasonics and filled. Time is of the essence with these procedures and all members of the team must be fully aware of their responsibilities and skilled in their execution.

When the tooth is ready to be replaced in its socket, the walls should be gently rinsed with saline to remove the blood clot. Additionally the tooth is rinsed to remove any residual cotton fibres or debris from the root-end filling material. The tooth is teased carefully and slowly into its original position in the socket, allowing for the slow escape of the blood that has built up in the socket. Slight pressure is applied to the buccal and lingual cortical plates to ensure adaptation. The occlusion is rechecked, and a splint is placed if necessary. Often only a periodontal pack is necessary. If a splint is used the tooth must be in physiological function. Convenient splints are made of soft, clear resin or nylon line that is acid-etched and cemented to the buccal surface. Splints are removed after 5–7 days.

The prognosis for intentionally replanted teeth is primarily dictated by the presence or absence of inflammatory and replacement resorption. Long-term studies provide mixed results with this technique, with 50–60% success over a 5–10-year period [8,64].

## REGENERATIVE PROCEDURES

A major factor influencing the prognosis of endodontic surgery is the complete loss of cortical bone overlying the root [70,155]. If the buccal or lingual cortical bone is lost or a naturally occurring dehiscence is revealed upon entry to the periradicular surgical site, the success rate is reduced (51,70,102, 123,146,155). When there is loss of the cortical plates both buccally and lingually, the success rate is reduced even further. In an attempt to improve the chance of success regenerative procedures have been advocated as a means of encouraging formation of bone. Regenerative procedures have been used widely in periodontal surgery. Regeneration of the periradicular tissues subsequent to surgery or due to the ravages of disease processes implies replacement of the various components of the tissue in their appropriate locations, amounts and relationships to each other [12]. There are a number of clinical situations in endodontic surgery where regenerative procedures might be suitable [133]. These include:

- apical periodontitis without communication to the alveolar crest;

- apical periodontitis with communication to the alveolar crest.
  - dehiscence;
  - proximal bone loss;
  - developmental grooves;
- root or furcation bone loss caused by perforations;
- cervical root resorption;
- oblique root fracture;
- ridge augmentation.

At present the prognosis for regenerative procedures in endodontic surgery in patients is inconclusive. However, animal studies [20,41,42,46], case reports [122] and empirical data would suggest that more favourable healing is likely when regenerative procedures are used. Unfortunately successful regeneration can only be demonstrated histologically. Clinically, measurements such as gain in probing attachment level, decrease in probing depth and increased filling of the osseous defect have been used to measure and compare results.

## Clinical techniques in regenerative procedures

In guided-tissue regeneration the type of healing that occurs after surgery is considered to be determined by the cells that first repopulate the root surface [100]; this has been supported by experimental work [78,79,113]. Membrane therapy has resulted in predictable formation of new attachment by preventing gingival connective tissue and gingival epithelium from contacting the root surface [58]. Regenerative membrane procedures aim to delay the advance of rapidly growing epithelial cells in order to allow the more slowly growing progenitor cells from the bone and periodontal ligament to repopulate the root surface and produce a new connective tissue attachment. The objectives of membrane application in endodontic surgery are the following [175]:

- To facilitate tissue regeneration by creating an optimum environment (stable and protected wound).
- To exclude undesirable, fast-proliferating cells that interfere with desired tissue regeneration.

A classification for guided-tissue regeneration (GTR) application in endodontic surgery based on

the location, extent and nature of the lesion has been proposed:

*Class I – bony defects located at the apex.*
*Class II – apical lesions with concomitant marginal lesions.*
*Class III – lateral or furcation lesions with or without a marginal lesion.*

Two main types of membrane have been used, absorbable and non-absorbable. The first commercially available membrane was an expanded polytetrafluoroethylene (ePTFE) non-absorbable membrane (GORE-TEX). The use of GORE-TEX membrane necessitated a second surgical procedure to remove it. With the development of absorbable membranes single visit surgical procedures became possible. Studies have subsequently shown that there is no significant difference in the healing with either type of membrane [27].

The absorbable membranes can be either natural materials such as collagen (Biomend or Bio-Gide) or synthetic polymers such as polyglactin. The natural materials are absorbed by enzymatic action while the synthetic materials are absorbed by hydrolysis. The use of an absorbable membrane (Bio-Gide) in combination with a bone substitute material (Bio-Oss) has been shown to stimulate substantial new bone and cementum formation with Sharpey's fibre attachment [30]. Histological evaluation suggests that the combined approach compares favourably with other treatment.

## SUCCESS AND FAILURE – AETIOLOGY AND EVALUATION

Although many studies have attempted to determine success–failure rates for periradicular surgery, none have been able to integrate fully all parameters of evaluation with techniques performed, materials used, patient compliance, and clinician expertise, variability and interpretative skills. Attempts at multivariate analysis have provided some trends and correlations, but even these findings may only be applicable to specifically controlled cases [146].

Success (complete healing) with periradicular surgery has been reported to range from very low levels to levels as high as 96.8% [142] using mixed

**Table 9.6** Factors influencing success or failure of periradicular surgery

*Valid causes for surgical failure*
Failure to debride the root canal space thoroughly
Failure to seal the root canal space adequately
Tissue irritation from toxic root canal or root-end fillings
Failure to manage root canal or root-end materials properly
Superimposition of periodontal disease
Longitudinal root fracture
Recurrent cystic lesion
Improper management of the supporting periodontium

*Uncertain causes for surgical failure*
Infected dentinal tubules
Infected periradicular lesion
Failure to use antibiotics when indicated
Accessory or lateral canals
Loss of alveolar bone
Root resorption
Timing of root canal filling (before or during surgery)
Type of root-end filling

**Table 9.7** Clinical evaluation of success and failure

*Clinical success*
No tenderness to percussion or palpation
Normal mobility and function
No sinusitis or paraesthesia
No sinus tract or periodontal pocket
No infection or swelling
Adjacent teeth respond normally to stimuli
Minimal to no scarring or discoloration
No subjective discomfort

*Clinical uncertainty*
Sporadic vague symptoms
Pressure sensation or feeling of fullness
Low grade discomfort on percussion, palpation or chewing
Discomfort with tongue pressure
Superimposed sinusitis focused on treated tooth
Occasional need to use analgesics

*Clinical failure*
Persistent subjective symptoms
Discomfort to percussion and/or palpation
Recurrent sinus tract or swelling
Evidence or irreparable tooth fracture
Excessive mobility or progressive periodontal breakdown
Inability to chew on the tooth

populations, frequently less than ideal percentages of review examinations and short follow-up periods. With longer follow-up periods of up to eight years, a success rate of 91.5% has been achieved [143], which correlates closely with other long-term prospective studies (91.2%) [186]. Whilst significant variability in results makes comparisons of studies questionable, the identification of factors that have contributed to the success or failure of periradicular surgery is essential, and these should be integrated into all phases of case assessment and treatment [90]. Often the aetiology of failure may be difficult to identify, and may encompass the integration of multiple factors. For periradicular surgery, most failures can be attributed to specific causes. At the same time, when failure cannot be explained, speculation may lead to uncertain aetiological factors and treatment. Table 9.6 lists aetiological factors often cited as valid or uncertain in the failure of periradicular surgery.

Evaluation of success or failure following root-end surgery is limited to clinical and radiological examinations. Clinical criteria for success or failure are used most commonly and are integrated with the radiological findings. Clinically patients are classified into one of three categories at the time of review examinations (Table 9.7). Patient assessment, however, must be made after integrating both clinical and radiological parameters of evaluation (Table 9.8). If the only goal of periradicular surgery is to retain the tooth in adequate clinical function [153], then many cases can be classified as successful. Many factors, however, such as case selection, evaluator bias, and patient factors can skew levels of success or failure. Likewise, many clinically symptom-free teeth may have histopathological changes at the root apices along with minimal or extensive radiological changes. Even in the presence of an apparently normal radiological appearance, a clinically symptom-free tooth may exhibit histopathological changes in the periradicular tissues. This is especially true adjacent to resected root surfaces which are difficult to assess radiologically.

## RETREATMENT OF SURGICAL PROCEDURES

Not all surgery is successful, but when a case has been identified as failing it is necessary to use all

**Table 9.8** Radiological evaluation of success and failure

*Radiological success*
Normal periodontal ligament width or slight increase
Normal lamina dura or elimination of radiolucency
Normal to fine-meshed osseous trabeculae
No resorption evident

*Radiological uncertainty*
Slight increase in periodontal ligament width
Slight increase in width of lamina dura
Size of radiolucency static or slight evidence of repair
Radiolucency is circular or asymmetrical
Extension of the periodontal ligament into radiolucency
Evidence of resorption

*Radiological failure*
Increased width of the periodontal ligament and lamina dura
Circular radiolucency with limited osseous trabeculae
Symmetrical radiolucency with funnel-shaped borders
Evidence of resorption

---

**Table 9.9** Causes of surgical failure

*Unsuspected*
Root fracture not readily visible
Post-hole perforation, especially on the buccal or lingual surface
Instrument perforation coronal to the resected root end
Persistent infection in the apically resected tubules
Corrosion of previously placed amalgam root-end filling

*Anatomical*
Fenestrations or dehiscences – loss of marginal bone
Aberrant root anatomy or canal space
Proximity of root of adjacent teeth
Proximity of maxillary sinus

*Technical*
Poor canal cleaning and filling
Inadequate root-end resection
Inadequate root-end preparation and filling
Toxicity of root-end filling material
Improper soft tissue management

---

tests and information available to determine the cause prior to further surgery. Table 9.9 lists some of the more common unsuspected, anatomical and technical causes for failure. Not all of these causes are amenable to further surgery, and a tooth may require extraction and prosthetic replacement.

Very few studies have evaluated the results of periradicular surgery that was performed subsequent to previous surgical failure [112,144]. Success rates of repeat surgery have been 50% or less with little subsequent alteration in healing after one year, but these figures relate to discontinued techniques. In a recent, systematic review and meta-analysis of the outcomes of resurgery [124] there was a near equal distribution of the cases between the three outcome groups: 35.7 % healed successfully, 26.3% healed with uncertain results and 38% did not heal.

The primary reason for failure following periradicular surgery is the presence of infected debris in uncleaned and filled canal space [145,146]. The primary cause for failure with root canal treatment has been identified as coronal leakage due to poor quality of the coronal restoration [134,150]. Therefore, it is essential to access, clean and fill as much of the canal space as possible and to seal thoroughly the coronal aspects of the root canal system before resorting to surgical intervention. Failing to adhere to this will inevitably result in failure.

## REFERENCES

1. Abedi HR, Van Mierlo BL, Wilder-Smith P, Torabinejad M (1995) Effects of ultrasonic root-end cavity preparation on the root apex. *Oral Surgery, Oral Medicine, Oral Pathology, Oral Radiology, Endodontics* **80**, 207–213.
2. Ainamo J, Löe H (1966) Anatomical characteristics of gingiva. A clinical and microscopic study of the free and attached gingiva. *Journal of Periodontology* **37**, 5–13.
3. Aktener BO, Pehlivan Y (1993) Sealing ability of cermet ionomer cement as a retrograde filling material. *International Endodontic Journal* **26**, 137–141.
4. Al-Ajam ADK, McGregor AJ (1993) Comparison of the sealing capabilities of Ketac-silver and extra high copper alloy amalgam when used as retrograde root canal filling. *Journal of Endodontics* **19**, 353–356.
5. Alhadainy HA, Elsaed HY, Elbaghdady YM (1993) An electrochemical study of the sealing ability of different retrofilling materials. *Journal of Endodontics* **19**, 508–511.
6. Altonen M, Mattila K (1976) Follow-up study of apicoectomized molars. *International Journal of Oral Surgery* **5**, 33–40.
7. American Association of Endodontists (1998) *Glossary – Contemporary Terminology for Endodontics*, 6th edn. Chicago, IL, USA: American Association of Endodontists.

8. Andreasen JO (1992) *Atlas of Replantation and Transplantation of Teeth*. Fribourg, Switzerland: Mediglobe, pp. 99–109.

9. Andreasen JO, Munksgaard EC, Fredebo L, Rud J (1993) Periodontal tissue regeneration including cementogenesis adjacent to dentin-bonded retrograde composite filling in humans. *Journal of Endodontics* **19**, 151–153.

10. Andreasen JO, Rud J, Munksgaard EC (1989) Retrograde root obturations using resin and a dentin bonding agent: a preliminary histologic study of tissue reactions in monkeys. *Danish Dental Journal* **93**, 195–197.

11. Arens DE, Adams WR, DeCastro RA (1981) *Endodontic Surgery*. Hagerstown, MD, USA: Harper & Row, pp. 31–55.

12. Aukhil I (1991) Biology of tooth-cell adhesion. *Dental Clinics of North America* **35**, 459–467.

13. Barnes IE (1991) *Surgical Endodontics. A Colour Manual*. Oxford, UK: Butterworth-Heinemann.

14. Barry GN, Heyman RA, Elias A (1975) Comparison of apical sealing methods. A preliminary report. *Oral Surgery, Oral Medicine, Oral Pathology* **39**, 806-811.

15. Beatty R (1986) The effect of reverse filling preparation design on apical leakage. *Journal of Dental Research* **65**, 259. Abstract 805.

16. Bellizzi R, Loushine R (1991) *A Clinical Atlas of Endodontic Surgery*. Chicago, IL, USA: Quintessence, pp. 13–15.

17. Benenati FW, Roane JB, Biggs JT, Simon JH (1986) Recall evaluation of iatrogenic root perforations repaired with amalgam and gutta-percha. *Journal of Endodontics* **12**, 161–166.

18. Bennett CR (1984) *Monheim's Local Anesthesia and Pain Control in Dental Practice*, 7th edn, St. Louis, MO, USA: Mosby, pp. 181–182.

19. Biggs JT, Benenati FW, Sabala CL (1988) Treatment of iatrogenic root perforations with associated osseous lesions. *Journal of Endodontics* **14**, 620–624.

20. Bohning BP, Davenport WD, Jeansonne BG (1999) The effect of guided tissue regeneration on the healing of osseous defects in rat calvaria. *Journal of Endodontics* **25**, 81–84.

21. Bostanci HS, Arpak MN, Gunhan O (1990) New attachment formation following periodontal surgery in a dog. *Journal of Nihon University School of Dentistry* **32**, 159–166.

22. Boyko GA, Brunette DM, Melcher AH (1980) Cell attachment to demineralized root surfaces in vitro. *Journal of Periodontal Research* **15**, 297–303.

23. Brännström M (1984) Smear layer: pathological and treatment considerations. *Operative Dentistry* **Supplement 3**, 35–42.

24. Brännström M, Glantz PO, Nordenvall KJ (1979) The effect of some cleaning solutions on the morphology of dentin prepared in different ways: an in vivo study. *Journal of Dentistry for Children* **46**, 19–23.

25. Buckley JA, Ciancio SG, McMullen JA (1984) Efficacy of epinephrine concentration in local anesthesia during periodontal surgery. *Journal of Periodontology* **55**, 653–657.

26. Byers M, Wheeler EF, Bothwell M (1992) Altered expression of NGF and P75 NGF-receptor by fibroblasts of injured teeth preceeds sensory nerve sprouting. *Growth Factors* **6**, 41–52.

27. Caffesse RG, Mota LF, Quinones CR, Morrison EC (1997) Clinical comparison of resorbable and non-resorbable barriers for guided periodontal tissue regeneration. *Journal of Clinical Periodontology* **24**, 747–752.

28. Callis PD, Santini A (1987) Tissue response to retrograde root fillings in the ferret canine: a comparison of glass ionomer cement and gutta-percha with sealer. *Oral Surgery, Oral Medicine, Oral Pathology* **64**, 475–479.

29. Cambruzzi JV, Marshall FJ (1983) Molar endodontic surgery. *Journal of the Canadian Dental Association* **49**, 61–65.

30. Camelo M, Nevins ML, Lynch SE, Schenk RK, Simion M. Nevins M (2001) Periodontal regeneration with an autogenous bone-Bio-Oss composite graft and a Bio-Gide membrane. *International Journal of Periodontics & Restorative Dentistry* **21**, 109–119.

31. Carr GB (1994) Surgical endodontics. In: Cohen S, Burns R (eds), *Pathways of the Pulp* 6th edn. St. Louis, MO, USA: Mosby-Year Book, pp. 531–567.

32. Carrigan PJ, Morse DR, Furst ML, Sinai IH (1984) A scanning electron microscopic evaluation of human dentinal tubules according to age and location. *Journal of Endodontics* **10,** 359–363.

33. Chong BS, Owadally ID, Pitt Ford TR, Wilson RF (1994) Antibacterial activity of potential retrograde root filling materials. *Endodontics and Dental Traumatology* **10**, 66–70.

34. Chong BS, Pitt Ford TR, Watson TF (1993) Light-cured glass ionomer cement as a retrograde root seal. *International Endodontic Journal* **26**, 218–224.

35. Chong BS, Hudson MB, Pitt Ford TR (2002) Improving the success of apicectomies using Mineral Trioxide Aggregate – preliminary results. *International Endodontic Journal* **35**, 108. Abstract R95.

36. Ciancio SG, Bourgault PC (1989) *Clinical Pharmacology for Dental Professionals*, 3rd edn, Chicago, IL, USA: Year Book Medical, pp. 146–148.

37. Codelli GR, Fry HR, Davis JW (1991) Burnished versus nonburnished application of citric acid to human diseased root surfaces: the effect of time and method of application. *Quintessence International* **22**, 277–283.

38. Craig KR, Harrison JW (1993) Wound healing following demineralization of resected root ends in periradicular surgery. *Journal of Endodontics* **19**, 339–347.

39. Crigger M, Renvert S, Bogle G (1983) The effect of topical citric acid application on surgically exposed periodontal attachment. *Journal of Periodontal Research* **18**, 303–305.

40. Crooks WG, Anderson RW, Powell BJ, Kimbrough WF (1994) Longitudinal evaluation of the seal of IRM root

end fillings. *Journal of Endodontics* **20**, 250–252.

41. Dahlin C, Gottlow J, Linde A, Nyman S (1990) Healing of maxillary and mandibular bone defects using a membrane technique. An experimental study in monkeys. *Scandinavian Journal of Plastic and Reconstructive Surgery and Hand Surgery* **24**, 13–19.

42. Dahlin C, Linde A, Gottlow J, Nyman S. (1988) Healing of bone defects by guided tissue regeneration. *Plastic and Reconstructive Surgery* **81**, 672–676.

43. DeGrood ME, Oguntebi BR, Cunningham CJ, Pink R (1995) A comparison of tissue reactions to Ketac-Fil and amalgam. *Journal of Endodontics* **21**, 65–69.

44. Doornbusch H, Broersma L, Boering G, Wesselink PR (2002) Radiographic evaluation of cases referred for surgical endodontics. *International Endodontic Journal* **35**, 472–477.

45. Dorn SO, Gartner AH (1990) Retrograde filling materials: a retrospective success–failure study of amalgam, EBA, and IRM. *Journal of Endodontics* **16**, 391–393.

46. Douthitt JC, Gutmann JL, Witherspoon DE (2001) Histologic assessment of healing after the use of a bioresorbable membrane in the management of buccal bone loss concomitant with periradicular surgery. *Journal of Endodontics* **27**, 404–410.

47. Dumsha TC, Gutmann JL (1985) Clinical guidelines for intentional replantation. *Compendium of Continuing Education in Dentistry* **6**, 604–608.

48. Finn MD, Schow RS, Schneiderman ED (1992) Osseous regeneration in the presence of four common hemostatic agents. *Journal of Oral and Maxillofacial Surgery* **50**, 608–612.

49. Finne K, Nord PG, Persson G, Lennartsson B (1977) Retrograde root filling with amalgam and Cavit. *Oral Surgery, Oral Medicine, Oral Pathology* **43**, 621–626.

50. Fong CD (1993) A sonic instrument for retrograde preparation. *Journal of Endodontics* **19**, 374–375.

51. Forssell H, Tammisalo T, Forssell K (1988) A follow-up study of apicectomized teeth. *Proceedings of the Finnish Dental Society* **84**, 85–93.

52. Frank AL, Glick DH, Patterson SS, Weine FS (1992) Long-term evaluation of surgically placed amalgam fillings. *Journal of Endodontics* **18**, 391–398.

53. Fuss Z, Assooline LS, Kaufman AY (1996) Determination of location of root perforations by electronic apex locators. *Oral Surgery, Oral Medicine, Oral Pathology, Oral Radiology, Endodontics* **82**, 324–329.

54. Fuss Z, Trope M (1996) Root perforations: classification and treatment choices based on prognostic factors. *Endodontics and Dental Traumatology* **12**, 255–264.

55. Gangarosa LP, Halik FJ (1967) A clinical evaluation of local anaesthetic solutions containing graded epinephrine concentrations. *Archives of Oral Biology* **12**, 611–621.

56. Gilheany PA, Figdor D, Tyas MJ (1994) Apical dentin permeability and microleakage associated with root end resection and retrograde filling. *Journal of Endodontics* **20**, 22–26.

57. Goldberg M (1984) Structures de l'email et de la dentine: effets d'agents demineralisants et incidences sur le collage de biomateriaux. *Actualites Odonto-Stomatologiques* **147**, 411–434.

58. Gottlow J, Nyman S, Karring T, Lindhe J (1984) New attachment formation as the result of controlled tissue regeneration. *Journal of Clinical Periodontology* **11**, 494–503.

59. Gutmann JL (1984) Principles of endodontic surgery for the general practitioner. *Dental Clinics of North America* **28**, 895–908.

60. Gutmann JL (1986) Surgical procedures in endodontic practice. In: Levine N (ed.) *Current Treatment in Dental Practice.* Philadelphia, PA, USA: Saunders, pp. 194–201.

61. Gutmann JL (1992) Clinical, radiographic and histologic perspectives on success and failure in endodontics. *Dental Clinics of North America* **36**, 379–392.

62. Gutmann JL (1993) Parameters of achieving quality anesthesia and hemostasis in surgical endodontics. *Anesthesia and Pain Control in Dentistry* **2**, 223–226.

63. Gutmann JL, Harrison JW (1985) Posterior endodontic surgery: anatomical considerations and clinical techniques. *International Endodontic Journal* **18**, 8–34.

64. Gutmann JL, Harrison JW (1994) *Surgical Endodontics.* St. Louis, MO, USA: Ishiyaku EuroAmerica.

65. Gutmann JL, Pitt Ford TR (1993) Management of the resected root end: a clinical review. *International Endodontic Journal* **26**, 273–283.

66. Gutmann JL, Saunders WP, Nguyen L, Guo IY, Saunders EM (1994) Ultrasonic root-end preparation: part 1. SEM analysis. *International Endodontic Journal* **27**, 318–324.

67. Halse A, Molven O, Grung B (1991) Follow-up after periapical surgery: the value of the one-year control. *Endodontics and Dental Traumatology* **7**, 246–250.

68. Hasse AL, Heng MK, Garret NR (1986) Blood pressure and electocardiographic response to dental treatment with use of local anesthesia. *Journal of the American Dental Association* **113**, 639–642.

69. Hickel R (1988) Erste klinische Ergebnisse von retrograden Wurzelfüllungen mit Cermet-Zement. *Deutsche Zahnärztliche Zeitschrift* **43**, 963–965.

70. Hirsch JM, Ahlström U, Henrikson PÅ, Heyden G, Petersen LE (1979) Periapical surgery. *International Journal of Oral Surgery* **8**, 173–185.

71. Ichesco WR, Ellison RL, Corcoran JF, Krause DC (1991) A spectrophotometric analysis of dentinal leakage in the resected root. *Journal of Endodontics* **17**, 503–507.

72. Ingle JI, Bakland LK (1994) *Endodontics*, 4th edn. Malvern, PA, USA: Williams & Wilkins, pp. 689–763.

73. Jastak JT, Yagiela JA (1983) Vasoconstrictors and local anesthesia: a review and rationale for use. *Journal of the American Dental Association* **107**, 623–630.

74. Jeansonne BG, Boggs WS, Lemon RR (1993) Ferric sulfate hemostasis: effect on osseous wound healing. II. With curettage and irrigation. *Journal of Endodontics* **19**, 174–176.

75. Jesslén P, Zetterqvist L, Heimdahl A (1995) Long-term results of amalgam versus glass ionomer cement as apical sealant after apicectomy. *Oral Surgery, Oral Medicine, Oral Pathology, Oral Radiology, Endodontics* **79**, 101–103.

76. Johnson SA (1991) Periradicular wound healing following the use of IRM as a root-end filling material. Master's Thesis, Baylor University, Texas, USA.

77. Kadohiro G (1984) A comparative study of the sealing quality of zinc-free amalgam and Diaket when used as a retrograde filling material. *Hawaii Dental Journal* **15**, 8–9.

78. Karring T, Nyman S, Gottlow J, Laurell L (1993) Development of the biological concept of guided tissue regeneration – animal and human studies. *Periodontology 2000* **1**, 26–35.

79. Karring T, Nyman S, Lindhe J (1980) Healing following implantation of periodontitis affected roots into bone tissue. *Journal of Clinical Periodontology* **7**, 96–105.

80. Keesling GR, Hinds EC (1963) Optimal concentration of epinephrine in lidocaine solutions. *Journal of the American Dental Association* **66**, 337–340.

81. Kellert M, Chalfin H, Solomon C (1994) Guided tissue regeneration: an adjunct to endodontic surgery. *Journal of the American Dental Association* **125**, 1229–1233.

82. Khoury F, Schulte A, Becker R, Hahn T (1987) Prospektive Vergleichsstudie zwischen prä- und intraoperativer Wurzelfüllung. *Deutsche Zahnärztliche Zeitschrift* **42**, 248–250.

83. Khoury F, Staehle HJ (1987) Retrograde Wurzelfüllungen aus Glasionomerzement. *Deutsche Zeitschrift fur Mund-, Kiefer-, und Gesichts-Chirurgie* **11**, 351–355.

84. Kim S, Pecora G, Rubinstein RA (2001) *Color Atlas of Microsurgery in Endodontics*. St. Louis, MO, USA: Mosby.

85. Knoll-Köhler E, Förtsch G (1992) Pulpal anesthesia dependent on epinephrine dose in 2% lidocaine. *Oral Surgery, Oral Medicine, Oral Pathology* **73**, 537–540.

86. Knoll-Köhler E, Frie A, Becker J, Ohlendorf D (1989) Changes in plasma epinephrine concentration after dental infiltration anesthesia with different doses of epinephrine. *Journal of Dental Research* **68**, 1098–1101.

87. Lee SJ, Monsef M, Torabinejad M (1993) Sealing ability of a mineral trioxide aggregate for repair of lateral root perforations. *Journal of Endodontics* **19**, 541–544.

88. Lemon RR (1992) Nonsurgical repair of perforation defects. Internal matrix concept. *Dental Clinics of North America* **36**, 439–457.

89. Lemon RR, Steele PJ, Jeansonne BG (1993) Ferric sulfate hemostasis: effect on osseous wound healing. I. Left in situ for maximum exposure. *Journal of Endodontics* **19**, 170–173.

90. Lin LM, Pascon EA, Skribner J, Gängler P, Langeland K (1991) Clinical, radiographic, and histologic study of endodontic treatment failures. *Oral Surgery, Oral Medicine, Oral Pathology* **71**, 603–611.

91. Lloyd A (1995) The combined effects of angulation of root-end resection using sonic retro-tips or burs on the linear leakage patterns of root-end filling materials. MScD thesis Cardiff: University of Wales College of Medicine.

92. Lloyd A, Jaunberzins A, Dummer PM, Bryant S (1996) Root-end cavity preparation using the MicroMega Sonic Retro-prep Tip™. SEM analysis. *International Endodontic Journal* **29**, 295–301.

93. Luks S (1956) Root end amalgam technic in the practice of endodontics. *Journal of the American Dental Association* **53**, 424–428.

94. Maalouf EM, Gutmann JL (1994) Biological perspectives on the non-surgical management of periradicular pathosis. *International Endodontic Journal* **27**, 154–162.

95. MacDonald A, Moore BK, Newton CW, Brown CE (1994) Evaluation of an apatite cement as a root end filling material. *Journal of Endodontics* **20**, 598–604.

96. Malamed SF (1990) *Handbook of Local Anesthesia*, 3rd edn. St. Louis, MO, USA: Mosby-Year Book, pp. 25–35.

97. Mälmstrom M, Perkki K, Lundquist K (1982) Apicectomy: a retrospective study. *Proceedings of the Finnish Dental Society* **78**, 26–31.

98. Martell B, Chandler NP (2002) Electrical and dye leakage comparison of three root-end restorative materials. *Quintessence International* **33**, 30–34.

99. Mattila K, Altonen M (1968) A clinical and roentgenological study of apicoectomized teeth. *Odontologisk Tidskrift* **76**, 389-408.

100. Melcher AH (1976) On the repair potential of periodontal tissues. *Journal of Periodontology* **47**, 256–260.

101. Meyers JP, Gutmann JL (1994) Histological healing following surgical endodontics and its implications in case assessment: a case report. *International Endodontic Journal* **27**, 339–342.

102. Mikkonen M, Kullaa-Mikkonen A, Kotilainen R (1983) Clinical and radiologic re-examination of apicoectomized teeth. *Oral Surgery, Oral Medicine, Oral Pathology* **55**, 302–306.

103. Mizunuma T (1986) Relationship between bond strength of resin to dentin and structural change of dentin collagen during etching – influence of ferric chloride to structure of the collagen. *Journal of the Japanese Society of Dental Materials* **5**, 54–64.

104. Molven O, Halse A, Grung B (1987) Observer strategy and the radiographic classification of healing after endodontic surgery. *International Journal of Oral and Maxillofacial Surgery* **16**, 432–439.

105. Molven O, Halse A, Grung B (1991) Surgical management of endodontic failures: indications and treatment results. *International Dental Journal* **41**, 33–42.

106. Molven O, Halse A, Grung B (1996) Incomplete healing (scar tissue) after periapical surgery – radiographic findings 8 to 12 years after treatment. *Journal of Endodontics* **22**, 264–268.

107. Moorehead FB (1927) Root-end resection. *Dental Cosmos* **69**, 463–467.

108. Nedderman TA, Hartwell GR, Portell FR (1988) A comparison of root surfaces following apical root resection with various burs: scanning electron microscope evaluation. *Journal of Endodontics* **14,** 423–427.

109. Nencka D, Walia HD, Austin BP (1995) Histologic evaluation of the biocompatibility of Diaket. *Journal of Dental Research* **74,** 101. Abstract 716.

110. Nery EB, Eslami A, Van Swol RL (1990) Biphasic calcium phosphate ceramic combined with fibrillar collagen with and without citric acid conditioning in the treatment of periodontal osseous defects. *Journal of Periodontology* **61,** 166–172.

111. Nicholls E (1962) Treatment of traumatic perforations of the pulp cavity. *Oral Surgery, Oral Medicine, Oral Pathology* **15,** 603–612.

112. Nordenram Å, Svärdström G (1970) Results of apicectomy. *Swedish Dental Journal* **63,** 593–604.

113. Nyman S, Gottlow J, Karring T, Lindhe J (1982) The regenerative potential of the periodontal ligament. An experimental study in the monkey. *Journal of Clinical Periodontology* **9,** 257–265.

114. O'Connor RP, Hutter JW, Roahen JO (1995) Leakage of amalgam and super-EBA root-end fillings using two preparation techniques and surgical microscopy. *Journal of Endodontics* **21,** 74–78.

115. Olsen FK, Austin BP, Walia H (1994) Osseous reaction to implanted ZOE retrograde filling materials in the tibia of rats. *Journal of Endodontics* **20,** 389–394.

116. Olson AK, MacPherson MG, Hartwell GR, Weller N, Kulild JC (1990) An in vitro evaluation of injectable thermoplasticized gutta-percha, glass ionomer, and amalgam when used as retrofilling materials. *Journal of Endodontics* **16,** 361–364.

117. Oswald RJ (1979) Procedural accidents and their repair. *Dental Clinics of North America* **23,** 593–616.

118. Oynick J, Oynick T (1978) A study of a new material for retrograde fillings. *Journal of Endodontics* **4,** 203–206.

119. Özata F, Erdilek N, Tezel H (1993) A comparative sealability study of different retrofilling materials. *International Endodontic Journal* **26,** 241–245.

120. Pashley DH (1984) Smear layer: physiological considerations. *Operative Dentistry* **Supplement 3,** 13–29.

121. Passanezi E, Alves ME, Janson WA, Ruben MP (1979) Periosteal activation and root demineralization associated with horizontal sliding flap. *Journal of Periodontology* **50,** 384–386.

122. Pecora G, Kim S, Celletti R, Davarpanah M (1995) The guided tissue regeneration principle in endodontic surgery: one-year postoperative results of large periapical lesions. *International Endodontic Journal* **28,** 41–46.

123. Persson G (1982) Periapical surgery of molars. *International Journal of Oral Surgery* **11,** 96–100.

124. Peterson J, Gutmann JL (2001) The outcome of endodontic resurgery: a systematic review. *International Endodontic Journal* **34,** 169–175.

125. Pileggi R, Dermody J, McDonald NJ, DiAndreth M, Turng BF, Minah GE (1995) Apical leakage of ultrasonically cut retro-preparations: a bacterial evaluation. *Journal of Dental Research* **74,** 101 (abstract 718).

126. Pinto VS, Zuolo ML, Mellonig JT (1995) Guided bone regeneration in the treatment of a large periapical lesion: a case report. *Practical Periodontics and Aesthetic Dentistry* **7,** 76–82.

127. Pitt Ford TR, Andreasen JO, Dorn SO, Kariyawasam SP (1994) Effect of IRM root end fillings on healing after replantation. *Journal of Endodontics* **20,** 381–385.

128. Pitt Ford TR, Andreasen JO, Dorn SO, Kariyawasam SP (1995) Effect of super-EBA as a root end filling on healing after replantation. *Journal of Endodontics* **21,** 13–15.

129. Pitt Ford TR, Roberts GJ (1990) Tissue response to glass ionomer retrograde root fillings. *International Endodontic Journal* **23,** 233–238.

130. Polson AM, Proye GT (1983) Fibrin linkage: a precursor for new attachment. *Journal of Periodontology* **54,** 141–147.

131. Powis DR, Folleras T, Merson SA, Wilson AD (1982) Improved adhesion of a glass ionomer cement to dentin and enamel. *Journal of Dental Research* **61,** 1416–1422.

132. Prodger TE, Symonds M (1977) ASPA adhesion study. *British Dental Journal* **143,** 266–270.

133. Rankow HJ, Krasner PR (1996) Endodontic applications of guided tissue regeneration in endodontic surgery. *Journal of Endodontics* **22,** 34–43.

134. Ray HA, Trope M (1995) Periapical status of endodontically treated teeth in relation to the technical quality of the root filling and the coronal restoration. *International Endodontic Journal* **28,** 12–18.

135. Regan JD, Witherspoon DE, Gutmann JL (1998) Prevention, identification and management of tooth perforations. *Endodontic Practice* **1,** 24–43.

136. Regan JD, Gutmann JL, Witherspoon DE (2002) Comparison of Diaket and MTA When used as root-end filling materials to support regeneration of the periradicular tissues. *Int End J* **35,** 840–847.

137. Register AA (1973) Bone and cementum induction by dentin, demineralized in situ. *Journal of Periodontology* **44,** 49–54.

138. Register AA, Burdick FA (1975) Accelerated reattachment with cementogenesis to dentin, demineralized in situ. I. Optimum range. *Journal of Periodontology* **46,** 646–655.

139. Reit C (1987) Decision strategies in endodontics: on the design of a recall program. *Endodontics and Dental Traumatology* **3,** 233–239.

140. Ririe CM, Crigger M, Selvig KA (1980) Healing of periodontal connective tissues following surgical wounding and application of citric acid in dogs. *Journal of Periodontal Research* **15,** 314–327.

141. Roberts DH, Sowray JH (1987) *Local Analgesia in Dentistry,* 2nd edn. Bristol, UK: Wright, pp. 84–88.

142. Rubinstein RA, Kim S (1999) Short-term observation of the results of endodontic surgery with the use of a surgical operation microscope and Super-EBA as root-end filling material. *Journal of Endodontics* **25,** 43–48.

143. Rubinstein RA, Kim S (2002) Long-term follow-up of cases considered healed one year after apical microsurgery. *Journal of Endodontics* **28**, 378–383.

144. Rud J, Andreasen JO (1972) Operative procedures in periapical surgery with contemporaneous root filling. *International Journal of Oral Surgery* **1**, 297–310.

145. Rud J, Andreasen JO (1972) A study of failures after endodontic surgery by radiographic, histologic and stereomicroscopic methods. *International Journal of Oral Surgery* **1**, 311–328.

146. Rud J, Andreasen JO, Möller Jensen JE (1972) A multivariate analysis of the influence of various factors upon healing after endodontic surgery. *International Journal of Oral Surgery* **1**, 258–271.

147. Rud J, Andreasen JO, Rud V (1989) Retrograde root filling utilizing resin and a dentin bonding agent: frequency of healing when compared to retrograde amalgam. *Danish Dental Journal* **93**, 267–273.

148. Rud J, Rud V, Munksgaard EC (1989) Retrograde root filling utilizing resin and a dentin bonding agent: indication and applications. *Danish Dental Journal* **93**, 223–229.

149. Ruse ND, Smith DC (1991) Adhesion to bovine dentin – surface characterization. *Journal of Dental Research* **70**, 1002–1008.

150. Saunders WP, Saunders EM (1994) Coronal leakage as a cause of failure in root-canal therapy: a review. *Endodontics and Dental Traumatology* **10**, 105–108.

151. Saunders WP, Saunders EM, Gutmann JL (1994) Ultrasonic root-end preparation: part 2. Microleakage of EBA root-end fillings *International Endodontic Journal* **27**, 325–329.

152. Scott JN, Zelikow R (1980) Replantation – a clinical philosophy. *Journal of the American Dental Association* **101**, 17–19.

153. Seltzer S (1988) *Endodontology: Biologic Considerations in Endodontic Procedures*, 2nd edn. Philadelphia, PA, USA: Lea & Febiger, pp. 439–470.

154. Sinai IH (1977) Endodontic perforations: their prognosis and treatment. *Journal of the American Dental Association* **95**, 90–95.

155. Skoglund A, Persson G (1985) A follow-up study of apicoectomized teeth with total loss of the buccal bone plate. *Oral Surgery, Oral Medicine, Oral Pathology* **59**, 78–81.

156. Sommer RF (1946) Essentials for successful root resection. *American Journal of Orthodontics and Oral Surgery* **32**, 76–100.

157. Stashenko P (1990) Role of immune cytokines in the pathogenesis of periapical lesions. *Endodontics and Dental Traumatology* **6**, 89–96.

158. Sterrett JD, Delaney B, Rizkalla A, Hawkins CH (1991) Optimal citric acid concentration for dentinal demineralization. *Quintessence International* **22**, 371–375.

159. Sultan M, Pitt Ford TR (1995) Ultrasonic preparation and obturation of root-end cavities. *International Endodontic Journal* **28**, 231–238.

160. Sumi Y, Hattori H, Hayashi K, Ueda M (1996) Ultrasonic root-end preparation: clinical and radiographic evaluation of results. *Journal of Oral and Maxillofacial Surgery* **54**, 590–593.

161. Tang HM, Torabinejad M, Kettering JD (2002) Leakage evaluation of root end filling materials using endotoxin. *Journal of Endodontics* **28**, 5–7.

162. Tetsch P (1974) Development of raised temperatures after osteotomies. *Journal of Maxillofacial Surgery* **2**, 141–145.

163. Tetsch P (1986) *Wurzelspitzenresektionen.* Munchen, Germany: Carl Hanser Verlag, p. 99.

164. Tidmarsh BG, Arrowsmith MG (1989) Dentinal tubules at the root ends of apicected teeth: a scanning electron microscopic study. *International Endodontic Journal* **22**, 184–189.

165. Torabinejad M (1995) Investigation of mineral trioxide aggregate for root-end filling. PhD thesis. London: University of London.

166. Torabinejad M, Higa RK, McKendry DJ, Pitt Ford TR (1994) Dye leakage of four root end filling materials: effects of blood contamination. *Journal of Endodontics* **20**, 159–163.

167. Torabinejad M, Hong CU, Lee SJ, Monsef M, Pitt Ford TR (1995) Investigation of mineral trioxide for root-end filling in dogs. *Journal of Endodontics* **21**, 603–608.

168. Torabinejad M, Wilder-Smith P, Kettering JD, Pitt Ford TR (1995) Comparative investigation of marginal adaptation of mineral trioxide aggregate and other commonly used root-end filling materials. *Journal of Endodontics* **21**, 295–299.

169. Torabinejad M, Pitt Ford TR, McKendry DJ, Abedi HR, Miller DA, Kariyawasam SP (1997) Histologic assessment of mineral trioxide aggregate as a root-end filling in monkeys. *Journal of Endodontics* **23**, 225–228.

170. Torabinejad M, Watson TF, Pitt Ford TR (1993) Sealing ability of a mineral trioxide aggregate when used as a root end filling material. *Journal of Endodontics* **19**, 591–595.

171. Trice FB (1959) Periapical surgery. *Dental Clinics of North America* **3**, 735–748.

172. Trope M, Tronstad L (1985) Long-term calcium hydroxide treatment of a tooth with iatrogenic root perforation and lateral periodontitis. *Endodontics and Dental Traumatology* **1**, 35–38.

173. Troullos ES, Goldstein DS, Hargreaves KM, Dionne RA (1987) Plasma epinephrine levels and cardiovascular response to high administered doses of epinephrine contained in local anesthesia. *Anesthesia Progress* **34**, 10–13.

174. Vertucci FJ, Beatty RG (1986) Apical leakage associated with retrofilling techniques: a dye study. *Journal of Endodontics* **12**, 331–336.

175. von Arx T, Cochran DL (2001) Rationale for the application of the GTR principle using a barrier membrane in endodontic surgery: a proposal of classification and literature review. *International Journal of Periodontics & Restorative Dentistry* **21**, 127–139.

176. Walia HD, Newlin S, Austin BP (1995) Electrochemical analysis of retrofilling microleakage in extracted

human teeth. *Journal of Dental Research* **74**, 101 (abstract 719).

177. Walia H, Strieff J, Gerstein H (1988) Use of a hemostatic agent in the repair of procedural errors. *Journal of Endodontics* **14**, 465-468.

178. Wang T, Nakabayashi N (1991) Effect of 2-(methacryloxy) ethyl phenyl hydrogen phosphate on adhesion to dentin. *Journal of Dental Research* **70**, 59–66.

179. Weine FS (1980) The case against intentional replantation. *Journal of the American Dental Association* **100**, 664–668.

180. Williams SS, Gutmann JL (1993) Healing response to Diaket-tricalcium phosphate root-end fillings. *Journal of Endodontics* **19**, 199 (abstract 61).

181. Witherspoon DE, Gutmann JL (1996) Haemostasis in periradicular surgery. *International Endodontic Journal* **29**, 135–149.

182. Wong WS, Rosenberg PA, Boyland RJ, Schulman A (1994) A comparison of the apical seals achieved using retrograde amalgam fillings and the Nd:YAG laser. *Journal of Endodontics* 20, 595–597.

183. Wuchenich G, Meadows D, Torabinejad M (1994) A comparison between two root end preparation techniques in human cadavers. *Journal of Endodontics* **20**, 279–282.

184. Zetterqvist L, Anneroth G, Nordenram A (1987) Glass-ionomer cement as retrograde filling material: an experimental investigation in monkeys. *International Journal of Oral and Maxillofacial Surgery* **16**, 459–464.

185. Zetterqvist L, Hall G, Holmlund A (1991) Apicectomy: a clinical comparison of amalgam and glass ionomer cement as apical sealants. *Oral Surgery, Oral Medicine, Oral Pathology* **71**, 489–491.

186. Zuolo ML, Ferreira MO, Gutmann JL (2000) Prognosis in periradicular surgery: a clinical prospective study. *International Endodontic Journal* **33**, 91–98.

# Endodontics in children

## C. Mason

Introduction 183

**Treatment of primary teeth** 183
   Indirect pulp capping 184
   Direct pulp capping 184
   Vital pulpotomy 185
   Formocresol pulpotomy 185
   Alternative pulpotomy medicaments 186
   Pulpectomy 187

**Treatment of immature permanent teeth** 188
   Treatment of vital teeth with open apices 188
   Treatment of non-vital teeth with open apices 189
   Surgical treatment 191

**References** 191

## INTRODUCTION

The basic aims of endodontic treatment in children are similar to those for the adult patient: prevention and treatment of apical periodontitis. The relief of pain, and the control of sepsis in the pulp and surrounding periradicular tissues are additional objectives. When deciding on a suitable treatment plan for primary teeth, consideration should be given to the maintenance of arch length; it is generally accepted that primary molar teeth in particular should be retained until they exfoliate naturally to avoid loss of space and crowding of the permanent dentition. Due to the morphological and physiological differences between primary and permanent teeth, techniques and medicaments for endodontic treatment vary.

Endodontic treatment for permanent teeth with immature roots also presents problems which require special techniques. Efforts should first be directed to maintaining pulp vitality, where possible, to allow maturation. Successful obturation of an immature root canal can be complicated and time-consuming.

## TREATMENT OF PRIMARY TEETH

Primary teeth differ morphologically from their permanent successors both in shape and size [14]. Primary molars have fine tapered roots which are flattened mesiodistally to enclose a ribbon-like root canal. Their pulp chambers are relatively larger, and their enamel and dentine are thinner than in permanent teeth. The single root canal may become partially calcified with age [31], to produce several intercommunicating canals, thus making instrumentation of the radicular pulp space difficult. Many lateral canals have been reported to exist in the furcation of primary molar teeth [78], and these may contribute to the early spread of infection from the pulp chamber to the inter-radicular area.

The diagnosis of pulp disease is especially difficult in young patients because they are usually unable to give an accurate account of their symptoms. The diagnosis is dependent on the combination of a good history, clinical and radiological examinations, and special tests. The clinical examination should include looking for abnormal tooth mobility, discharging sinus tracts and tenderness to pressure. In primary teeth and newly erupted permanent teeth, assessment of vitality has been shown to be an unreliable guide to the histological status of the pulp [42,51]. Tests carried out with an electric pulp tester involve a gradually increasing current applied to the tooth and rely on conduction along nerve pathways. False positive results are common, and care must be taken to avoid metal restorations. Extensively necrotic pulps may also still have intact nerve pathways. As with all non-invasive special investigations, the contralateral and adjacent teeth should be tested, preferably before the suspect tooth. This enables the young patient to have some experience of the sensation felt and may help to allay anxiety. Young patients may give a positive response in an attempt to please.

Recent developments in assessing pulp vitality include laser Doppler flowmetry. This was originally developed to measure blood flow in skin and other organs [33], and later applied to testing pulp vitality [26]. Advantages include non-invasiveness, no resultant pain and direct assessment of blood flow in the pulp. In addition, no reliance is placed on patients to relate their feelings, and this is especially of benefit in children. The present equipment is expensive and the technique is time-consuming; specific versions for routine dental use are not yet available.

Preoperative radiological examination is essential to eliminate local contraindications to root canal treatment, such as gross canal destruction, advanced internal or external root resorption, and marked alveolar bone loss.

General contraindications to treatment may include poor patient cooperation and lack of parental motivation. A history of a cardiac or renal condition where it is essential to avoid infection would indicate extraction of primary teeth rather than endodontic treatment. Patients who are immunocompromised, as a result of either disease or drug therapy, will also need careful assessment, and extraction of primary teeth is usually the treatment of choice.

The treatment techniques that have been advocated for use on primary teeth may be grouped as follows:

- indirect pulp capping;
- direct pulp capping;
- vital pulpotomy (one or two visits);
- pulpectomy (one or two visits).

In all cases, the administration of local anaesthesia and adequate tooth isolation, normally with rubber dam, are advised. For maxillary teeth, infiltration anaesthesia is usually satisfactory, whereas a block injection or intraligamentary infiltration is more likely to eliminate pain when pulp treatment is carried out on vital mandibular primary molar teeth.

## Indirect pulp capping

This is the term used to describe the placement of a dressing over residual hard carious dentine in an attempt to allow secondary dentine to be formed within the pulp chamber [70]. Pulpal exposure is therefore avoided in teeth with deep carious lesions when there is no clinical or radiological evidence of pulpal degeneration or periradicular disease. Contraindications to this method of treatment include a history of spontaneous pain, associated swelling, tenderness to biting, or mobility. Likewise, preoperative radiographs must be examined for root resorption, pulp calcifications or periradicular radiolucency, which if present, would necessitate more extensive treatment.

At the initial visit, all soft carious dentine is removed with a slow running bur or a hand excavator. The amelodentinal junction must be free from all softened and stained carious dentine. The area of dentine over the site of a potential pulpal exposure is covered with a layer of setting cement containing calcium hydroxide (e.g. Dycal, Caulk, Milford, DE, USA), and sealed with an overlying structural base of a quick-setting, reinforced zinc oxide–eugenol preparation (e.g. IRM, Dentsply, Konstanz, Germany). The final restoration can then be placed. A success rate of 92% for indirect pulp capping with calcium hydroxide in primary incisors followed for 42 months has been reported [6]. Hence, for primary teeth, regular review of vitality is preferable to subjecting the patient to subsequent re-entry into the tooth as was formerly advocated. Some operators prefer to use a zinc oxide–eugenol preparation alone for indirect pulp capping [35].

## Direct pulp capping

Direct pulp capping is generally not advocated for primary teeth. Inflammation within the pulp can persist and is followed by necrosis or internal resorption. The only possible application of the technique is when pulp tissue has been mechanically exposed as a result of cavity preparation [58]. Calcium hydroxide is placed on the exposure and encourages formation of a dentine bridge below the exposure site in an attempt to maintain pulp vitality. The technique should not be used for carious exposures. The exposure site should be gently irrigated with a non-irritant solution, e.g. saline, to remove any debris that may impede healing and also to keep the pulp moist. The capping material should be flowed gently over the exposure and allowed to set. Various capping materials have been employed. Calcium hydroxide, used alone or together with zinc oxide–eugenol, has been most widely investigated [65,73]. Other materials, e.g. antibiotic and steroid preparations, polycarboxylate cement and formocresol, have also been used, without notable success. The use of dentine bonding systems has been advocated by some authors and preliminary results have been promising [38,58]. The advantage is that a polymeric film can be layered over an exposure site without displacing the pulp and onto surrounding dentine where it permeates the tubules. Further work is required before these materials can be strongly recommended as capping agents. Following pulp capping and final restoration, the tooth should be monitored clinically and radiologically for any signs of subsequent pulp necrosis or resorption.

## Vital pulpotomy

This technique involves removal of the entire coronal pulp that has undergone irreversible inflammatory change or necrosis, leaving remaining vital tissue intact within the root canals. The cut radicular pulp stumps are covered with a medicament which will result in either healing or 'fixation' of the tissue beyond the interface of dressing and radicular pulp. Pulpotomy provides the most suitable method for treating carious exposures in primary teeth which have been without a history of swelling, sinus tract or any evidence of internal or external root resorption.

Electrosurgery may be used for pulpotomy procedures, as the main advantage is that the need for any potentially toxic medicament can be avoided. However, when electrosurgery was used to remove the entire coronal pulp and treat the remaining stumps, root resorption occurred [71]. An alternative method may be to remove the coronal pulp mechanically and treat the remaining pulp stumps electrosurgically [61], in order to avoid

excessive heat dissipation. Although a clinical and radiological success rate of 99% has been demonstrated at two years [43], the electrosurgical pulpotomy technique is still experimental. Lasers have been suggested as an alternative instrument but studies have shown carbonization, necrosis and inflammation of the pulp with little evidence of repair [34,58,69].

## Formocresol pulpotomy

Buckley [5] formulated a solution containing equal parts of formalin and tricresol. A commercial solution containing 19% formaldehyde, 35% cresol in a glycerine/water vehicle (Buckley's formocresol, Cosby laboratories, Burbank, CA, USA), was later developed as a suitable medicament for the treatment of pulpally exposed primary teeth. The aim of this treatment technique is to fix the coronal portion of the radicular pulp and maintain vitality of the remaining apical portion [72]. Formocresol acts through its aldehyde group and binds to the amino acids of protein and bacteria to prevent autolysis and hydrolysis so rendering tissue inert [40]. The use of formocresol for pulpotomy has recently been reviewed [58,75].

Over the years, there has been increasing concern about the toxicity, both local and systemic, of formocresol. Experimental evidence has shown that sufficient formocresol was absorbed systemically from multiple pulpotomy sites in one dog to induce early tissue injury in the kidneys and liver [52–54]. However, with the quantity normally used in man, the risk is much less and therefore negligible. A definite relationship between formocresol pulpotomies in primary teeth and enamel defects on their permanent successors has been demonstrated [57], but not confirmed in subsequent studies [50,60]. In addition, carcinogenic and mutagenic properties have been recognized, which together with local and systemic effects, have led to extensive investigation of the efficacy of a diluted solution. Clinical studies have confirmed that a 1:5 dilution is equally effective and should be used routinely [20,49]. The solution may be prepared by first making up a diluent solution of three parts glycerine with one part distilled water. To this is then added one part concentrated formocresol, and mixed thoroughly.

*One-visit formocresol pulpotomy*

Originally, a three- to five-stage procedure was described [72,75], but in recent years it has become preferable to complete the pulpotomy procedure in a single visit [59], provided adequate analgesia has been achieved. The one-visit formocresol pulpotomy (Fig. 10.1) entails the application of a pledget of cotton wool moistened with the medicament to the cut pulp stumps, after removal of the coronal pulp and arrest of haemorrhage. The pledget is left in situ for 3–5 min, although a 1-min application has been recommended [39]. Following this, the amputated pulp tissue appears black. A zinc oxide–eugenol dressing is then prepared and pressed into the chamber, before final restoration of the tooth with a stainless steel crown. It is unnecessary to incorporate formocresol into this zinc oxide–eugenol sub-base [2]. A clinical success rate of 94% in pulpotomized primary teeth using a one-fifth diluted formocresol solution followed up for 4–36 months has been achieved [20].

*Two-visit formocresol pulpotomy*

With this technique (Fig. 10.1), the formocresol pledget is sealed in the pulp chamber for a period of one week, and at the second visit the procedure is completed as for the one-visit pulpotomy. This may be preferable for uncooperative patients as appointment times are reduced, or in cases where a hyperaemic pulp is encountered, or inadequate analgesia has been achieved.

Whichever technique is used, the final restoration of choice is a full coverage stainless steel crown, as this minimizes the risks of fracture and microleakage, and hence enhances the prognosis.

## Alternative pulpotomy medicaments

*Glutaraldehyde*

Glutaraldehyde has been investigated as an alternative 'fixing' medicament to formocresol because of its low toxicity [67]. Glutaraldehyde is a larger

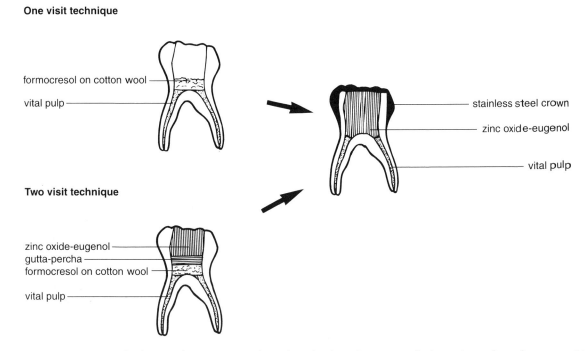

**One visit technique**

formocresol on cotton wool

vital pulp

stainless steel crown

zinc oxide-eugenol

vital pulp

**Two visit technique**

zinc oxide-eugenol
gutta-percha
formocresol on cotton wool

vital pulp

**Figure 10.1** Formocresol pulpotomy for a primary molar with vital pulp in the root canals. It may be performed as a one-visit or two-visit procedure.

molecule than formaldehyde, and as a result diffusion through the tissues is reduced. When 2% unbuffered glutaraldehyde was used, over 96% clinical success was reported after 42 months [24,25]. A 90% clinical success rate was achieved after one year, when 2% buffered glutaraldehyde had been applied for 5 min [22]. After two years there was a failure rate of 18%, as a result of internal resorption [21].

Although glutaraldehyde is potentially a possible replacement for formocresol, questions are still raised about its safety [75]. On a weight for weight basis there is little difference in toxicity between formocresol and glutaraldehyde [13].

## Ferric sulphate

Ferric sulphate is commonly used in dentistry for control of bleeding during surgery or for gingival retraction. When applied directly to pulp tissue, a ferric ion-protein complex is formed which blocks the cut vessels mechanically. Although not a fixative, having only bacteriostatic properties, ferric sulphate is used to control haemorrhage by gentle intermittent application. A zinc oxide–eugenol base is then used to cover the pulp stumps, prior to restoration. A better clinical success rate was reported after one year when 15.5% ferric sulphate was used compared with 1:5 diluted formocresol [12]. In a more recent study there was no difference between the two medicaments [17]. Following these promising results, this technique was subjected to further clinical investigation with a longer follow-up period, and performed well [18]. The shorter application time compared with formocresol has clear advantages when treating children.

## Calcium hydroxide

Although the application of pure calcium hydroxide to the cut pulp stumps after haemorrhage control was previously favoured for pulpotomy of primary teeth [3], the work of Magnusson [45] cast doubt on the use of this material in primary teeth. However, later studies would indicate that if a carefully controlled technique is used then calcium hydroxide may produce long-term results which are comparable with those obtained when formocresol is used [65,73]. Calcium hydroxide in its pure powder form is a clinically acceptable alternative when strict selection criteria are used [76]. The critical factor is

the level of inflammation in the pulp and attempts have been made to assess this objectively by measuring prostaglandin levels [77]. However, this work is still experimental.

## Mineral trioxide aggregate (MTA)

This material was shown to be more successful than calcium hydroxide in pulp capping [56]. More recently it was reported as an alternative to formocresol in pulpotomies in primary teeth [11].

## Bone morphogenic proteins (BMPs)

This family of growth factors was discovered by the observation that demineralized bone matrix could stimulate new bone when implanted in an ectopic site such as muscle [74]. Following the development of molecular biology, these factors could be isolated and their physiological roles investigated. A number of BMPs are capable of inducing reparative dentine and recombinant human BMPs have been used experimentally [55]. These materials would have clear advantages in pulpotomy techniques, producing a biological barrier without concern regarding toxicity.

## Pulpectomy

Non-vital primary teeth may be retained successfully when this technique is employed. Pulpal necrosis, alveolar swelling, inter-radicular or peri-radicular radiolucency are not contraindications to treatment; root canal treatment provides the most satisfactory method of retaining the restorable primary tooth where extraction remains the only other option. The whole procedure can be completed in one visit where there is no abscess, or over two visits when acute discharge is present. In this situation, a cotton pledget containing a medicament, e.g. formocresol, should be sealed into the pulp chamber for one week, after canal preparation, and prior to obturation. There is no consensus as to the preferred filling material, but absorbable materials based on zinc oxide–eugenol, calcium hydroxide and iodoform paste have been used [39].

Once any initial pain or swelling has been relieved, an access cavity is prepared under rubber dam isolation. The use of local anaesthesia is recommended as some vital tissue could still be encountered in one of the root canals. Any pulp tissue in the root canals is removed using fine barbed broaches, or files, and the canals are prepared with files to within 2 mm of the apices. Dilute sodium hypochlorite solution should be used to irrigate the canals and achieve chemical dissolution of any remaining pulp. Finally, the canals should be flushed thoroughly and dried. The chosen filling material should be mixed to a creamy consistency and carried into the canals using a pressure syringe, Lentulo spiral root canal filler, or, if mixed to a stiffer consistency, packed into the canal with a plugger. Various filling techniques including the Lentulo spiral filler and the Jiffy tube pressure syringe have been compared for filling root canals of primary teeth, and the Lentulo spiral performed best [1]. After root canal filling, the pulp chamber should be packed with a suitable cement, and the tooth restored with a stainless steel crown. Pulpectomies were compared using zinc oxide–eugenol and KRI paste in 139 primary molars [32]. Both pastes were introduced into root canals with a Lentulo spiral filler. The follow-up period extended between six months and seven years, with the overall success rate for KRI paste being better than that for zinc oxide–eugenol.

Pulpectomy can also be considered to be an alternative to current pulpotomy techniques when treating vital primary teeth with carious exposure, as it eliminates the need for potentially toxic aldehyde containing compounds, and can be completed in one visit.

## TREATMENT OF IMMATURE PERMANENT TEETH

Current treatment strategies for immature teeth in which the pulp has been exposed are conservative, and have as their ultimate objective the maintenance of vitality of the radicular pulp to allow root formation to be completed. It is essential to assess the restorability of the tooth and to assess the patient orthodontically.

### Treatment of vital teeth with open apices

Traumatic pulp exposure in an immature permanent tooth with a good blood supply leads initially to local haemorrhage in the tissue immediately beneath the exposure site, followed by superficial inflammation. The wound is subsequently covered with fibrin [41]. If the inflamed tissue is removed to a level where healthy pulp is encountered, a dressing of calcium hydroxide placed over the cut pulp will ultimately cause induction of hard tissue and dentine formation by newly differentiated odontoblasts [64].

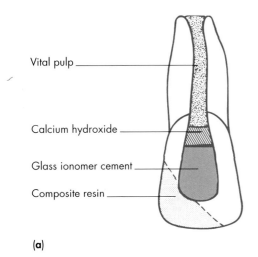

Vital pulp

Calcium hydroxide

Glass ionomer cement

Composite resin

(a)

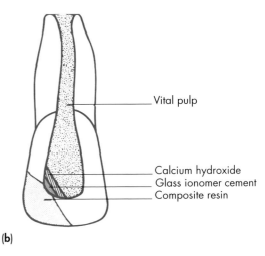

Vital pulp

Calcium hydroxide
Glass ionomer cement
Composite resin

(b)

**Figure 10.2** (**a**) Coronal pulpotomy for an immature incisor with extensive damage to the coronal pulp. (**b**) partial pulpotomy when pulp damage is superficial.

## Pulpotomy

This may be performed at various levels, depending on the size of the exposure and the condition of the pulp observed at the initial exposure site. The classic operation (Fig. 10.2) refers to the removal of the coronal pulp to the cervical region [46].

## Partial (or Cvek) pulpotomy

A more conservative approach to pulpotomy in those cases where a small exposure is found has been proposed [28]. In this technique (Fig. 10.2) the pulp immediately adjacent to the exposure site should be removed to a depth of 2 mm with an adequately cooled diamond bur in a turbine handpiece. This partial amputation is followed by irrigation with saline and arrest of haemorrhage with cotton-wool pledgets or blunt-ended paper points. If bleeding at the exposure site cannot be controlled, it is likely that inflamed pulp tissue remains; therefore a further deeper cut should be performed. Calcium hydroxide powder mixed with water to form a stiff paste (or a calcium hydroxide base material) is placed against the cut pulp tissue, before restoring the tooth with glass ionomer covered by composite resin retained by etched enamel. Within 6–8 weeks, calcific tissue is usually evident adjacent to the site of pulp amputation [4].

The size of the pulpal exposure and the interval between accident and treatment are not critical for healing, hence extensive exposures for long periods of time are no longer a contraindication to pulpotomy in immature permanent incisors [8]. A success rate of over 90% has been reported in other studies [19,23], where permanent teeth were treated by pulpotomy, with the time elapsing between trauma and treatment varying from one to 14 days.

The tooth should be kept under review clinically and radiologically at six months, and then at annual intervals to assess continued pulp vitality and normal root development. Calcification within the root canal may be observed, but this is no longer an indication for the removal of the remaining pulp tissue followed by root canal treatment.

## Partial pulpotomy in carious immature teeth

A pulp exposed by caries in a newly erupted permanent tooth is a problem for which extraction is occasionally the most appropriate solution; this depends on orthodontic considerations. If the preferred option is to retain the tooth, methods have been developed to maintain pulp vitality allowing continued root development. When calcium hydroxide was used for pulpotomy in immature posterior teeth with carious exposures a high frequency of pulpal healing was reported [47]. Removal of the superficial layer of the pulp beneath the exposure site, with a diamond bur in a turbine handpiece, is recommended. The wound is then dressed with calcium hydroxide following haemostasis, and sealed with zinc oxide–eugenol cement before an overlying restoration is placed. Although very promising, further corroborative studies are required [15,47].

## Treatment of non-vital teeth with open apices

The objective of endodontic treatment for non-vital teeth with immature roots is essentially the same as that for conventional root canal treatment, namely to produce a filling which seals the canal system. However, in immature incisor teeth, the root canal may diverge towards the apex and is oval in cross-section, with a greater labiopalatal than mesiodistal dimension. The apical foramen is patent to varying degrees from nearly closed, to a widely divergent or 'blunderbuss' type. The walls of the root canal are often very thin in the case of a newly erupted immature tooth, and may be further weakened during mechanical preparation of the root canal. In addition, a relatively short root presents an adverse crown : root ratio for the subsequent coronal restoration.

Theoretical considerations would suggest that continued root growth with histologically normal dentine and cementum is only possible in those cases where the epithelial root sheath of Hertwig has retained its function. Thus when a chronically infected immature tooth is treated, the only type of root-end closure that may be anticipated is calcific occlusion. This has been shown to be the result of dystrophic calcifications, formed within apical granulation tissue, which coalesce to form a corporate mass, continuous with the predentine at the root apex [10]. However, some teeth which do not respond to conventional vitality testing techniques are shown to have vital tissue towards the root apex when instrumentation is carried out within the root canal. For practical purposes, the treatment in each case is virtually identical, i.e. to clean the root canal and to deliver calcium hydroxide to within 1–2 mm of the root apex, so as to encourage either root growth or apical repair [62]. The tooth is opened on the palatal aspect to give adequate access to the root canal, and necrotic tissue removed with barbed broaches or files to within 1 mm of the root apex. The walls of the canals may then be gently cleaned using either hand files or an ultrasonically operated file. It is important at this stage to avoid disruption of the apical tissues so all instrumentation should be carefully controlled short of the apical foramen.

After irrigation with 2% sodium hypochlorite [48] followed by sterile water and drying with paper points, the root canal is filled with a thick aqueous slurry of calcium hydroxide, or a commercial product (e.g. Hypocal, Elman, New York, NY, USA, or Calasept, Scania Dental AB, Knivsta, Sweden). Calcium hydroxide is now widely recommended as the sole root canal dressing (Fig. 10.3) [29]. The quality of canal filling with calcium hydroxide should be checked radiologically, before sealing the access cavity with a fortified zinc oxide–eugenol cement. The patient should be reviewed at 1, 3, 6 and 12 months. The frequency of changing the calcium hydroxide dressing varies between authors: at one month and then six-monthly [27], or only if absorbed in the apical third [16,29, 37,79]. Recent work suggests that if the calcium hydroxide is changed more frequently, the length of time to form an apical barrier is reduced. Dressing changes are recommended at three-monthly intervals by these authors or if the temporary filling has failed [36,44]. Further prospective studies with large numbers of subjects are required to determine the optimum frequency. The better condensed the initial dressing, the less likely it will need to be replaced at each follow-up visit. The time taken for a mechanically detectable calcific barrier to form has been shown to vary between 9 and 18 months [7,68,79].

When a barrier appears to have formed radiologically, the tooth should be reisolated and opened, the dressing should be washed out and dried, prior to checking for apical closure by probing with a file. The root canal should be filled with gutta-percha and sealer, using a condensation technique that fills the canal both laterally and apically. The available filling techniques are customized gutta-percha points, lateral condensation, vertical condensation and thermoplastic delivery (Fig. 10.3) [29,30].

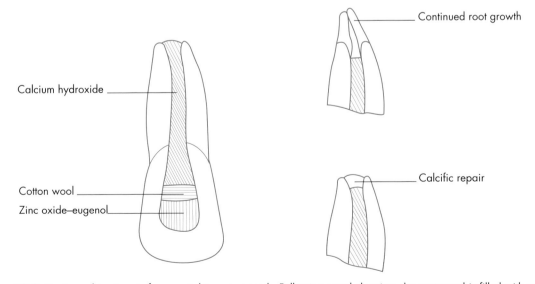

**Figure 10.3** Root canal treatment of a non-vital immature tooth. Following canal cleaning, the root canal is filled with calcium hydroxide. Either continued root growth or calcific repair may occur.

Since apical closure can be time-consuming using conventional calcium hydroxide therapy, alternative techniques have been investigated. Mineral trioxide aggregate (MTA) is a new material being used for pulp capping and apexification. The main components of MTA are calcium silicate and calcium oxide. The material has a long setting time (3–4 h), is uninhibited by moisture and has a compressive strength equal to IRM [63,66]; MTA is biocompatible and cementum has been shown to grow over its surface when used for root surface repair. The technique for apexification involves using calcium hydroxide for one week to disinfect the canal, followed by placement of MTA as an apical plug. The canal may be filled with gutta-percha one week later or when any apical area has healed [63,66].

The prognosis for root-filled immature teeth depends on the degree of immaturity of the root. The thinner the root canal walls, the more likely is fracture to occur [9].

## Surgical treatment

If attempts to induce root-end closure are ultimately unsuccessful, as for example when a persisting sinus tract is present, then a surgical approach is indicated. In an apprehensive child it may be necessary to carry this out under sedation or general anaesthesia; and consent for all eventualities should be obtained. Surgery may be necessary to look for a longitudinal root fracture; if present, the tooth would need to be extracted. When surgery is to be undertaken, the root canal is normally filled with gutta-percha beforehand, and the root canal filling cut back during surgery so that a root-end filling of MTA can be placed. Further details of endodontic surgery are given in Chapter 9.

## REFERENCES

1. Aylard SR, Johnson R (1987) Assessment of filling techniques for primary teeth. *Pediatric Dentistry* **9**, 195–198.
2. Beaver HA, Kopel HM, Sabes WR (1966) The effect of zinc oxide–eugenol on a formocresolized pulp. *Journal of Dentistry for Children* **33**, 381–396.
3. Berk H (1950) Effect of calcium-hydroxide methyl cellulose paste on the dental pulp. *Journal of Dentistry for Children* **17**, 65–68.
4. Brännström M, Nyborg H, Strömberg T (1979) Experiments with pulp capping. *Oral Surgery, Oral Medicine, Oral Pathology* **48**, 347–352.
5. Buckley JP (1904) A rational treatment for putrescent pulps. *Dental Review* **18**, 1193–1197.
6. Coll JA, Josell S, Nassof S, Shelton P, Richards MA (1988) An evaluation of pulpal therapy in primary incisors. *Pediatric Dentistry* **10**, 178–184.
7. Cvek M (1972) Treatment of non-vital permanent incisors with calcium hydroxide. I. Follow-up of periapical repair and apical closure of immature roots. *Odontologisk Revy* **23**, 27–44.
8. Cvek M (1978) A clinical report on partial pulpotomy and capping with calcium hydroxide in permanent incisors with complicated crown fracture. *Journal of Endodontics* **4**, 232–237.
9. Cvek M (1992) Prognosis of luxated non-vital maxillary incisors treated with calcium hydroxide and filled with gutta-percha. A retrospective clinical study. *Endodontics and Dental Traumatology* **8**, 45–55.
10. Dylewski JJ (1971) Apical closure of nonvital teeth. *Oral Surgery, Oral Medicine, Oral Pathology* **32**, 82–89.
11. Eidelman E, Holan G, Fuks AB (2001) Mineral trioxide aggregate vs. formocresol in pulpotomized primary molars: a preliminary report. *Pediatric Dentistry* **23**, 15–18.
12. Fei AL, Udin RD, Johnson R (1991) A clinical study of ferric sulfate as a pulpotomy agent in primary teeth. *Pediatric Dentistry* **13**, 327–332.
13. Feigal RJ, Messer HH (1990) A critical look at glutaraldehyde. *Pediatric Dentistry* **12**, 69–71.
14. Finn SB (1973) *Clinical Pedodontics*, 4th edn. Philadelphia, PA, USA: Saunders, p. 217.
15. Fong CD, Davis MJ (2002) Partial pulpotomy for immature permanent teeth, its present and future. *Pediatric Dentistry* **24**, 29–32.
16. Foreman PC, Barnes IE (1990) A review of calcium hydroxide. *International Endodontics Journal* **23**, 283–297.
17. Fuks AB, Holan G, Davis J, Eidelman E (1994) Ferric sulfate versus diluted formocresol in pulpotomized primary molars: preliminary report. *Pediatric Dentistry* **16**, 158–159 (Abstract).
18. Fuks AB, Holan G, Davis JM, Eidelman E (1997) Ferric sulfate versus dilute formocresol in pulpotomized primary molars: long-term follow up. *Pediatric Dentistry* **19**, 327–330.
19. Fuks AB, Bielak S, Chosak A (1982) Clinical and radiographic assessment of direct pulp capping and pulpotomy in young permanent teeth. *Pediatric Dentistry* **4**, 240–244.
20. Fuks AB, Bimstein E (1981) Clinical evaluation of diluted formocresol pulpotomies in primary teeth of school children. *Pediatric Dentistry* **3**, 321–324.
21. Fuks AB, Bimstein E, Guelmann M, Klein H (1990) Assessment of a 2 percent buffered glutaraldehyde solution in pulpotomized primary teeth of schoolchildren. *Journal of Dentistry for Children* **57**, 371–375.
22. Fuks AB, Bimstein E, Klein H (1986) Assessment of a 2% buffered glutaraldehyde solution in pulpotomized

primary teeth of school children: a preliminary report. *Journal of Pedodontics* **10**, 323–330.

23. Fuks AB, Chosack A, Klein H, Eidelman E (1987) Partial pulpotomy as a treatment alternative for exposed pulps in crown-fractured permanent incisors. *Endodontics and Dental Traumatology* **3**, 100–102.

24. Garcia-Godoy F (1983) Clinical evaluation of glutaraldehyde pulpotomies in primary teeth. *Acta Odontologica Pediatrica* **4**, 41–44.

25. Garcia-Godoy F (1986) A 42 month clinical evaluation of glutaraldehyde pulpotomies in primary teeth. *Journal of Pedodontics* **10**, 148–155.

26. Gazelius B, Olgart L, Edwall B, Edwall L (1986) Non-invasive recording of blood flow in human dental pulp. *Endodontics and Dental Traumatology* **2**, 219–221.

27. Ghose LJ, Baghdady VS, Hikmat YM (1987) Apexification of immature apices of pulpless permanent anterior teeth with calcium hydroxide. *Journal of Endodontics* **13**, 285–290.

28. Granath LE. Hagman G (1971) Experimental pulpotomy in human bicuspids with reference to cutting technique. *Acta Odontologica Scandinavica* **29**, 155–163.

29. Gutmann JL, Heaton JF (1981) Management of the open apex. 2. Non-vital teeth. *International Endodontic Journal* **14** 173–178.

30. Gutmann JL, Rakusin H (1987) Perspectives on root canal obturation with thermoplasticized injectable gutta-percha. *International Endodontic Journal* **20**, 261–270.

31. Hibbard ED, Ireland RL (1957) Morphology of the root canals of the primary molar teeth. *Journal of Dentistry for Children* **24**, 250–257.

32. Holan G, Fuks AB (1993) A comparison of pulpectomies using ZOE and KRI paste in primary molars: a retrospective study. *Pediatric Dentistry* **15**, 403–407.

33. Holloway GA (1983) Laser doppler measurement of cutaneous blood flow. In: Rolfe P (ed.) *Non-invasive Physiological Measurements*, Vol 2. London, UK: Academic Press, pp. 219–249.

34. Jukic S, Anic I, Koba K, Najzar-Fleger D, Matsumoto K (1997) The effect of pulpotomy using $CO_2$ and Nd:YAG lasers on dental pulp tissue. *International Endodontic Journal* **30**, 175–180.

35. King JB, Crawford JJ, Lindahl RL (1965) Indirect pulp capping: a bacteriologic study of deep carious dentine in human teeth. *Oral Surgery, Oral Medicine, Oral Pathology* **20**, 663–671.

36. Kinirons MJ, Srinivasan V, Welbury RR, Finucane D (2001) A study in two centres of variations in the time of apical barrier detection and barrier position in nonvital immature permanent incisors. *International Journal of Paediatric Dentistry* **11**, 447–451.

37. Kleier DJ, Barr ES (1991) A study of endodontically apexified teeth. *Endodontics and Dental Traumatology* **7**, 112–117.

38. Kopel HM (1997) The pulp capping procedure in primary molar teeth 'revisited'. *ASDC Journal of Dentistry for Children* **65**, 327–333.

39. Kopel HM (1994) Pediatric endodontics. In: Ingle JI,

Bakland LK (eds) *Endodontics*, 4th edn. Malvern, PA, USA: Williams and Wilkins pp. 835–867.

40. Loos PJ, Han SS (1971) An enzyme histochemical study of the effect of various concentrations of formocresol on connective tissues. *Oral Surgery, Oral Medicine, Oral Pathology* **31**, 571–585.

41. Luostarinen V (1971) Dental pulp response to trauma. An experimental study in the rat. *Suomen Hammaslaakariseuran Toimituksia* **67**, **Supplement 2**, 3–74.

42. McDonald RE (1956) Diagnostic aids and vital pulp therapy for deciduous teeth. *Journal of the American Dental Association* **53**, 14–22.

43. Mack RB, Dean JA (1993) Electrosurgical pulpotomy: a retrospective study. *Journal of Dentistry for Children* **60**, 107–114.

44. Mackie IC (1998) Management and root canal treatment of non-vital immature permanent incisor teeth (UK National Clinical Guidelines in Paediatric Dentistry). *International Journal of Paediatric Dentistry* **8**, 289–293.

45. Magnusson B (1970) Therapeutic pulpotomy in primary molars – clinical and histological follow up. 1. Calcium hydroxide paste as wound dressing. *Odontologisk Revy* **21**, 415–431.

46. Massler M, Malone AJ (1952) Fractured anterior teeth – diagnosis treatment and prognosis. *Dental Digest* **58**, 442–447.

47. Mejàre I, Cvek M (1993) Partial pulpotomy in young permanent teeth with deep carious lesions. *Endodontics and Dental Traumatology* **9**, 238–242.

48. Moorer WR, Wesselink PR (1982) Factors promoting the tissue dissolving capability of sodium hypochlorite. *International Endodontic Journal* **15**, 187–196.

49. Morawa AP, Straffon LH, Han SS, Corpron RE (1975) Clinical evaluation of pulpotomies using dilute formocresol. *Journal of Dentistry for Children* **42**, 360–363.

50. Mulder GR, Van Amerongen WE, Vingerling PA (1987) Consequences of endodontic treatment of primary teeth. Part II. A clinical investigation into the influence of formocresol pulpotomy on the permanent successor. *Journal of Dentistry for Children* **54**, 35–39.

51. Mumford JM (1967) Pain perception threshold on stimulating teeth and the histological condition of the pulp. *British Dental Journal* **123**, 427–433.

52. Myers DR, Pashley DH, Whitford GM, McKinney RV (1983) Tissue changes induced by the absorption of formocresol from pulpotomy sites in dogs. *Pediatric Dentistry* **5**, 6–8.

53. Myers DR, Pashley DH, Whitford GM, Sobel RE, McKinney RV (1981) The acute toxicity of high doses of systemically administered formocresol in dogs. *Pediatric Dentistry* **3**, 37–41.

54. Myers DR, Shoaf HK, Dirksen TR, Pashley DH, Whitford GM, Reynolds KE (1978) Distribution of 14C-formaldehyde after pulpotomy with formocresol. *Journal of the American Dental Association* **96**, 805–813.

55. Nakashima M (1994) Induction of dentin formation on canine amputated pulp by recombinant human bone morphogenic proteins (BMP)-2 and -4. *Journal of Dental Research* **73**, 1515–1522.

56. Pitt Ford TR, Torabinejad M, Abedi HR, Bakland LK, Kariyawasam SP (1996) Using mineral trioxide aggregate as a pulp-capping material. *Journal of the American Dental Association* **127**, 1491–1494.

57. Pruhs RJ, Olen GA, Sharma PS (1977) Relationship between formocresol pulpotomies on primary teeth and enamel defects on their permanent successors. *Journal of the American Dental Association* **94**, 698–700.

58. Ranly DM, Garcia-Godoy F (2000) Current and potential pulp therapies for primary and young permanent teeth. *Journal of Dentistry* **28**, 153–161.

59. Redig DF (1968) A comparison and evaluation of two formocresol pulpotomy techniques using Buckley's Formocresol. *Journal of Dentistry for Children* **35**, 22–30.

60. Rolling I, Poulsen S (1978) Formocresol pulpotomy of primary teeth and occurrence of enamel defects on the permanent successors. *Acta Odontologica Scandinavica* **36**, 243–247.

61. Ruemping DR, Morton TH, Anderson MW (1983) Electrosurgical pulpotomy in primates – a comparison with formocresol pulpotomy. *Pediatric Dentistry* **5**, 14–18.

62. Rule DC, Winter GB (1966) Root growth and apical repair subsequent to pulpal necrosis in children. *British Dental Journal* **120**, 586–590.

63. Schmitt D, Lee J, Bogen G (2001) Multifaceted use of ProRoot MTA root canal repair material. *Pediatric Dentistry* **23**, 326–330.

64. Schröder U, Granath LE (1971) On internal dentine resorption in deciduous molars treated by pulpotomy and capped with calcium hydroxide. *Odontologisk Revy* **22**, 179–188.

65. Schröder U, Szpringer-Nodzak M, Janicha J, Wacinska M, Budny J, Mlosek K (1987) A one-year follow-up of partial pulpotomy and calcium hydroxide capping in primary molars. *Endodontics and Dental Traumatology* **3**, 304–306.

66. Schwartz RS, Mauger M, Clement DJ, Walker WA (1999) Mineral Trioxide Aggregate: a new material for endododontics. *Journal of the American Dental Association* **130**, 967–975.

67. S-Gravenmade EJ (1975) Some biochemical considerations of fixation in endodontics. *Journal of Endodontics* **1**, 233–237.

68. Sheehy EC, Roberts GJ (1997) Use of calcium hydroxide for apical barrier formation and healing in non-vital immature permanent teeth: a review. *British Dental Journal* **183**, 241–246.

69. Shoji S, Nakamura M, Horiuchi H (1985) Histopathological changes in dental pulps irradiated by $CO_2$ laser: a preliminary report on laser pulpotomy. *Journal of Endodontics* **11**, 379–384.

70. Shovelton DS (1972) The maintenance of pulp vitality. *British Dental Journal* **133**, 95–101.

71. Shulman ER, McIver FT, Burkes EJ (1987) Comparison of electrosurgery and formocresol as pulpotomy techniques in monkey primary teeth. *Pediatric Dentistry* **9**, 189–194.

72. Sweet CA (1930) Procedure for treatment of exposed and pulpless deciduous teeth. *Journal of the American Dental Association* **17**, 1150–1153.

73. Turner C, Courts FJ, Stanley HR (1987) A histological comparison of direct pulp capping agents in primary canines. *Journal of Dentistry for Children* **54**, 423–428.

74. Urist M (1965) Bone formation by autoinduction. *Science* **150**, 893–899.

75. Waterhouse PJ (1995) Formocresol and alternative primary molar pulpotomy medicaments: a review. *Endodontics and Dental Traumatology* **11**, 157–162.

76. Waterhouse PJ, Nunn JH, Whitworth JM (2000) An investigation of the relative efficacy of Buckley's formocresol and calcium hydroxide in primary molar vital pulp therapy. *British Dental Journal* **188**, 32–36.

77. Waterhouse PJ, Whitworth JM, Nunn JH (1999) Development of a method to detect and quantify Prostaglandin E2 in pulpal blood from cariously exposed, vital primary molar teeth. *International Endodontic Journal* **32** 381–387.

78. Winter GB (1962) Abscess formation in connexion with deciduous molar teeth. *Archives of Oral Biology* **7**, 373–379.

79. Yates JA (1988) Barrier formation time in non-vital teeth with open apices. *International Endodontic Journal* **21**, 313–319.

# Endodontic aspects of traumatic injuries

## H. E. Pitt Ford and T. R. Pitt Ford

Introduction  195

History, examination and immediate management  195

Types of injury  197

Effects of trauma on the dental tissues  197

Management of primary teeth  197
   Fractures  197
   Luxation injuries  198
   Discoloration of primary teeth  198

Management of permanent teeth  198
   Fractures  198
   Luxation injuries  202

Root canal treatment of immature teeth  206

Auto-transplantation of an immature premolar into the incisor space  207

Complications  208
   External inflammatory root resorption  208
   Cervical external inflammatory root resorption  208
   External replacement root resorption  209
   Barrier formation coronal to the apex  210
   Previous injury  210
   Root canal retreatment  210
   Discoloration  210
   Avoidance of cervical root fracture  210

Orthodontic treatment  211

References  211

## INTRODUCTION

This chapter is principally concerned with the endodontic aspects of traumatic injuries of the teeth, and does not attempt to cover traumatology comprehensively. For this reference should be made to a textbook on traumatology or to current guidelines [10,23,28]. Because most general practitioners see only a small number of patients with traumatic injuries, it may be appropriate to refer the more complex injuries to a colleague with specialist experience.

When a tooth has been damaged through trauma, a good history and thorough examination are essential to ensure a correct diagnosis and the best outcome. The status of the pulp of all involved teeth must be assessed, and their vitality maintained wherever possible. Many injured teeth are immature, and their development and maturation depend on maintaining pulp vitality. Vital teeth may not respond to sensitivity testing immediately after an accident.

## HISTORY, EXAMINATION AND IMMEDIATE MANAGEMENT

A dental injury should always be treated as an emergency. Management of any severe bleeding or respiratory problems takes priority. Any period of unconsciousness, amnesia, headache, nausea or vomiting may indicate cerebral involvement, and the patient should be referred immediately for medical examination and appropriate care [41].

A full account of when, where and how the injury occurred must be recorded. The circumstances of the accident may have legal implications and a photograph may be especially useful. The time interval between injury and presentation can influence the choice of treatment, and may be critical to the success of replantation of avulsed teeth. The place may suggest possible contamination of open wounds and the need for tetanus prophylaxis. The way the injury occurred may give some indication of the type and extent of the injury. Any previous injury or treatment should be recorded. The medical history must be reviewed as this may influence treatment planning, for example if the patient suffers from a cardiac, immunological or blood disorder. Antibiotic or other prophylaxis may be required [1,60].

The clinical examination should include assessment of the soft tissues and facial skeleton. Disturbances to the occlusion are investigated as these may indicate jaw fracture or condylar displacement. Any soft tissue injury is noted and the possible presence of a foreign body considered; radiographic examination may be necessary to locate this. Injuries to the oral mucosa are investigated, especially bleeding from the gingival sulcus; lacerations may occur with displaced teeth; bleeding from a non-lacerated gingival margin may indicate periodontal damage. The probing depths of the gingival sulci are recorded. It should always be remembered that the effect of an injury may not be confined to the visibly affected teeth, and adjacent apparently unaffected teeth should always be included in the examination and investigations. Infractions, fractures, pulpal exposures, mobility or displacement are noted along with any colour changes. A dark discoloration immediately after the injury indicates haemorrhage within the pulp space. There may be potential for repair and therefore this is not an indication for root canal treatment. If, however the tooth becomes dark some months after the injury this usually indicates pulp necrosis. Yellow discoloration some time after the injury is associated with pulp calcification and is not an indication for root canal treatment, even if there is no response to sensitivity testing. Lost pieces of fractured teeth should be accounted for, in case they are embedded in soft tissue, or have been swallowed or inhaled. Thermal sensitivity of the teeth may be a consequence of exposed dentine or pulp. Mobility and percussion testing should be carried out as they may indicate damage to the supporting tissues.

Reactions to pulp sensitivity testing should be recorded; some injured teeth may have the potential to recover but may not respond for up to two years after trauma [45]; the results of tests provide a baseline for later comparison. A negative response to sensitivity testing should not therefore be taken as an indication for root canal treatment. Blood flow in severely luxated teeth has been shown some time ahead of their pulps responding to electric pulp testing [45]. In assessing vitality of luxated teeth it is not unusual for the findings to be contradictory and misleading [12].

Radiographic examination of permanent teeth should include a paralleling-technique periapical film of each affected tooth using a film holder to standardize projections for later comparison. For luxation injuries a further film with the tube rotated horizontally is often helpful [7]. If a root fracture is suspected in the maxillary incisor region an occlusal radiograph should be taken. If an immature tooth has been non-vital for some time, its development will have been arrested, leaving the pulp space larger than would be expected. For primary teeth an occlusal film alone is usually sufficient.

Inconsistencies between the history and the injuries sustained, particularly if accompanied by late presentation, should alert the practitioner to the possibility of non-accidental injury.

Following a thorough clinical and radiographic examination, a diagnosis is made for each injured tooth. The importance of this cannot be overstated. The outcome of treatment is dependent on a correct diagnosis and inappropriate treatment may readily be initiated at this stage. The prognosis should be considered and the value, or otherwise, of prolonged endodontic treatment determined. New treatment methods, such as with the recent introduction of mineral trioxide aggregate (MTA Pro root, Dentsply, Weybridge, UK), have resulted in more practical and less demanding endodontic procedures for patients who have sustained dental injury. Also methods of strengthening the cervical region of immature teeth reduce the risk of loss through fracture (see below). A tooth is the best space maintainer and its retention preserves alveolar bone for later restorations.

Soft tissue injuries should be cleaned and sutured if necessary, and any tooth fragments embedded in the lips removed. Exposed dentine is covered and pulp exposures treated; displaced teeth are repositioned and splinted when appropriate. If a permanent tooth has been avulsed, the socket is irrigated with saline to remove blood clot, and the tooth replanted and splinted. These injuries are covered in more detail later.

If the patient is very upset, it may be better to delay non-urgent treatment until a subsequent visit. In the case of a traumatically exposed pulp, inflammation has been shown to not extend beyond 3–4 mm after several days [33].

## TYPES OF INJURY

Trauma may cause the following damage to the teeth:

- infraction of enamel;
- fracture of enamel;
- fracture of enamel and dentine;
- fracture of enamel and dentine with pulp exposure;
- crown–root fracture involving enamel, dentine cementum and pulp;
- intra-alveolar root fracture;
- concussion;
- subluxation;
- extrusive luxation;
- lateral luxation;
- intrusive luxation;
- avulsion.

Sudden contact of upper and lower teeth caused by, for example, a blow to the mandible can result in damage to posterior teeth. These injuries are rare but can result in a range of damage, from minimal loss of hard tissue to vertical crown–root fracture or avulsion.

## EFFECTS OF TRAUMA ON THE DENTAL TISSUES

Many traumatized teeth are immature. These teeth have large pulp spaces and short, wide dentinal tubules. Infection may therefore readily spread to the pulp if the crown is fractured. This may lead to loss of vitality, as may severance or crushing of the apical vessels during luxation injuries. The pulp of an avulsed tooth may also become infected via the apex. Teeth depend on a vital pulp in order to develop their potential maturity and strength. A tooth that loses its vitality while immature is always prone to fracture, especially in the cervical region or of the root [17].

The cementum on the root surface may be damaged by luxation injuries; the natural repair mechanism involves limited surface resorption. However, where there is extensive damage to the cementum, ankylosis associated with replacement resorption is a frequent complication. If infection from the pulp complicates damage to cementum, then external inflammatory root resorption may be very rapid, particularly in immature teeth [32].

## MANAGEMENT OF PRIMARY TEETH

When a primary tooth is injured a major consideration is avoidance of damage to the successional tooth. This may occur either mechanically at the time of injury, during treatment, or as a result of infection. Young children may not be very cooperative, particularly after a traumatic injury when the soft tissues are sore, swollen and bruised, therefore immediate treatment may need to be limited.

### Fractures

#### Crown fractures

Enamel fractures should be smoothed, while fractures into dentine should be covered. If the pulp has been exposed and if there is sufficient cooperation, a partial pulpotomy and restoration may be carried out with a view to preserving pulp vitality; this does not need to be done at the emergency visit. Otherwise extraction of the tooth may be indicated. The technique of pulpotomy is covered in the section on permanent teeth. Root canal treatment of primary teeth has been covered in Chapter 10. An infected primary tooth should not be left untreated as the infection may cause damage to the permanent successor (Fig. 11.1).

#### Intra-alveolar root fracture

This is less common in primary teeth than in permanent teeth. Active intervention is rarely required. If the coronal fragment is very loose and at risk of being inhaled or grossly displaced, or pulp necrosis and infection develop, extraction is usually indicated; however, the apical fragment is normally left in situ to resorb naturally and to avoid surgical damage to the developing permanent successor.

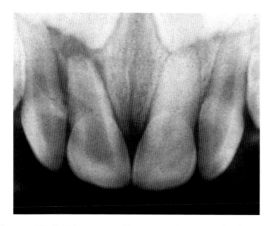

**Figure 11.1** Primary maxillary central incisors that have suffered a traumatic injury. The maxillary left incisor has responded with calcification of the pulp space, while the right incisor has developed an abscess.

## Luxation injuries

In general a conservative approach to management is adopted with primary teeth. Laterally luxated primary teeth are frequently repositioned naturally in time by occlusal forces. If a laterally luxated tooth interferes with the occlusion, the luxation is mild and there is no risk to the permanent successor, it may be carefully repositioned [10]. If the root apex is directed palatally towards the developing permanent tooth then it should be extracted atraumatically. If a tooth is very mobile and in danger of inhalation, or if occlusal interference is too great, it should be extracted. Intruded teeth will usually re-erupt albeit sometimes over several months.

Replantation of avulsed primary teeth is not normally carried out because of the potential risk of direct physical damage to the developing permanent tooth, or damage from later infection of the pulp of the primary tooth.

## Discoloration of primary teeth

Pulp damage is a frequent complication of injuries, and as a result primary teeth may discolour. Immediate discoloration indicates bleeding in the pulp and the possibility of repair. Later darkening of the tooth signifies pulp necrosis and if there is associated infection, root canal treatment or extraction is indicated. Later yellow discoloration indicates

pulp canal obliteration and no intervention is required (Fig. 11.1).

## MANAGEMENT OF PERMANENT TEETH

### Fractures

*Infractions and fracture of enamel*

Infraction of enamel rarely requires operative treatment, but the pulpal status should be monitored. Infection may very rarely enter the pulp through enamel infractions. There is no effective treatment to avoid this. Fractures of enamel may be either smoothed or repaired with composite resin.

The likelihood of pulp canal obliteration or pulp necrosis occurring is low for both enamel infractions and enamel fractures [55]. The chance of pulp damage is increased if there is associated luxation of the tooth [49].

*Fracture of enamel and dentine*

In children, trauma to anterior teeth commonly affects sound teeth, which frequently have large pulps and wide dentinal tubules. Any injury that exposes dentine can, therefore, result in damage to the pulp. Fractures involving dentine open up numerous dentinal tubules. If left untreated, bacterial plaque will grow on the exposed surface and cause pulpal inflammation, which may lead to pulp necrosis. The early placement of a restoration prevents permanent pulp damage and relieves sensitivity. The use of composite resin retained by etched enamel and a dentine bonding agent restores the appearance and does not hinder subsequent monitoring of pulp vitality (Fig. 11.2). This has been shown to seal more effectively than conventional glass ionomer cement [43]. Restoration of the contour of the tooth may be left until a later visit. In recent years fractured fragments have been successfully reattached with composite resin retained by etched enamel.

The likelihood of pulp canal obliteration or pulp necrosis occurring is low following fractures involving dentine, provided the dentine tubules are effectively covered [55,63]. The chance of pulp

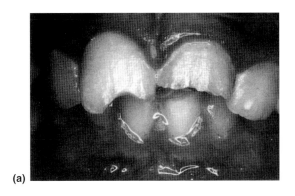

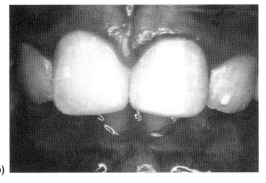

**Figure 11.2** (**a**) Fractured incisal edges of maxillary central incisors exposing dentine. (**b**) Restoration of incisal edges using composite resin retained by etched enamel.

damage is increased if there is associated luxation of the tooth [49,50].

*Fracture of enamel and dentine with pulp exposure*

*Immature teeth.* If this type of injury occurs in a young patient whose tooth is immature, then treatment is directed at maintaining pulp vitality to allow continued tooth maturation; this considerably improves the long-term prognosis of the tooth by reducing the risk of subsequent root fracture [17]. Permanent incisor teeth have been shown to reach maturity at the age of about 13 years. The pulp can usually be treated conservatively as it has a good blood supply and rarely becomes necrotic [16,34]. Partial pulpotomy is the treatment of choice [16,29,30,33]. The advantages of partial pulpotomy over pulp capping are that inflamed pulp tissue and adjacent infected dentine are removed, and that the pulp dressing is placed in a cavity where it can be covered by a protective base. If the

restoration is lost, the cavity dressing should not be displaced.

Local anaesthesia is necessary to carry out a pulpotomy. The tooth is isolated with rubber dam to exclude salivary contamination; retention of rubber dam on an immature tooth is facilitated by a suitable clamp (e.g. Ash EW, Dentsply). If the tooth is partially erupted or very crowded a split dam technique may be used, with a caulking agent (e.g. Ora-Seal, Ultradent Products, Salt Lake City, UT, USA). A small cavity approximately $2 \times 2$ mm is cut in the fractured dentine surface at the exposure site, with the periphery of the cavity floor in dentine (Fig. 11.3). Pulp removal is usually confined to the superficial 2 mm since infection does not normally extend beyond this level. The pulp is best removed with a bur in the turbine handpiece using copious water spray; this causes less damage than a bur at low speed or use of an excavator [20,29,30]. Haemorrhage is arrested using a cotton pellet soaked in

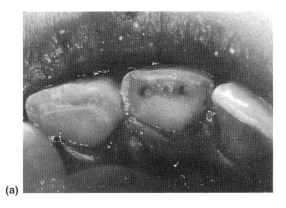

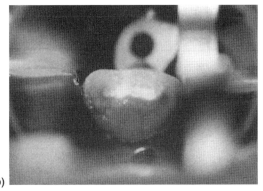

**Figure 11.3** (**a**) Maxillary right central incisor with a fracture involving the pulp. (**b**) After placement of medicament in the partial pulpotomy preparation.

saline and the wound is covered with mineral trioxide aggregate [47,48,53]. Over this is placed a layer of resin modified glass ionomer cement, before restoring the tooth with composite resin. Should the resin be lost the restoration within the cavity should remain intact. Alternatively the cavity may be restored with a calcium hydroxide base (either a slurry which is subsequently compressed and dried with cotton wool or a hard setting base material) and IRM (Dentsply). A hard tissue barrier should form beneath the dressing [20,29,47,48,53] (Fig. 11.3). The coronal contour should be restored with etch-retained composite resin.

The tooth should be reviewed after six months, and then at least annually for several years, to ensure continued pulp vitality by regular pulp testing, and continued root development by examination of radiographs. Should the restoration fail, it must be replaced immediately in order to prevent infection of the pulp via the pulpotomy site, as the hard tissue barrier is usually porous [33]. This treatment has a high success rate; the pulp may be expected to remain vital and healthy [16,29,33]. There is no need for root canal treatment subsequent to pulpotomy, unless necrosis and infection develop [20].

*Mature teeth.* Where crown fracture of a mature tooth involves the pulp, conservative treatment by partial pulpotomy should still be considered as the first treatment option. However, where the entire clinical crown has been lost, pulpal extirpation, root canal filling and construction of a post crown is usually indicated.

### Crown–root fracture involving enamel, dentine, cementum and pulp

In this type of extensive tooth fracture, the coronal fragment is usually retained by a limited amount of periodontal ligament. These teeth may have a poor prognosis, especially if the fracture line is a long way subgingival on the palatal aspect. When the patient first presents, the coronal fragment is often loose and painful to bite on. It is usually necessary to give local anaesthesia to allow removal of the fragment and to assess the extent of the fracture. If time does not allow this, the fragment may be bonded temporarily to the tooth to minimize discomfort.

Where the fracture does not extend far sub-gingivally, it is often possible to restore the tooth without crown lengthening. Otherwise periodontal surgery to expose the margin of the fracture, or orthodontic extrusion, will need to be considered.

In an immature tooth, where the fracture does not extend far subgingivally, pulpotomy should be carried out (as described above). Where loss of the root is more extensive, the tooth will be difficult to restore and is likely to have a poor long-term prognosis. While its loss will be planned for in the longer term it may be possible to carry out a pulpotomy (as above), restoring the supragingival contour with composite resin and retain the tooth while the dentition continues to develop.

In a mature tooth where the fracture is superficial, pulpotomy may still be the first line of treatment, or it may be more appropriate to carry out root canal treatment and restore the tooth with a post crown. If the fracture is deeper, it will be difficult to isolate the tooth for root canal treatment, and orthodontic extrusion of the root followed by crown lengthening will need to be considered before restoration by a post crown [10,35]. When the fracture is very deep, there may be too little root remaining to support a restoration even after orthodontic extrusion; such teeth are also more likely to fail subsequently [27]. Where the prognosis is very poor, extraction of the remaining root should be considered.

### Intra-alveolar root fracture

Intra-alveolar root fractures are relatively uncommon, and fortunately often occur without the complication of bacterial contamination from the mouth. The coronal fragment may be mobile with the fulcrum coronal to the apex, and may be extrusively or laterally luxated. The tooth should be examined carefully for any periodontal injury whereby the gingival sulcus communicates with the fracture; this substantially reduces the prognosis.

Diagnosis of intra-alveolar root fracture is made by radiological examination with two films taken at different vertical angles. Root fractures are more frequently observed on an occlusal film than a film taken with a paralleling technique (Fig. 11.4).

The apical fragment almost without exception remains vital, and does not require treatment. This

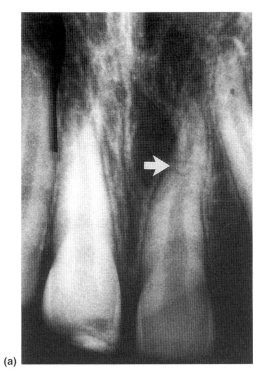
(a)

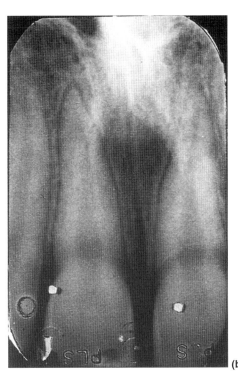
(b)

**Figure 11.4** (a) Part of an occlusal radiograph more easily demonstrates an intra-alveolar root fracture (arrowed) of the left maxillary central incisor than (b) a paralleling technique radiograph of the same tooth, on which the fracture is very difficult to observe.

is therefore in effect a luxation injury of the coronal fragment. If there is no mobility, no immediate treatment is required and the root should heal with hard tissue; the pulp is likely to remain vital. Teeth that have fractures remote from the gingival sulcus have the best long-term prognosis (Fig. 11.4). If the fracture is close to the neck of the tooth, the prognosis will be poorer, but extraction need not be indicated, unless there is a communication between the gingival sulcus and the fracture line. Teeth with a transverse fracture have a poorer long-term prognosis than those with an oblique fracture because of the risk of future displacement [21] (Fig. 11.5).

If the tooth is displaced or mobile, immediate treatment consists of repositioning the coronal fragment and splinting if the coronal fragment is very mobile, typically for approximately four weeks. Recent work has failed to show a correlation between splinting method or duration and healing, and suggested that teeth with no or slight loosening may not require splinting. No displacement of the coronal fragment and preserved vitality of the pulp are highly indicative of fracture healing [18,21,59]. The splint should allow physiological movement to avoid ankylosis. The patient is advised to use a chlorhexidine mouthwash, and the tooth reviewed at the time of intended splint removal. Pulp sensitivity is checked. Where there is no response, the tooth should be reviewed again at three-monthly intervals. Where no vital response is obtained, provided there is no tenderness to palpation, nor a sinus tract, pulp testing should be carried out at three- and then six-monthly intervals either until a response occurs, or evidence of pulp necrosis appears.

The most favourable response is uniting of the two fragments by hard tissue laid down both in the root canal and on the root surface. A less favourable but still satisfactory outcome is continued pulp vitality in the coronal fragment but no union of the fragments. The sharp edges at the fracture line become rounded by remodelling, and connective

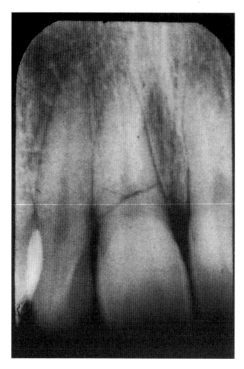

**Figure 11.5** Radiograph of a right maxillary central incisor with a horizontal root fracture close to the gingival margin. The pulp responded to electric pulp testing one year after trauma, however the long-term prognosis is poor.

tissue and/or bone lie between the fragments; the space between the fragments may increase with continued alveolar growth in younger patients. Often the pulp in the coronal fragment calcifies and radiologically shows an obliterated pulp space [6]; the pulp may not respond to sensitivity testing [4,11,62]. Pulp canal obliteration is not an indication for root canal treatment [10,37].

Pulp necrosis occurs in approximately 20% of intra-alveolar root-fractured teeth and is associated with initial coronal displacement, lack of pulp sensitivity after the accident, coronal position of the root fracture, a communication with the gingival sulcus, maturity of the root and coronal fracture [6,11,18,21,59,62]. Pulp necrosis is invariably confined to the coronal fragment [10,11]. As well as the loss of response to thermal and electrical stimuli, there is frequently a radiolucency in the bone around the tooth at the fracture line (Fig. 11.6). Root canal treatment should be carried out in the coronal fragment alone unless there is definite evidence to implicate the apical fragment. Following cleaning and shaping

of the canal in the coronal fragment, a well-packed dressing of calcium hydroxide is placed to allow healing at the fracture site. When soft tissue healing has taken place, after about one month, MTA may be placed in the first 2 or 3 mm at the fracture line, followed by back filling with gutta-percha [53] (see section on root filling of immature teeth for method). Alternatively the calcium hydroxide may be replaced as required, as described below for treatment of an immature tooth, until a hard tissue barrier forms at the fracture line. The root canal may then be filled with gutta-percha (Fig. 11.6). If there is an inadequate hard tissue stop at the apical end of the coronal fragment, the first millimetre or two may be packed with calcium hydroxide to avoid gutta-percha being extruded at the fracture site. This treatment has a high success rate [15,38]. It is not normally practical to attempt to do root canal treatment of both fragments. If the apical fragment is non-vital surgical removal is indicated.

## Luxation injuries

A luxation injury is characterized by damage to the supporting tissues of the tooth; the tooth may be displaced. There may be interruption of the vessels and nerves at the apex. The prognosis for pulp recovery is reduced if there is a concomitant crown fracture as this is a possible route for entry of bacteria. Luxation injuries are the most common type of dental injury [9].

### Concussion

This is an injury to the supporting tissues without loosening or displacement of the tooth. Lasting pulp damage is rare, especially in an immature tooth, although the tooth may not respond to sensitivity testing for some months.

### Subluxation

The tooth is loosened in its socket but not displaced. With subluxation there is unlikely to be severance of the blood vessels supplying the pulp, giving a good possibility of pulp survival. Pulp survival rate is 90% for immature teeth and 75% for mature teeth [7]. It is essential to allow the pulp time for recovery before deciding to remove it.

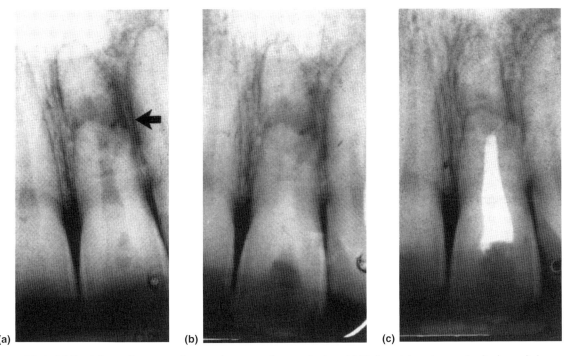

**Figure 11.6** (a) The left maxillary central incisor has a root fracture in the mid-third, and there is a periradicular radiolucency at the fracture line (arrowed). (b) The root canal of the coronal fragment has been cleaned, shaped and filled with calcium hydroxide. (c) One year later the root canal has been filled by lateral condensation of gutta-percha.

## Extrusive luxation

If this is severe the pulpal vessels and nerves are usually severed. In an immature tooth that is repositioned soon after injury, revascularization, followed by obliteration of the pulp space, is the likely outcome; in a mature tooth pulp necrosis is more common [7]. External inflammatory root resorption may occur following pulp necrosis.

## Lateral luxation

The tooth is displaced laterally and the apex may be locked into bone. This can be diagnosed by percussion, when the tooth gives a high ringing tone. This crushing injury causes damage to the supporting structures. The labial plate of bone may also be fractured. Pulpal healing may be expected in 70% of immature teeth [7] (Fig. 11.7). Revascularization will take some weeks but return of functioning nerve fibres may take a year or more [46]; therefore root canal treatment should not be undertaken unless there is positive evidence of pulpal infection.

In mature teeth that have suffered a severe luxation injury pulpal healing is unlikely, and therefore root canal treatment is indicated, except in cases where follow-up can be assured to observe for possible recovery. Damage to the supporting structures makes both inflammatory and replacement external root resorption frequent complications of lateral luxation [7].

A laterally luxated tooth may need to be disimpacted from its new position, using local anaesthesia if necessary, to allow correct repositioning. If the apex is displaced labially this is most readily achieved from behind the patient, by pressing with the thumb on the impacted apex. The tooth may be splinted with a flexible splint for 2–3 weeks (Fig. 11.8). The patient is recommended to use a chlorhexidine mouthwash during the early stages of healing. Radiographs are taken at one month to check for signs of disease, especially external inflammatory root resorption. If there are signs of this, the pulp should be removed promptly and the pulp space disinfected. Root canal treatment should then be carried out (see later). If no signs of disease

203

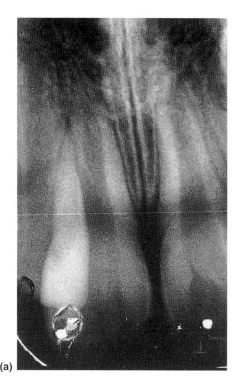

(a)

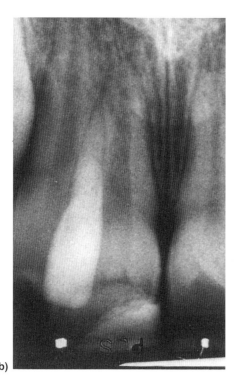

(b)

**Figure 11.7** (a) The immature right central incisor was luxated. (b) one year later the root has continued to form.

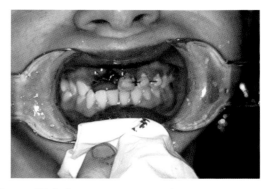

**Figure 11.8** Emergency treatment after a traumatic injury. The right maxillary incisor was avulsed and lost. The left central incisor was luxated and has been repositioned and splinted.

are observed, the patient is reviewed again after 2, 3, 6 months and 1 year. Pulp sensitivity is assessed at each period using thermal and electric tests; electric pulp testing often does not produce a response in the early period after luxation injury. Concurrent with return of sensitivity, there may be evidence of pulp canal obliteration (Fig. 11.9), which is very common in laterally luxated teeth [8]. This causes a yellowish coronal discoloration and the tooth may cease to respond to sensitivity testing. This is not an indication for root canal treatment.

In about 4% of luxated teeth periapical radiolucency, together with discoloration and absence of sensitivity, is a temporary phenomenon and disappears as healing progresses [3].

### Intrusive luxation

This is a severe injury; the tooth is forced into its socket, so crushing the supporting structures and the blood vessels and nerve fibres that supply the pulp. The tooth is likely to be wedged in the supporting bone, therefore displaying a lack of mobility and a ringing note on percussion. Radiographs will show obliteration of the periodontal ligament space. Many immature teeth will re-erupt spontaneously, but if there is no evidence of this after three weeks, rapid orthodontic repositioning should be undertaken. Access to the clinical crown must be available for endodontic treatment should this become necessary. Severe intrusions may require surgical repositioning. Pulp necrosis is a very frequent com-

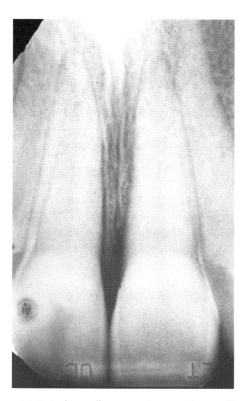

**Figure 11.9** Both maxillary central incisors have suffered luxation injuries and have responded with calcification of the pulp spaces.

plication of intrusion; 60% of immature teeth become non-vital [7]. Immature teeth should therefore be observed for signs of pulp vitality returning or complications developing. The regime for reviewing intrusions is similar to that for other luxations. If evidence of pulp necrosis or infection appear, root canal treatment should be undertaken (see below). Mature teeth do not re-erupt and almost without exception become non-vital; treatment consists of pulp extirpation, disinfection of the pulp space, dressing with calcium hydroxide for a short period and subsequent root canal filling [23].

Radiographs should be taken frequently to check for the presence of external inflammatory root resorption. Another complication of intrusion is a high incidence of replacement resorption [7], as a result of damage to the cementum. This can be diagnosed by percussion and radiologically. Intrusion is a severe injury, which may be best referred for specialist care.

*Avulsion*

The tooth is completely displaced from its socket, and should be replaced as soon as possible, preferably at the site of the accident. Immature avulsed teeth, which have been replanted immediately or correctly stored until emergency treatment can be obtained, have a reasonable prognosis for pulp revascularization and periodontal healing; mature teeth do not revascularize [23]. Both external inflammatory and replacement resorption are frequent complications [13,57].

The avulsed tooth needs careful handling while it is out of the mouth to prevent damage to the periodontal ligament. It should not be allowed to dry out, and if necessary is best kept in cold milk. The patient should be taken immediately to an experienced practitioner. If the tooth has been dry for more than one hour the prognosis is considerably reduced. The medical history must be considered as to whether replantation is appropriate, or whether any special precautions may be required. The tetanus status should be checked if the accident took place outside. The tooth is examined, without touching the root to avoid damage to the periodontal ligament, and dirt rinsed off with saline; under no circumstances should it be scrubbed or severe periodontal ligament damage will occur. It is helpful to note the length of the tooth for future endodontic treatment. It may be necessary to take a radiograph of the socket to check that no part of the root remains. Local anaesthesia may not always be needed; the socket is syringed with saline to remove any clot, and the tooth gently repositioned into its socket; the position is then confirmed radiographically. The tooth is splinted for 7–10 days, using a flexible splint. For optimal healing it is essential to avoid infection, therefore in the days following replantation the patient should use a chlorhexidine mouthwash. Splinting for longer periods should be avoided to reduce the risk of ankylosis.

With immature teeth there is a good chance of pulp revascularization, so the pulp should not be electively removed; revascularization will allow root formation and maturation to continue, and reduce the risk of subsequent fracture of the tooth [17]. However, there is a risk that infection present on the root surface or on the apical surface of the pulp at the time of replantation may initiate, or perpetuate, inflammatory resorption, which can rapidly destroy the thin wall of the immature root. If this or any other positive sign of infection does occur, the pulp space should be cleaned and disinfected, and root canal treatment undertaken (see below). Otherwise regular clinical and radiological reviews should be undertaken at approximately 1, 2, 3, 6 months and 1 year; the patient should be asked to return immediately should any problems develop.

With mature teeth the chances of pulp revascularization are so low that the necrotic pulp should be extirpated through a conventional access cavity at the time of splint removal. The cleaned and shaped root canal is initially filled with a dressing of calcium hydroxide prior to root canal filling with gutta-percha. There appears to be no benefit in leaving calcium hydroxide in the tooth for a prolonged period [25]. Calcium hydroxide should not be inserted within one week of injury, to allow periodontal healing to take place at the apex.

## ROOT CANAL TREATMENT OF IMMATURE TEETH

The teeth most commonly injured are the incisors. The apices of these teeth are not normally closed until about the age of 13 years, although in a two-dimensional radiograph they may appear closed much earlier than this. It is necessary to produce an apical barrier against which a root filling can be packed. This may be done in one of two ways. A plug of MTA may be inserted at the apex, as soon as soft tissue healing has taken place. This will set hard and form a mechanical barrier, over which cementum will subsequently grow. Alternatively, the formation of a biological hard tissue barrier may be encouraged prior to inserting a root filling. In either case the elimination of infection from the root canal space is essential.

Local anaesthesia is given so that a rubber dam clamp can be placed securely on the tooth and in case the pulp is still partially vital; an Ash EW clamp will fit most anterior teeth. Sometimes it is not possible to clamp the affected tooth as it may be insufficiently erupted or the teeth may be very crowded. It may then be helpful to use a split rubber dam technique, with Ora-seal caulking

(Ultradent) to prevent sodium hypochlorite from entering the mouth. The access cavity on the palatal surface of the crown should be sufficiently large, and sufficiently incisally placed, to allow adequate access to the wide root canal. However, since both sodium hypochlorite and calcium hydroxide dissolve organic matter it is not necessary to have straight-line access to the whole root canal. Indeed to attempt this would often be to weaken the neck of the tooth excessively. The cervical constriction apical to the cingulum should be reduced [12]. Instrumentation should be carried out to 1–2 mm short of the radiographic apex, unless necrotic tissue is encountered at this level when instruments should be taken further. The length of the root canal is estimated by taking a radiograph with a file of known length in place. If the canal is very wide it may be helpful to wedge the file in place with a pledget of cotton wool.

Filing of the root canal walls must be avoided as the canal walls are already thin; instead the pulp space should be cleaned by copious irrigation with a solution of sodium hypochlorite [31]. After thorough cleaning, a stiff paste of calcium hydroxide is packed into the canal with root canal pluggers [44]. Calcium hydroxide is alkaline and has an antibacterial effect, and thus allows healing to take place. The quality of the calcium hydroxide filling should be checked radiologically before closure of the access cavity with an effective temporary filling (e.g. IRM, Dentsply) (Fig. 11.10). Calcium hydroxide has the same radiolucency as dentine. It is essential that the temporary filling does not break down during the course of treatment, or the canal space will become recontaminated. The tooth should be reviewed after one month, and a radiograph taken. If infection has been controlled and soft tissue healing has taken place, MTA may be inserted into the apical few millimetres. The calcium hydroxide is removed and the canal irrigated and dried; MTA powder is mixed with sterile water to a stiff paste and inserted into the root canal using measured root canal pluggers. Alternatively, the material may be injected into the canal. A Messing gun (Produits Dentaires, Vevey, Switzerland) is appropriate for this. A radiograph is taken. As the material takes 3–4 h to set, it can readily be removed if at this stage its position needs adjustment; it can be washed out thoroughly with water. Alternatively, if it is not far enough, it may be moistened to soften it and further

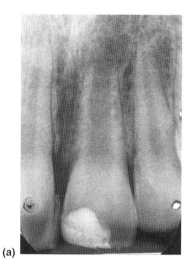 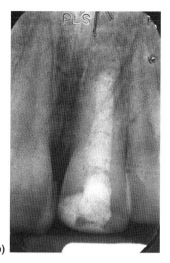 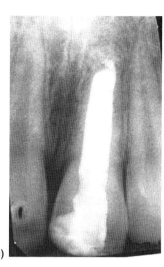

(a)          (b)          (c)

**Figure 11.10** (a) The left maxillary central incisor is non-vital after a traumatic injury; the root canal is much wider than that of the right central incisor, signifying that the tooth has been non-vital for some time. (b) The root canal has been cleaned, shaped and filled with a non-setting calcium hydroxide preparation. Fourteen months later a hard tissue barrier has formed at the apex. (c) The tooth has been root filled using the Obtura system of injected gutta-percha.

plugging undertaken. When in the correct position, a cotton pellet is inserted into the canal and the access cavity sealed. At a subsequent visit the canal may be back-filled with gutta-percha. Cementum has been shown to grow over the MTA at the apex [53].

Alternatively, when the patient returns for review of the calcium hydroxide dressing, the radiograph is used to ascertain whether the density of calcium hydroxide in the apical part of the root canal has reduced. This is usually caused by inflammation of the periapical tissues. If the calcium hydroxide is still well condensed the tooth should be reviewed after a further two months. If not, the entire calcium hydroxide dressing should be removed, the canal irrigated with sodium hypochlorite solution and dried, and the calcium hydroxide replaced; this should be reviewed again after one month. When a dressing repeatedly disappears or a large periapical radiolucency fails to heal, a cause such as infection in the tissues beyond the apex or a longitudinal root fracture needs to be considered, and the treatment plan reassessed. Surgery may be required or the tooth may need to be extracted. With most teeth, further reviews are carried out at 3, 6 and 12 months, provided that there are no problems. After one year a hard tissue barrier should have formed, which may be visible radiologically [14,60]. The tooth should be isolated and the dressing removed so that the presence of a barrier can be verified with a file (e.g. ISO size 25). If there is an apical stop, the root canal should be filled by a suitable gutta-percha technique (Fig. 11.10).

The type of barrier formed is dependent on the state of the apical pulp stump at the time of root canal treatment. Where the apical pulp stump and Hertwig's root sheath are undamaged, continued root formation may take place, but if it has been destroyed a calcific barrier is expected [26,36]. Histological examination of barriers shows that they resemble cellular cementum and appear to be continuous with the cementum [22].

Obturation of these teeth may be challenging, owing to the large canal diameter and divergent root canal walls [12]. An injectable gutta-percha system such as the Obtura 2 (Obtura-Spartan, Fenton, MO, USA) may be used (Fig. 11.10) or customized gutta-percha cones may be fabricated.

## AUTO-TRANSPLANTATION OF AN IMMATURE PREMOLAR INTO THE INCISOR SPACE

This may be undertaken in a patient who requires extraction of premolars as a part of orthodontic treatment. It has a high success rate but relies on careful case selection and meticulous surgical technique. The premolar must be immature, preferably with the root length nearly complete and the apex open. The desired outcome is that the pulp of the transplanted tooth should revascularize, and remain vital. This is followed by pulp canal obliteration. Apical to the part of the root which had formed by the time of transplantion the root should grow and mature normally. Should the pulp become necrotic, root canal treatment is complicated and is best referred to a specialist.

## COMPLICATIONS

### External inflammatory root resorption

This may occur if infection develops in the pulp space and there is damage to the adjacent cementum;

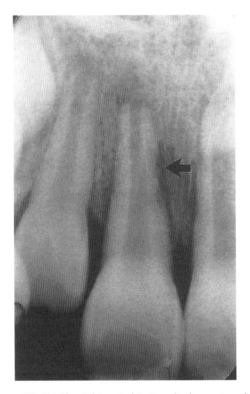

**Figure 11.11** The right central incisor displays external inflammatory root resorption on the mesial aspect (arrowed); there is a radiolucency of the bone adjacent to that in the tooth. The pulp of the tooth was necrotic as a consequence of a luxation injury.

this is common in the more severe luxation injuries [40,56]. Bacteria and their toxins may track along the dentinal tubules to the surface of the root, where the resultant inflammatory reaction attracts osteoclasts, which may destroy a large part of the root within a few weeks (Fig. 11.11). Inflammatory resorption is diagnosed radiologically as a localized area of tooth resorption with a radiolucent area in the adjacent bone. This may occur particularly rapidly in immature teeth, which have thin roots and wide dentinal tubules. It is therefore very important to take frequent radiographs and to disinfect the pulp space promptly if this type of resorption is seen. This will halt the resorption and the periodontal structures should heal [32].

The root canal must be thoroughly cleaned with sodium hypochlorite to kill bacteria. Calcium hydroxide is then inserted and will create an unsuitable environment for the continued survival of bacteria in the pulp space or dentinal tubules; it also raises the pH, which discourages osteoclastic activity [32]. Should the coronal seal subsequently fail, bacteria may re-enter the root canal and potentially stimulate further resorption.

### Cervical external inflammatory root resorption

Sometimes a late complication of trauma, particularly luxation, is inflammatory resorption close to the neck of the tooth (Fig. 11.12). This may occur in vital as well as root-filled teeth and is often unrelated to the pulpal status, as infection has come from the damaged root surface [56]. The resorption spreads around the root canal rather than into it. Cervical resorption may be difficult to differentiate radiologically from internal resorption. However, if two views are taken at different horizontal angles, the lesion in cervical resorption will be seen to change position; it should be possible to distinguish the outline of the root canal superimposed upon it. Root canal treatment, or retreatment, is not the appropriate method of dealing with the problem. Where the condition is limited and surgical access is good, surgical repair of the defect may be undertaken. In the case of a vital tooth, only if it is considered that surgical repair will expose the pulp, should root canal treatment be undertaken first. If the condition is extensive or surgical access is poor, extraction is usually indicated.

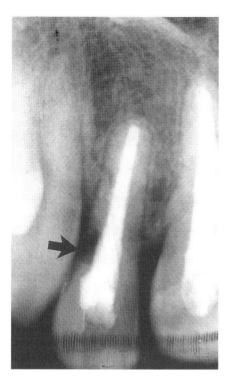

**Figure 11.12** Cervical external inflammatory resorption (arrowed) has occurred on the distal surface of the right lateral incisor approximately three years after trauma. If surgical access is good, the defect may be repaired, or the tooth may need to be extracted as in this example.

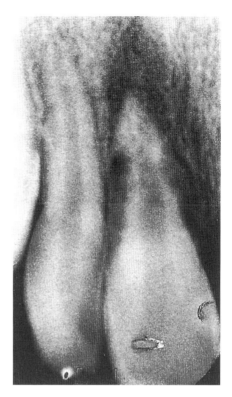

**Figure 11.13** The right central incisor displays replacement resorption on the mesial and distal root surfaces; there is a moth-eaten appearance. The tooth had been replanted two hours after avulsion one year previously.

It has been suggested that cervical resorption may be associated with bleaching of non-vital teeth [19]. However, this procedure should not cause damage if the dentine tubules of the root are protected and if sodium perborate and water are used rather than hydrogen peroxide [51,52].

## External replacement root resorption

This may occur when there is damage to the periodontal structures as in severe luxation injuries and especially with avulsions if the periodontal ligament is allowed to dry out [40,56]. Replacement resorption can be detected at follow-up appointments as the tooth gives a ringing note to percussion testing and lacks mobility. Radiologically the periodontal ligament space is difficult to detect in affected parts. The condition can often only be observed on radiographs much later when the root has a moth-eaten appearance (Fig. 11.13). Because the cementum

barrier is damaged in replacement resorption, the body treats the tooth as bone, and the tooth is gradually resorbed during physiological bone turnover and replaced by bone. In a healthy tooth, the cementum resists osteoclastic activity. Being a physiological process, replacement resorption cannot be treated, therefore carrying out root canal treatment is of no benefit. The tooth will ultimately be lost, but the time taken is variable and depends on the rate of bone turnover. In some young patients it can progress rapidly, and during the growth phase can cause the ankylosed tooth to appear to sink into the jaw as the surrounding alveolar bone grows with further eruption of the adjacent teeth [2]. Between the ages of 6 and 12 years, although infraocclusion may occur, it is preferable not to extract the tooth, provided it is free of infection, as more bone will develop if the root is left in situ. It may be appropriate to restore the incisal edge to improve its appearance. If desired, the crown may be removed and the root retained to preserve the alveolar bone provided there is no inflammation present. In older patients the tooth can be left until symptoms arise from later infection.

## Barrier formation coronal to the apex

If vital tissue remains at the apex, and if the calcium hydroxide is placed short of the apex, a calcific barrier may form coronal to the apex. This may be desirable if the apical portion remains vital. However if subsequent infection occurs, treatment will be required: if the barrier is near the apex, apical surgery may be the treatment of choice; if it is more coronal, it will be necessary to instrument through the barrier. In this case it is very important to have excellent access and vision to avoid perforation. This treatment is best referred to a specialist.

## Previous injury

Sometimes a patient presents with a new injury to an already traumatized tooth and the history of the presenting injury may fail to correlate with the findings of the clinical and radiological examinations and special tests. The patient should be questioned specifically about a previous injury.

## Root canal retreatment

If a patient presents with signs or symptoms related to a root-filled immature tooth and there are technical deficiencies in the previous treatment, root canal retreatment is indicated, and is more successful than surgery which is often complicated by a short root with thin walls. Root canal retreatment is covered in Chapter 13. If the technical quality of the previous treatment is very good, the possibility of recent root fracture must be considered.

## Discoloration

Because non-vital teeth tend to discolour, many patients request to have their teeth bleached. This may be done, under rubber dam, by removing the smear layer from the access cavity and inserting a thick paste of sodium perborate and water. A dressing is placed over this and the patient recalled

after one week. At this visit the treatment may be repeated if required, or the cavity restored with composite resin. Care must be taken that the root filling is removed to the cervical constriction but not far beyond, to reduce the risk of cervical external resorption, which has been reported following bleaching [19]. Alternatively a veneer or crown may be necessary.

## Avoidance of cervical root fracture

Non-vital immature teeth have thin roots with weak dentine walls, and are especially at risk of root fracture at the neck of the tooth [17] (Fig. 11.14). This risk may be much reduced if composite resin is bonded into the neck of the tooth. The root filling is either inserted short of the neck of the tooth or cut back to a suitable level; the access cavity is etched

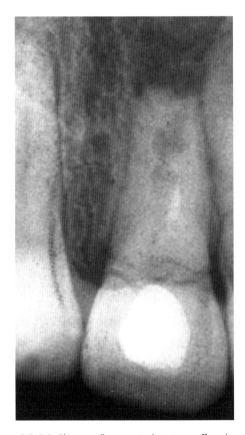

**Figure 11.14** The maxillary central incisor suffered a cervical root fracture before root canal treatment was completed.

and a bonding agent applied. Composite resin is then inserted into the neck of the tooth. If a post is planned then provision should be made for this [39,58].

## ORTHODONTIC TREATMENT

Orthodontists are very concerned about causing resorption of root-filled previously traumatized teeth during tooth movement. However, there is no scientific evidence to show that these teeth are more at risk than vital ones [42,54]. It is essential that the root canal treatment has been carried out properly prior to orthodontic movement and that infection has been eliminated; where there is any concern about the technical quality of the root canal filling, the root canal treatment should be redone first. There is no hard evidence to support the clinical practice of delaying permanent filling of root canals of teeth containing calcium hydroxide until the completion of orthodontic treatment. This practice incurs increased risk of the temporary restoration being lost and the canal reinfected. It also causes additional inconvenience and stress to the patient, as well as risking further complication if the tooth is repeatedly opened to replace calcium hydroxide [24].

## REFERENCES

1. American Heart Association (1997) Prevention of Bacterial Endocarditis. www.americanheart.org/Scientific/statements/1997/079701.html
2. Andersson L, Malmgren B (1999) The problem of dentoalveolar ankylosis and subsequent replacement resorption in the growing patient. *Australian Endodontic Journal* **25**, 57–61.
3. Andreasen FM (1986) Transient apical breakdown and its relation to color and sensibility changes after luxation injuries to teeth. *Endodontics and Dental Traumatology* **2**, 9–19.
4. Andreasen FM (1989) Pulpal healing after luxation injuries and root fracture in the permanent dentition. *Endodontics and Dental Traumatology* **5**, 111–131.
5. Andreasen FM, Andreasen JO (1985) Diagnosis of luxation injuries: the importance of standardized clinical, radiographic and photographic techniques in clinical investigations. *Endodontics and Dental Traumatology* **1**, 160–169.
6. Andreasen FM, Andreasen JO, Bayer T (1989) Prognosis of root-fractured permanent incisors – prediction of healing modalities. *Endodontics and Dental Traumatology* **5**, 11–22.
7. Andreasen FM, Vestergaard Pedersen B (1985) Prognosis of luxated permanent teeth – the development of pulp necrosis. *Endodontics and Dental Traumatology* **1**, 207–220.
8. Andreasen FM, Yu Z, Thomsen BL, Andersen PK (1987) Occurrence of pulp canal obliteration after luxation injuries in the permanent dentition. *Endodontics and Dental Traumatology* **3**, 103–115.
9. Andreasen JO (1970) Etiology and pathogenesis of traumatic dental injuries. A clinical study of 1,298 cases. *Scandinavian Journal of Dental Research* **78**, 329–342.
10. Andreasen JO, Andreasen FM (1994) *Textbook and Color Atlas of Traumatic Injuries to the Teeth,* 3rd edn. Copenhagen: Munksgaard.
11. Andreasen JO, Hjorting-Hansen E (1967) Intraalveolar root fractures: radiographic and histologic study of 50 cases. *Journal of Oral Surgery* **25**, 414–426.
12. Barnett F (2002) The role of endodontics in the treatment of luxated permanent teeth. *Dental Traumatology* **18**, 47–56.
13. Boyd DH, Kinirons MJ, Gregg TA (2000) A prospective study of factors affecting survival of replanted permanent incisors in children. *International Journal of Paediatric Dentistry* **10**, 200–205.
14. Cvek M (1972) Treatment of non-vital permanent incisors with calcium hydroxide. I. Follow-up of periapical repair and apical closure of immature roots. *Odontologisk Revy* **23**, 27–44.
15. Cvek M (1974) Treatment of non-vital permanent incisors with calcium hydroxide. IV. Periodontal healing and closure of the root canal in the coronal fragment of teeth with intra-alveolar fracture and vital apical fragment. A follow-up. *Odontologisk Revy* **25**, 239–246.
16. Cvek M (1978) A clinical report on partial pulpotomy and capping with calcium hydroxide in permanent incisors with complicated crown fracture. *Journal of Endodontics* **4**, 232–237.
17 Cvek M (1992) Prognosis of luxated non-vital maxillary incisors treated with calcium hydroxide and filled with gutta-percha. A retrospective clinical study. *Endodontics and Dental Traumatology* **8**, 45–55.
18. Cvek M, Andreasen J, Borum MK, (2001) Healing of 208 intra-alveolar root fractures in patients aged 7–17 years. *Dental Traumatology* **17**, 53–62.
19. Cvek M, Lindvall AM (1985) External root resorption following bleaching of pulpless teeth with oxygen peroxide. *Endodontics and Dental Traumatology* **1**, 56–60.
20. Cvek M, Lundberg M (1983) Histological appearance of pulps after exposure by a crown fracture, partial pulpotomy, and clinical diagnosis of healing. *Journal of Endodontics* **9**, 8–11.
21. Cvek M, Mejare I, Andreasen JO (2002) Healing and prognosis of teeth with intra-alveolar fractures involving the cervical part of the root. *Dental Traumatology* **18**, 57–65.
22. Cvek M, Sundström B (1974) Treatment of non-vital permanent incisors with calcium hydroxide. V.

Histologic appearance of roentgenographically demonstrable apical closure of immature roots. *Odontologisk Revy* **25**, 379–392.

23. Dental Practice Board for England and Wales (1999 *Treatment of Avulsed Teeth in Children; Treatment of Traumatically Intruded Permanent Incisor Teeth in Children; Management and Root Canal Treatment of Non-vital Immature Permanent Incisor Teeth*. National clinical guidelines and policy document. Eastbourne: Dental Practice Board.

24. Drysdale C, Gibbs SL, Pitt Ford TR (1996) Orthodontic management of root filled teeth. *British Journal of Orthodontics* **23**, 255–260.

25. Dumsha T, Hovland EJ (1995) Evaluation of long-term calcium hydroxide treatment in avulsed teeth – an in vivo study. *International Endodontic Journal* **28**, 7–11.

26. Feiglin B (1985) Differences in apex formation during apexification with calcium hydroxide paste. *Endodontics and Dental Traumatology* **1**, 195–199.

27. Feiglin B (1986) Problems with the endodontic–orthodontic management of fractured teeth. *International Endodontic Journal* **19**, 57–63.

28. Flores MT, Andreasen JO, Bakland LK *et al* (2001) Guidelines for the evaluation and management of traumatic dental injuries. *Dental Traumatology* **17**, 1–4, 49–52, 97–102, 145–148, 193–198.

29. Fuks AB, Chosack A, Klein H, Eidelman E (1987) Partial pulpotomy as a treatment alternative for exposed pulps in crown-fractured permanent incisors. *Endodontics and Dental Traumatology* **3**, 100–102.

30. Granath LE, Hagman G (1971) Experimental pulpotomy in human bicuspids with reference to cutting technique. *Acta Odontologica Scandinavica* **29**, 155–163.

31. Gutmann JL, Heaton JF (1981) Management of the open apex. 2. Non-vital teeth. *International Endodontic Journal* **14**, 173–178.

32. Hammarström LE, Blomlöf LB, Feiglin B, Lindskog SF (1986) Effect of calcium hydroxide treatment on periodontal repair and root resorption. *Endodontics and Dental Traumatology* **2**, 184–189.

33. Heide S, Kerekes K (1986) Delayed partial pulpotomy in permanent incisors of monkeys. *International Endodontic Journal* **19**, 78–89.

34. Heide S, Mjör I (1983) Pulp reactions to experimental exposures in young permanent monkey teeth. *International Endodontic Journal* **16**, 11–19.

35. Heithersay GS (1973) Combined endodontic–orthodontic treatment of transverse root fractures in the region of the alveolar crest. *Oral Surgery, Oral Medicine, Oral Pathology* **36**, 404–415.

36. Heithersay GS (1975) Calcium hydroxide in the treatment of pulpless teeth with associated pathology. *Journal of the British Endodontic Society* **8**, 74–93.

37. Jacobsen I, Kerekes K (1977) Long-term prognosis of traumatized permanent anterior teeth showing calcifying processes in the pulp cavity. *Scandinavian Journal of Dental Research* **85**, 588–598.

38. Jacobsen I, Kerekes K (1980) Diagnosis and treatment of pulp necrosis in permanent anterior teeth with root fracture. *Scandinavian Journal of Dental Research* **88**, 370–376.

39. Katebzadeh N, Dalton BC, Trope M (1998) Strengthening immature teeth during and after apexification. *Journal of Endodontics* **24**, 256–259.

40. Kinirons MJ, Boyd DH, Gregg TA (1999) Inflammatory and replacement resorption in reimplanted permanent incisor teeth: a study of the characteristics of 84 teeth. *Endodontics and Dental Traumatology* **15**, 269–272.

41. Kopel HM, Johnson R (1985) Examination and neurologic assessment of children with oro-facial trauma. *Endodontics and Dental Traumatology* **1**, 155–159.

42. Levander E, Malmgren O (1988) Evaluation of the risk of root resorption during orthodontic treatment: a study of upper incisors. *European Journal of Orthodontics* **10**, 30–38.

43. MacGuire A, Murray JJ, Al-Majed I (2000) A retrospective study of treatment provided in the primary and secondary care services for children attending a dental hospital following complicated crown fracture in the permanent dentition. *International Journal of Paediatric Dentistry* **10**, 182–190.

44. Metzger Z, Solomonov M, Mass E (2001) Calcium hydroxide retention in wide root canals with flaring apices. *Dental Traumatology* **17**, 86–92.

45. Odor TM, Pitt Ford TR, McDonald F (1998) Use of laser Doppler flowmetry for pulp testing – preliminary findings. *International Endodontic Journal* **31**, 189–220 (Abstract).

46. Olgart L, Gazelius B, Lindh-Strömberg U (1988) Laser Doppler flowmetry in assessing vitality in luxated permanent teeth. *International Endodontic Journal* **21**, 300–306.

47. Pitt Ford TR, Shabahang S (2002) Management of incompletely formed roots. In: Walton R, Torabinejad M (eds) *Principles and Practice of Endodontics* Philadelphia, USA: Saunders, pp. 388–404.

48. Pitt Ford T, Torabinejad M, Abedi H, Bakland LK, Kariawasam SP (1996) Using mineral trioxide aggregate as a pulp-capping material. *Journal of the American Dental Association* **127**, 1491–1494.

49. Ravn JJ (1981) Follow-up study of permanent incisors with enamel-dentin fractures after acute trauma. *Scandinavian Journal of Dental Research* **89**, 355–365.

50. Robertson A, Andreasen FM, Andreasen JO, Noren JG (2000) Long-term prognosis of crown-fractured permanent incisors. The effect of stage of root development and associated luxation injury. *International Journal of Paediatric Dentistry* **10**, 191–199.

51. Rotstein I, Mor C, Friedman S (1993) Prognosis of intracoronal bleaching with sodium perborate preparation in vitro: 1-year study. *Journal of Endodontics* **19**, 10–12.

52. Rotstein I, Zalkind M, Mor C, Tarabeah A, Friedman S (1991) In vitro efficacy of sodium perborate preparations used for intracoronal bleaching of discolored non-vital teeth. *Endodontics and Dental Traumatology* **7**, 177–180.

53. Shabahang S, Torabinejad M (2000) Treatment of teeth with open apices using mineral trioxide aggregate.

*Practical Periodontics and Aesthetic Dentistry* **12**, 315–320.

54. Spurrier SW, Hall SH, Joondeph DR, Shapiro PA, Riedel RA (1990) A comparison of apical root resorption during orthodontic treatment in endodontically treated and vital teeth. *American Journal of Orthodontics and Dentofacial Orthopedics* **97**, 130–134.

55. Stalhane I, Hedegard B (1975) Traumatized permanent teeth in children aged 7–15 years. Part II. *Swedish Dental Journal* **68**, 157–169.

56. Tronstad L (1988) Root resorption – etiology, terminology and clinical manifestations. *Endodontics and Dental Traumatology* **4**, 241–252.

57. Trope M (2002) Clinical management of the avulsed tooth: present strategies and future directions. *Dental Traumatology* **18**, 1–11.

58. Trope M, Maltz DO, Tronstad L (1985) Resistance to fracture of restored endodontically treated teeth. *Dental Traumatology* **1**, 108–111.

59. Welbury RR, Kinirons MJ, Day P, Gregg TA (2002) Outcomes of root fractured permanent incisors. *Paediatric Dentistry* **24**, 98–102.

60. Working Party of the British Society for Antimicrobial Chemotherapy (2001) *British National Formulary* British Medical Association, London, pp. 255–256.

61. Yates JA (1988) Barrier formation time in non-vital teeth with open apices. *International Endodontic Journal* **21**, 313–319.

62. Zachrisson BU, Jacobsen I (1975) Long-term prognosis of 66 permanent anterior teeth with root fracture. *Scandinavian Journal of Dental Research* **83**, 345–354.

63. Zadik D, Chosack A, Eidelman E (1979) The prognosis of traumatized permanent anterior teeth with fracture of the enamel and dentin. *Oral Surgery, Oral Medicine, Oral Pathology* **47**, 173–175.

# Marginal periodontitis and the dental pulp

## J. H. Simon and A. L. Frank

Anatomy  215

Effect of necrotic pulp on the periodontium  215

Effect of marginal periodontitis on the pulp  216

Classification  217
  Primary endodontic lesion  217
  Primary endodontic lesion with secondary periodontal
    involvement  217
  Primary periodontal lesion  221
  Primary periodontal lesion with secondary endodontic
    involvement  222
  Combined lesions  226
  Retrospective classification  226
  Prognosis  226

Complications due to radicular anomalies  227
  Diagnosis  227
  Treatment  228

Anatomical redesigning  228
  Indications  228
  Contraindications for anatomical redesigning  228
  Root amputation  229
  Tooth resection  231
  Bicuspidization  233

References  234

## ANATOMY

From the beginning pulp and periodontium are intimately related. The pulp develops from the dental papilla while the periodontal ligament and cementum are derived from the dental follicle. They are separated only by Hertwig's epithelial root sheath prior to root formation. However, there is a common area at the future apical foramen.

As development progresses there is a direct vascular communication between the pulp and periodontium through the apical foramen and accessory (lateral) canals. There are many studies documenting the incidence and location of accessory canals in animal and human teeth [10,13,16,20, 23,26,28,31]. Another area of communication is the dentinal tubules that have been denuded of cementum by development, disease or periodontal treatment. The cervical area may be unprotected by acellular cementum developmentally. This area becomes important because of the effects of bleaching and resorptive defects. Other areas of dentinal communication may be in developmental grooves both palatogingival and apical [36]. The base of these grooves is often not covered by cementum and the presence of accessory canals has been observed.

## EFFECT OF NECROTIC PULP ON THE PERIODONTIUM

When the pulp becomes necrotic either totally or partially, there is a direct inflammatory (vascular) response by the periodontal ligament at the apical foramen and/or at the opening of accessory canals [33]. All the aetiological factors of pulp disease may leach through the openings and trigger an inflammatory vascular response in the periodontal ligament. Endotoxin, spirochetes, other bacteria, yeasts and viruses can exit into the periodontal ligament [4,12,17,19,38,39,40,42]. Many of these are similar pathogens to those that cause marginal periodontitis.

In an experimental study, small and large defects were created on root surfaces of extracted lateral incisors with open or mature apices. The canals were either infected or filled with calcium hydroxide, and replanted. It was concluded that intrapulpal infection promoted marginal epithelial downgrowth on the denuded dentine surface after 20 weeks [8].

The effects of endodontic pathogens on marginal periodontal wound healing on dentinal surfaces surrounded by healthy periodontal ligament have been assessed [21]. The significant differences were that in infected teeth the defect was covered by 20% more epithelium and the non-infected had 10% more connective tissue covering. They concluded that the pathogens in a necrotic canal stimulate epithelial downgrowth along denuded dentine surfaces with marginal communication. Thus endodontic infections in patients with marginal periodontitis may augment propagation of the periodontitis.

The magnitude and rate of radiological proximal bone loss in relation to endodontic infection in periodontally involved teeth was measured in a retrospective longitudinal study on 175 single-rooted endodontically treated teeth [20]. After observing for a minimum of three years, it was found that in patients with marginal periodontitis the teeth with failing root canal treatment lost more attachment radiologically than teeth with no periapical lesions or healing lesions. A three-fold increase in bone loss in teeth with periapical disease was reported.

The effect of endodontic infection on periodontal probing depth and the presence of furcation involvement in mandibular molars has been investigated [18]. In 100 patients who had molars with periapical lesions on both roots, the periodontal probing depth was significantly greater than around teeth without periapical lesions. It was suggested that root canal infection in molars involved with marginal periodontitis may potentiate periodontitis progression by spreading pathogens through accessory canals and dentinal tubules. It was concluded that endodontic infection in mandibular molars was associated with more attachment loss in the furca, and is thus a risk factor in patients with marginal periodontitis.

The profiles of periodontal pathogens in pulp and periodontal diseases affecting the same tooth was studied by means of 16S RNA gene directed polymerase chain reaction samples from 31 teeth [32]. Specific polymerase chain reaction methods were used to detect *Actinobacillus actinomycetemcomitans, Bacteroides forsythicus, Eikenella corrodens, Fusobacterium nucleatum, Porphyromonas gingivalis Prevotella intermedia* and *Treponena denticola*. The pathogens were found in all endodontic samples. In chronic apical periodontitis and chronic marginal periodontitis the same pathogens were found. It was concluded that periodontal pathogens often accompany endodontic infections and support the concept that endo/perio interrelationships are a critical pathway for both diseases. In addition foreign bodies and materials may also pass into the periapical tissues. Extrinic foreign bodies, including foreign lipids, cellulose granulomas and iatrogenic materials, can cause a direct inflammatory response.

## EFFECT OF MARGINAL PERIODONTITIS ON THE PULP

The effect of periodontal inflammation on the pulp is an area of controversy. Conflicting studies abound [2,3,6,7,11,14,15,27,30,34,37,41,43]. There are a number of studies that have concluded that marginal periodontitis has no effect on the pulp at least until it involves the apex. On the other hand there are studies that conclude that the effect of marginal periodontitis on the pulp is degenerative, i.e. an increase in calcifications, fibrosis and collagen resorption and also a direct inflammatory affect. It is our view that the pulp is not directly affected by marginal periodontitis until recession has opened an accessory canal to the oral environment. At this time pathogens from the oral cavity penetrate the accessory canal to the pulp and a direct inflammatory response leads to necrosis. However, as long as the accessory canal is covered by tissue, necrosis does not follow. It has been stated that as long as the apical vasculature is intact, the pulp will maintain its vitality. This concept is shown in teeth with primary marginal periodontitis and secondary endodontic disease (necrosis).

The effect of periodontal treatment on the pulp is similar during scaling, curettage or surgery. If vessels in accessory canals are severed and/or the canals are opened to the oral environment, a pathway is created for pathogenic invasion and secondary necrosis of the pulp to occur.

## CLASSIFICATION

There have been many ways to classify so-called endo-perio lesions [1,5,7,34,35]. The simplest is to call them endodontic, periodontal or a combination of the two. They can also be classified by treatment depending on whether endodontic, periodontal or a combination of both treatments is necessary. However, these do not explain how the lesions form. The following classification is preferred because it explains the theoretical pathways of lesion formation [35]:

- primary endodontic lesion;
- primary endodontic lesion with secondary periodontal involvement;
- primary periodontal lesion;
- primary periodontal lesion with secondary endodontic involvement;
- combined lesions.

### Primary endodontic lesion

An acute exacerbation of a chronic apical lesion on a tooth with a necrotic pulp may drain coronally through the periodontal ligament into the gingival sulcus area (Fig. 12.1a). This situation may mimic a periodontal abscess. However, it is only periodontal in that it passes through the periodontal ligament area (Figs 12.2–12.6). In reality, it is a sinus tract resulting from pulp disease. Thus it is essential that a gutta-percha cone is inserted into the sinus tract and one or more radiographs taken to determine the origin of the lesion. When the sinus tract is probed, it is narrow and lacks width. A similar situation occurs where drainage from the apex of a molar tooth extends coronally into the furcation area (Fig 12.7). Direct extension of inflammation from the pulp may also occur into the furcation area of a non-vital tooth when a lateral canal is present (Fig. 12.8).

Primary endodontic lesions usually heal following root canal treatment; the sinus tract extending into the gingival sulcus or furcation area disappears at an early stage once the necrotic pulp has been treated. It is important to recognize that failure of any periodontal treatment will occur when the presence of a necrotic pulp has not been diagnosed, and therefore not treated.

### Primary endodontic lesion with secondary periodontal involvement

If after a period of time a suppurating primary endodontic lesion remains untreated, it may then

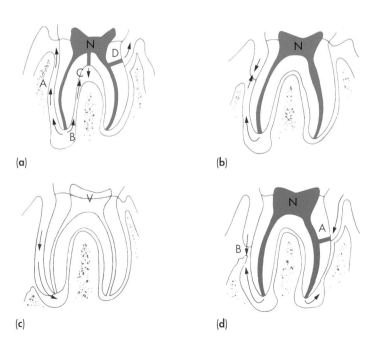

(a)  (b)  (c)  (d)

**Figure 12.1** Classification of endodontic-periodontal lesions. (**a**) Primary endodontic lesions: pathway extending from apex to gingival sulcus via periodontium (A); apex to furcation (B); lateral canal to furcation (C); lateral canal to pocket (D). (**b**) Primary endodontic lesion with secondary periodontal involvement. (**c**) Primary periodontal lesion extending to the apex. (**d**) Primary periodontal lesion with secondary endodontic involvement via a lateral canal (A). Combined lesion from coalescence of separate lesions (B). N = Necrotic pulp. V = Vital pulp.

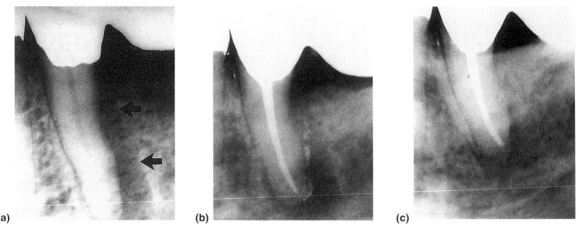

(a)      (b)      (c)

**Figure 12.2** Primary endodontic lesion. Mandibular premolar with a radiolucency along the distal surface of the root. (a) Pretreatment, the lesion (arrowed) drained through the gingival sulcus. (b) Immediately after treatment, root canal sealer can be observed in the sinus tract. (c) Six months later, there is evidence of considerable healing and bone filling.

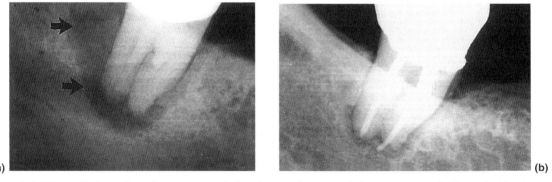

(a)                                        (b)

**Figure 12.3** (a) Mandibular molar with a narrow probable distal pocket and radiolucency (arrowed). (b) Marked healing apparent at one-year recall confirming that the original 'pocket' was of endodontic origin.

become secondarily involved with marginal periodontal breakdown (Fig. 12.1b). Plaque forms at the gingival margin of the sinus tract and leads to marginal periodontitis. When plaque or calculus is encountered with a probe, the treatment and prognosis of the tooth are altered; the tooth now requires both endodontic and periodontal treatment. If the endodontic treatment is adequate, the prognosis depends on the severity of the marginal periodontal damage and the efficacy of periodontal treatment. With endodontic treatment alone, only part of the lesion will heal to the level of the secondary periodontal lesion. In general, healing of the tissues only damaged by suppuration from the pulp space can be anticipated.

Primary endodontic lesions with secondary periodontal involvement may also occur as a result of root perforation during root canal treatment, or where pins or posts have been misplaced during coronal restoration (Fig. 12.9). Symptoms may be acute, with periodontal abscess formation associated with pain, swelling, exudation of pus, pocket formation and tooth mobility. A more chronic response may sometimes occur without pain, and involves the sudden appearance of a pocket with bleeding on probing or exudation of pus. When the root perforation is situated close to the alveolar crest, it may be possible to raise a flap and repair the defect with an appropriate filling material, and then to replace the flap apically, so exteriorizing the

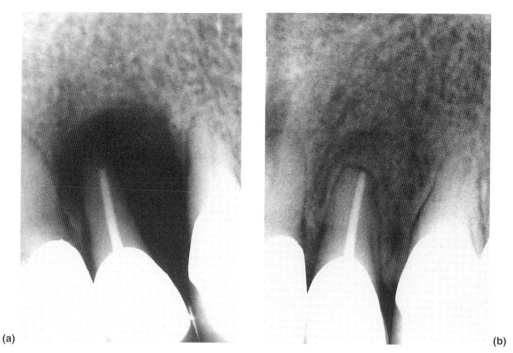

(a)  (b)

**Figure 12.4** (a) Immediately after root canal filling a non-vital lateral incisor with extensive loss of surrounding bone. (b) Radiograph taken one year later showing healing, and confirming lesion was of endodontic origin.

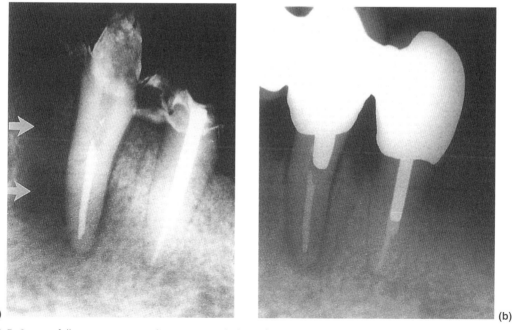

(a)  (b)

**Figure 12.5** Success following treatment of a primary endodontic lesion. (a) Immediate post-treatment radiograph of a mandibular canine showing mesial radiolucency (arrowed). (b) Radiograph at 15 months showing healing.

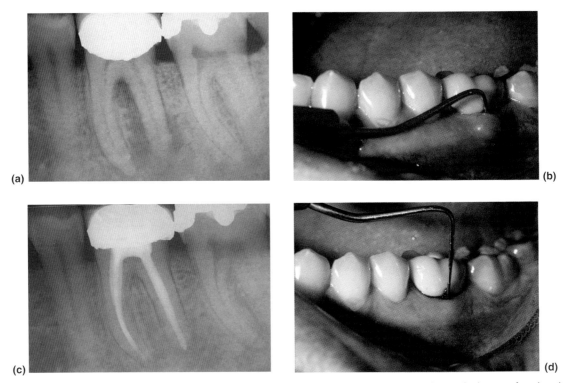

**Figure 12.6** Mandibular molar where apical lesion extends into furcation. **(a)** Preoperative radiograph showing furcal and distal radiolucency. **(b)** Clinical photograph of gingival swelling and a periodontal probe in the furcation. **(c)** A one-year recall radiograph with furcal and distal radiolucencies healed. **(d)** Clinical photograph showing minimal pocket depth on the buccal. Only root canal treatment was performed.

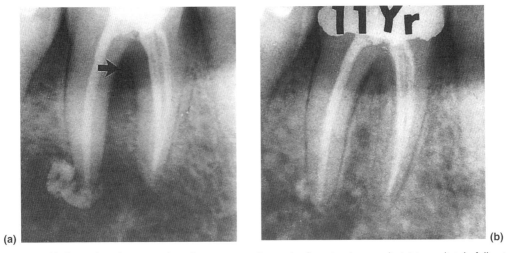

**Figure 12.7** Mandibular molar where apical involvement extends into the furcation (arrowed). **(a)** Immediately following root canal treatment, excess sealer is present at the apex of the distal root. **(b)** Radiograph 11 years later showing healing apically and in the furcation.

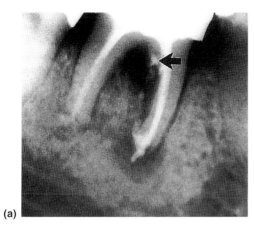
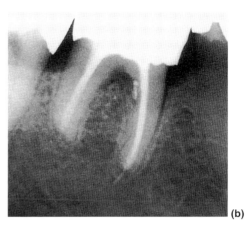

**Figure 12.8** Primary endodontic lesion with a lateral canal in the furcation. (**a**) Post-treatment radiograph demonstrates a filled lateral canal opening into the furcation (arrowed). (**b**) After 18 months total healing of lesions at the apex and adjacent to the lateral canal is demonstrated.

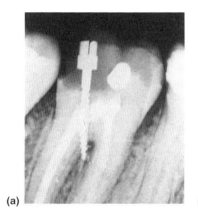
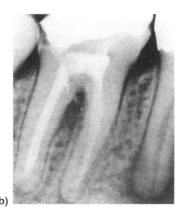
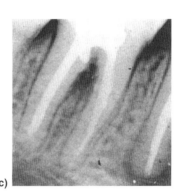

**Figure 12.9** Primary endodontic lesion with secondary periodontal involvement. (**a**) A Dentatus screw has perforated the furcation of a mandibular second molar. (**b**) After six months, bone loss is evident in the furcation and a pocket has formed. (**c**) The perforation has been treated from within the tooth and the pocket has been curetted. No pocket is probable clinically and some new bone has formed in the furcation.

repaired perforation. In deeper perforations, or in the roof of the furcation, immediate internal repair of the perforation has a better prognosis than management of an infected one. Amalgam has been widely used but the long-term results have been disappointing. Recent work with mineral trioxide aggregate has demonstrated cemental healing following immediate repair [29]; delayed repair was not as good but indicates potential for further investigation.

Root fractures may also present as primary endodontic lesions with secondary periodontal involvement. These typically occur on root-treated teeth (Fig. 12.10), often with post crowns in situ.

The signs may range from a local deepening of a periodontal pocket to more acute periodontal abscess formation. Root fractures have also become an increasing problem with molar teeth that have been treated by root resection. In a study of 100 patients, a total of 38 teeth failed during the ten-year period of observation, and 47% of the failures were due to root fractures, with the vast majority being in mandibular molar teeth [25].

**Primary periodontal lesion**

These lesions (Fig. 12.1c) are caused by marginal periodontitis, which progresses apically along the

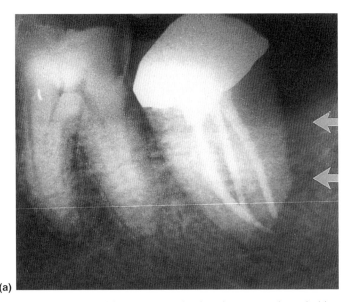

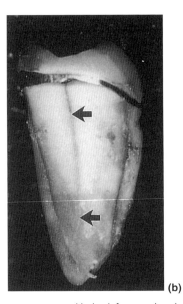

(a)                                                                    (b)

**Figure 12.10** Longitudinal fracture. (**a**) A distal pocket (arrowed), probable to the apex on a mandibular left second molar, persisted following root canal treatment, necessitating extraction. (**b**) Following extraction, a longitudinal fracture on the distal root surface (arrowed) was evident extending the length of the tooth. Fused roots prevented 'anatomical redesigning'.

root surface until the apical region is approximated. In primarily periodontally involved teeth, pulp-testing procedures reveal a clinically normal pulp response (Figs 12.11 and 12.12). In addition one would anticipate a probable pocket that has width, possibly becoming progressively shallower as the probe is moved laterally. There is an accumulation of plaque and frequently calculus.

The prognosis in this situation depends wholly upon the stage of marginal periodontitis and the efficacy of periodontal treatment. The clinician must also be aware of the radiological appearance of marginal periodontitis associated with developmental radicular anomalies (see later).

## Primary periodontal lesion with secondary endodontic involvement

The apical progression of a periodontal pocket can continue until the apex is reached; the vital pulp may become necrotic as a result of infection entering via a lateral canal or the apical foramen (Fig. 12.1d). In single rooted teeth the prognosis is usually hopeless, which is the opposite of that for the primary endodontic lesion. In molar teeth not all the roots may suffer the same loss of supporting

tissues to the apex, in which case the possibility of root resection should be considered.

The treatment of marginal periodontitis can lead to secondary endodontic involvement. Lateral canals and dentinal tubules may be opened to the oral environment by curettage, scaling or surgical

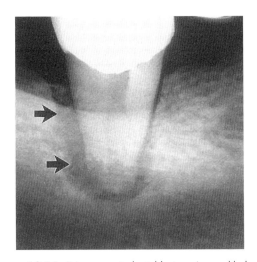

**Figure 12.11** Primary periodontal lesion. A mandibular molar presented with a probable pocket distally (arrowed). Pulp testing gave a vital response indicating a lesion of periodontal origin; the tooth was extracted.

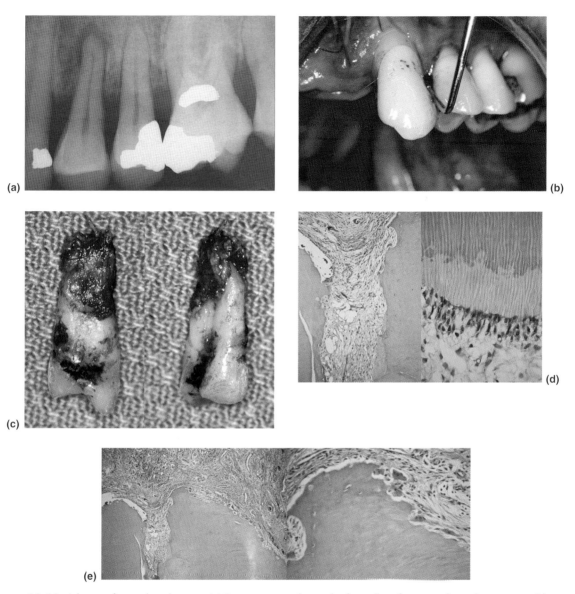

**Figure 12.12** A lesion of periodontal origin. (**a**) Preoperative radiograph of maxillary first premolar with a periapical lesion but no obvious endodontic cause. (**b**) Clinical photograph with periodontal probe in place. (**c**) Two views of the extracted tooth. The pulp tested normal to sensitivity testing procedures. Note mesial anatomical groove along the root. (**d**) Micrographs showing vital pulp in the tooth. (**e**) Micrographs showing inflammatory resorption and periodontitis.

flap procedures (Figs 12.13 and 12.14). In addition, it is possible for a blood vessel within a lateral canal to be severed by a curette during treatment. Controversy exists as to whether progressive periodontitis has any effect on the vitality of the pulp. Pulp changes resulting from marginal periodontitis involves the main apical foramen [24]. Provided that the blood supply through the apex is intact, the pulp has a strong capacity for survival (Fig. 12.11). A strong relationship between the cultivable microorganisms from the root canals of human caries-free teeth with advanced periodontitis and from their periodontal pockets has been shown [22], with the microorganisms in the pocket a possible source of root canal infection. Support for this concept has come from research in which cultured samples

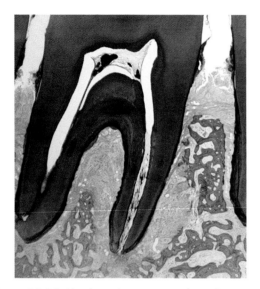

**Figure 12.13** Histological examination shows that furcation involvement can be severe in advanced marginal periodontitis. The pulp can become affected through a lateral canal.

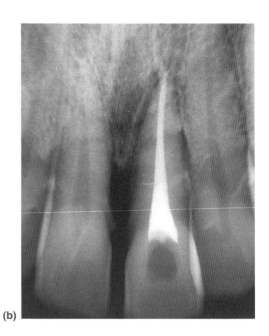

(b)

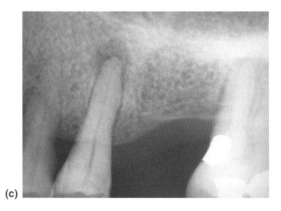

(c)

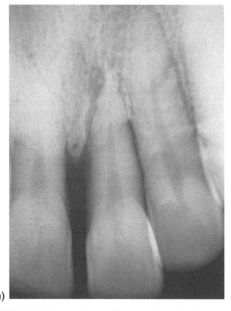

(a)

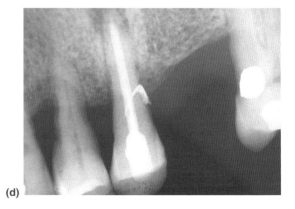

(d)

**Figure 12.14** Marginal periodontitis with endodontic involvement. (**a**) Radiograph of an unrestored tooth with generalized periodontitis and a necrotic pulp. (**b**) After endodontic treatment a communication with the oral environment through a lateral canal has been demonstrated. (**c**) A similar situation on a premolar with generalized periodontitis and a necrotic pulp. (**d**) A lateral canal has been filled, indicating how the pulp became necrotic.

obtained from the pulp tissue and radicular dentine of human periodontally involved teeth showed bacterial growth in 87% of the teeth [2,3]. It was suggested that the reservoir of bacteria in the dentine and pulp tissue might contribute to the failure of periodontal treatment. The possibility might also exist that these teeth would develop pulp necrosis.

There is often a lack of relationship between marginal periodontitis and pulp involvement [37];

the histological status of the pulps of 100 periodontally involved teeth was the same as that for 22 control teeth with a normal periodontium [25]. Despite the conflict of opinion from various research studies [7,43], it would seem that, on a clinical basis at least, plaque-associated marginal periodontitis rarely causes significant pathological changes in the pulp, and this remains true until the periodontal pocket reaches the apical foramen.

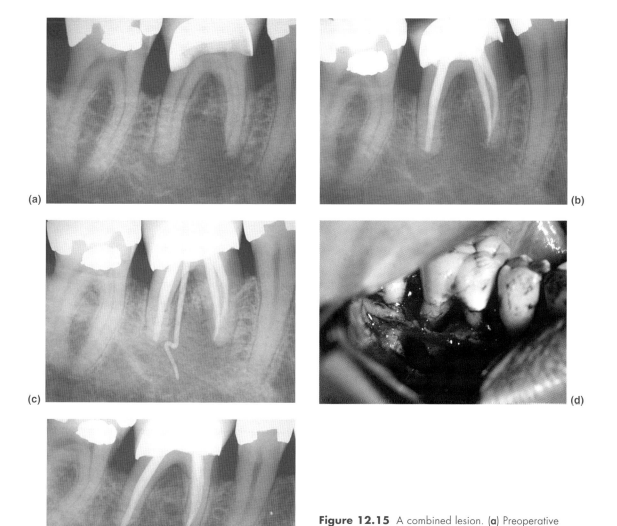

(a)

(b)

(c)

(d)

(e)

**Figure 12.15** A combined lesion. (**a**) Preoperative radiograph of a mandibular molar with a furcal lesion and necrotic pulp. (**b**) After endodontic treatment. (**c**) Recall radiograph with a gutta-percha point in the gingival sulcus. (**d**) Periodontal surgery and treatment were performed on the cervical and furcal areas. (**e**) One year after both endodontic and periodontal treatment, the lesions healed.

## Combined lesions

Combined lesions (Fig. 12.1d) occur where an endodontic lesion progressing coronally becomes continuous with a plaque-infected periodontal pocket progressing apically [35]. The degree of attachment loss in the type of lesion is invariably large and the prognosis guarded. The prognosis is particularly poor in single rooted teeth, but the situation may be salvaged in molars by sectioning the tooth, where not all the roots are as severely involved. Healing of apical periodontitis may be anticipated following successful endodontic treatment. The periodontal aspects then may (or may not) respond to periodontal treatment, depending on the severity of involvement (Figs 12.15 and 12.16). A similar radiological appearance may result from a longitudinally fractured tooth. If a sinus tract is present, it may be necessary to raise a flap to help determine the exact cause of the lesion. A fracture that has penetrated to the pulp space, with resultant necrosis, may also be labelled a true combined lesion and yet not be amenable to successful treatment (Fig. 12.10).

## Retrospective classification

The classifying of primary endodontic and primary periodontal lesions presents little clinical difficulty. In a primarily endodontically involved tooth the pulp is infected and non-vital; however, in a tooth with a primary periodontal defect the pulp is vital and responsive to testing. This is not true in the differential classification of primary endodontic lesions with secondary periodontal involvement, or primary periodontal lesions with secondary endodontic involvement, or the combined lesions. All of these three entities are clinically and radiologically very similar. If the lesion is diagnosed and treated as primarily endodontic because of lack of evidence of marginal periodontitis, and there is soft-tissue healing on clinical probing and bony healing on a recall radiogragh, a valid retrospective diagnosis can then be made. The degree of healing that has taken place following root canal treatment will determine the retrospective classification. At that stage, in the absence of adequate healing, further periodontal treatment would be indicated.

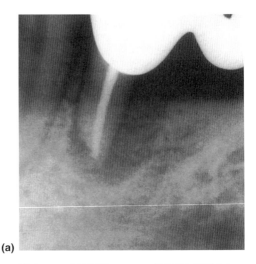

**(a)**

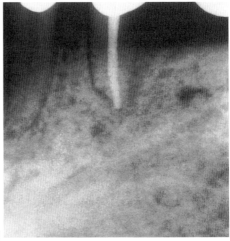

**(b)**

**Figure 12.16** Combined endodontic-periodontal lesion, in which healing will occur to the level of the marginal periodontal breakdown. **(a)** Immediate postoperative radiograph after root canal treatment of a non-vital premolar, which received periodontal curettage. **(b)** Recall radiograph at two years demonstrated stable healing.

## Prognosis

The prognosis of each classification has been discussed along with aetiology. To assist in their comparative understanding, each will be repeated in the following summary.

### *Primary endodontic lesion*

Treatment – root canal treatment.
Prognosis – good.

*Primary periodontal lesion*

Treatment – periodontal treatment.
Prognosis – depends on periodontal treatment and patient response.

*Combined lesions*

Treatment – endodontic and periodontal treatment.
Prognosis – dependent on periodontal treatment and patient response.

## COMPLICATIONS DUE TO RADICULAR ANOMALIES

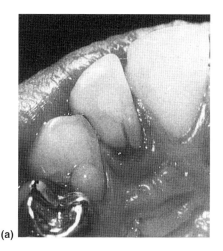

(a)

Observation of extracted teeth and clinical cases has disclosed a particular group that fails to respond to treatment. These are directly associated with an invagination or a longitudinal developmental radicular groove, which can lead to untreatable localized marginal periodontitis (Fig. 12.17). These grooves usually begin in the central fossa of maxillary central or lateral incisors crossing over the cingulum, and continuing apically down the root for varying distances. Such a groove is apparently the result of an attempt of the tooth germ to form another root. This fissure-like channel may provide a nidus for plaque and an avenue for the progression of marginal periodontitis.

From the time the tooth develops with this anomalous root defect, the potential for isolated marginal periodontitis exits. As long as the epithelial attachment remains intact, the periodontium remains healthy. However, once this attachment is breached and the groove becomes involved, a self-sustaining infrabony pocket can be formed along its entire length. Radiologically the area of bone destruction follows the course of the groove.

### Diagnosis

The clinical diagnosis of this condition is all important. The patient may have the symptoms of a periodontal abscess or a variety of endodontic conditions. If the condition is purely periodontal, it can be diagnosed by visually following the groove to the gingival sulcus and by probing the depth of the pocket, which is usually tubular in form and

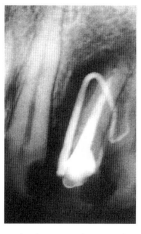

(b)

**Figure 12.17** Radicular anomaly. (**a**) A lingual groove on the lateral incisor was probable to the apex. (**b**) Root canal treatment did not improve the situation and the defect remained probable to a gutta-percha point.

localized to this one area, as opposed to a more generalized periodontal problem. The tooth will be responsive to pulp-testing procedures. Bone destruction that follows the groove longitudinally may be apparent radiologically. If this entity is also associated with an endodontic problem, the patient may present clinically with any of the spectrum of endodontic symptoms, and pulp testing will not produce a response.

The prognosis for root canal treatment will be guarded, depending upon the apical extent of the groove. The dentist must look for the groove because it may have been altered by a previous restoration on the palatal surface. The appearance of a teardrop-shaped area on the radiograph should immediately arouse suspicion. The developmental groove may actually be visible on the radiograph; if so, it will appear as a dark longitudinal line. This condition must be differentiated from a longitudinal fracture, which may give a similar radiological appearance.

### Treatment

In essence, since this lesion is a self-sustaining infrabony pocket, scaling and root planing alone may be inadequate. Although the acute nature of the problem may be alleviated initially, the reason for the inflammation must be eradicated by burring out the groove and surgical management of the tissues, or in advanced cases by extraction.

## ANATOMICAL REDESIGNING

To assist in periodontal treatment and in certain endodontic situations, anatomical redesigning may become necessary. Such redesigning, which includes root amputation, resection and bicuspidization techniques, develops a periodontally maintainable environment for the remaining root(s). The ten-year survival rate is approximately 68% [9].

*Root amputation* is the removal of one or more roots from a multirooted tooth, leaving the majority of the crown and any existing restoration intact.

*Tooth resection* involves the removal of one or more roots of a tooth along with their coronal part(s); it is sometimes referred to as hemisection.

*Bicuspidization* is the separation of a multirooted tooth by a vertical cut through the furcation.

### Indications

There are a number of indications for root amputation or tooth resection:

- Advanced marginal periodontitis. The pattern of alveolar bone loss in marginal periodontitis may be unequal on the different roots of a molar tooth. If left untreated, the adjacent healthier root support could eventually become involved by direct extension of the periodontal lesion and the prognosis of the tooth would deteriorate. Removal of the offending root(s)

would allow the well-supported part of the tooth to be retained as a functional tooth with healthy tissues and a normal radiological appearance.
- Close root proximity. The distobuccal root of the maxillay first molar and the mesiobuccal root of the second molar often tend to flare towards each other. Marginal periodontitis in these areas may lead to angular bone loss, which is difficult to treat and also provides the patient with a particular problem of plaque control management. Selective root removal will allow the re-establishment of a proper embrasure area.
- Furcation involvement.
- Extensive root caries or root resorption.
- Root fracture or perforation.
- Inability to perform root canal treatment. The canal may be calcified, a broken instrument present, or a ledge may have been created as a result of procedural errors.

The indications for bicuspidization are:

- Gross perforation in the furcation. The length of the remaining roots must be favourable.
- Close root proximity. This prevents periodontal treatment or patient home maintenance; it can be improved by root separation.

### Contraindications for anatomical redesigning

- Poor patient motivation and plaque control. This is particularly so if there has been inadequate improvement following initial periodontal treatment.
- Unfavourable bony support. This relates to all remaining roots of the involved tooth, particularly if it is an abutment for a fixed prosthesis.
- Fused roots. These prevent root removal. A special clinical situation with a more favourable prognosis exits when there is only apical fusion and adequate interradicular bone, allowing for surgical root removal.
- Short thin roots.
- A long root trunk. The furcation area is situated so far apically that considerable supporting bone would need to be sacrificed.

- Surrounding anatomy. This may preclude the formation of a functional band of attached gingiva around the ramaining roots.
- Non-negotiable canals. The canals are sclerosed or blocked by a broken instrument, and root-end surgery is impossible.
- Non-restorable tooth.

## Root amputation

This form of treatment relates primarily to maxillary molar teeth and the most common root to be removed by amputation is the distobuccal of the first molar. Whenever possible, root canal treatment and sealing of the pulp chamber with a permanent restorative material extending into the coronal part of the root to be resected should be carried out, prior to root removal (Fig. 12.18). Coronal reshaping

and buccolingual narrowing should also be completed to bring occlusal forces over the solid roots that remain.

The need for root removal may become apparent during diagnosis and treatment planning of the case, as a solution to treating roots with extensive periodontal breakdown. Root canal treatment is completed on the tooth in question with a permanent restorative material placed in the pulp chamber and coronal part of the root to be amputated, as soon as the patient's plaque control has reached a satisfactory level and the inflammatory phase has been resolved. Full-thickness mucoperiosteal flaps are reflected to expose the furcation area. Careful exploration with a furcation periodontal probe is required to make sure that the furcation has not been exposed on all three surfaces. If so, tooth resection would be required, leaving one root in

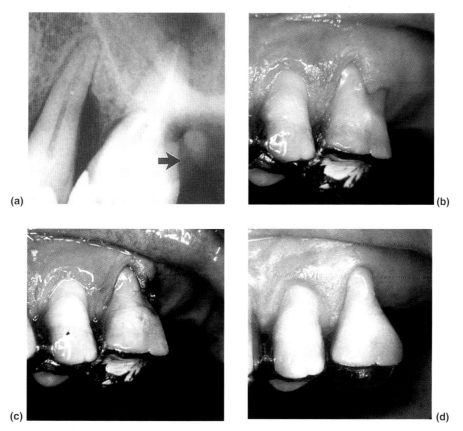

(a)  (b)  (c)  (d)

**Figure 12.18** (a) Marginal periodontal involvement of the distobuccal root (arrowed) of the maxillary first molar necessitated its amputation. (b) Prior to amputation. (c) Following amputation. (d) The remaining tooth after being smoothed and polished.

situ, or the tooth would need to be extracted. The cut in the root is made with a long thin bur, which is long enough to reach from one side of the root to the other. Care must be taken to maintain the correct angulation of the bur, so as not to damage the remaining root(s) or the crown. The bur is held at a 45° angle to the tooth at the level of the furcation. Removal of some of the buccal cortical plate of bone may be required so that the separated root can be gently elevated out of its socket, without undue pressure being applied to the adjacent tooth or bone. Once the root has been removed, the area of the stump should be reshaped with burs, so that it blends imperceptibly into the remaining tooth structure. Enough clearance should also be left between the undersurface of the crown and the gingival tissue to allow for adequate plaque control. The tooth surface should finally be finished with fine burs and then polished.

A re-evaluation of the periodontal situation is carried out some three months after root removal. If mucogingival and osseous deformities remain in this quadrant of the mouth, definitive periodontal surgery should then be carried out.

An alternative method of treatment allows for root amputation to be carried out at the time of periodontal surgery; this has the advantage of allowing for only one surgical procedure. The disadvantage is that bony healing has yet to occur, and the extent to which this will progress cannot always be predicted; this may result in more radical reshaping in the area than might otherwise be required. In this approach, a cavity is cut over the pulp stump with a suitable bur and an appropriate dressing placed over the exposed pulp. Definitive root canal treatment is carried out at a later stage after the periodontal dressings have been removed [36]. It is more difficult to control root canal irrigants, prevent microbial contamination of the pulp space, and fill the orifice of the resected root.

Situations may present where it is reasonable to amputate the root of a mandibular molar. If such a tooth presents with a periodontally-involved mesial root and it is part of a multiunit bridge or splinted crowns, its amputation should be considered. The buccolingual dimension of the occlusal aspect of the tooth and pontics should be reduced to minimize and redirect the occlusal forces if possible (Fig. 12.19). Another situation where an amputation

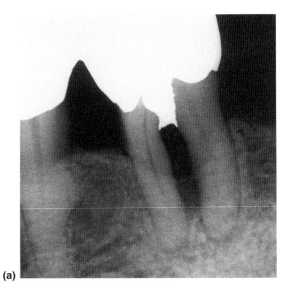

(a)

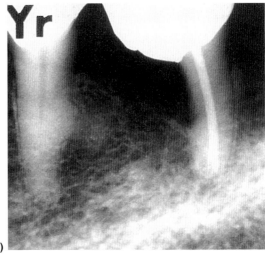

(b)

**Figure 12.19** (a) A perforation with periodontal breakdown in the furcation of a mandibular molar; the tooth was part of a 4-unit splint. The mesial root was amputated and the coronal restoration recontoured and reduced buccolingually. (b) Recall at 13 years demonstrated long-term stability.

could be considered is when the periodontally involved root of a crowned tooth is adjacent to another crowned tooth. They could be firmly splinted to each other to avoid longitudinal fracture of the remaining root (Fig. 12.20); broad interproximal contact without splinting is not sufficient (Fig. 12.21). Maxillary molars do not normally present a similar problem because of the support provided

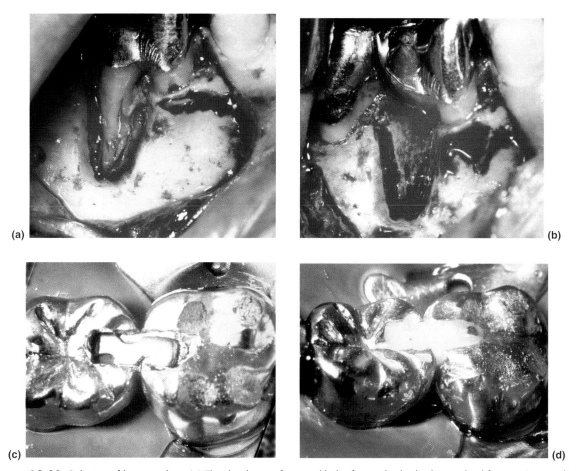

**Figure 12.20** Splinting of lower molars. (**a**) The distal root of a mandibular first molar had a longitudinal fracture (arrowed) necessitating removal. (**b**) Following amputation of the root and contouring of the remaining structure. (**c**) An occlusal preparation was made for a metal splint. (**d**) A restorative filling material has been used to keep the splint in place.

by the two remaining roots. The remaining coronal portion of the amputated root should be physiologically contoured to allow for maintenance of periodontal health. The canal at the amputation site should be prepared and filled with a suitable restorative material to prevent the accumulation of plaque and development of caries. It is best to place the filling internally prior to root removal. If this is not feasible, a filling should be placed into the resected root end during the surgical procedure.

## Tooth resection

Tooth resection is often the treatment of choice in deep furcation involvements. It is also the treatment

of choice where teeth are to be included in a fixed prosthesis [1]. A considerable advantage is achieved if the initial crown preparation is completed first. This then serves as a guide to entering the furcation.

Full-thickness mucoperiosteal flaps are reflected and the tooth is sectioned using a long tapered bur. In maxillary molars, depending on the degree of furcation involvement, it may be possible to retain two roots, providing the furcation is not open between them, such as mesial and palatal, or distal and palatal, or the two buccal roots. If the furcation proves to be open mesially, buccally and distally, only the best supported root is retained. Sometimes this can only be judged by sectioning all three roots and assessing them individually [16]. The fissure

231

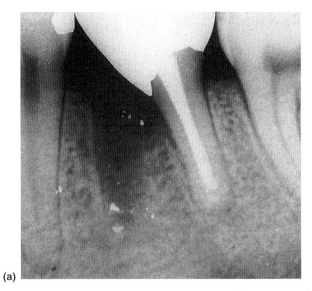
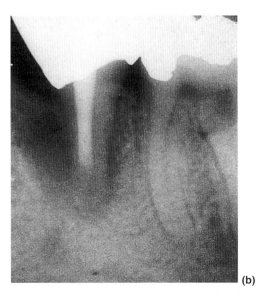

(a)  (b)

**Figure 12.21** Broad interproximal contact is not sufficient support following amputation. (**a**) A crown was prepared on the distal root of the first molar to provide broad interproximal contact with the adjacent tooth. (**b**) Although successful for four years, a longitudinal fracture then occurred; a diffuse radiolucency can be seen around the root. The tooth had to be extracted.

bur is positioned in the long axis of the tooth at the most coronal level of the involved furcation. Initial cuts are made in the crown in the direction of the adjacent furcation. The same step is then followed from the adjacent furcation towards the initial cut. The bur is then alternated between the two cuts until they are joined. Mandibular molars are sectioned buccolingually into two halves. As a general rule it is important to make the cut at the expense of the part which is to be removed (Fig. 12.22a). This minimizes the risk of overcutting the retained section. When sectioning has been completed, the involved part of the tooth is extracted with forceps. In finishing the preparation it is important to remove the overhang of the crown that may be left at the roof of the furcation and to blend the cut surface into the retained portion of the tooth. This should be checked radiologically. When the vertical cut to the furcation ends in close proximity to or at the level of bone, it is necessary to remove approximately 1 mm of the bone with a sharp scalpel in order to expose some intact cementum beyond the cut surface (Fig. 12.22b). It is not advisable to end the restoration within the cut, leaving raw-cut dentine exposed because of the potential for later marginal caries (Fig. 12.23). The biological width of the periodontium

must be maintained. This will facilitate the preparation for the restoration to follow (Fig. 12.24). There may be situations where it is necessary to consider occlusal factors, as in amputation, and reduce the size of the occlusal table. Root fracture is a common cause of failure [25].

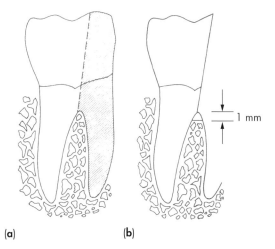

(a)  (b)

**Figure 12.22** Resection. (**a**) The cut should be made at the expense of the part to be removed. (**b**) The restoration should not leave the raw cut exposed; 1 mm of the bone should be removed to facilitate preparation.

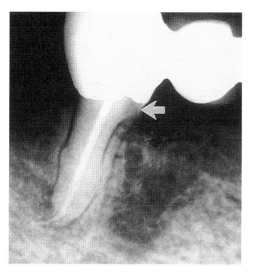

**Figure 12.23** The lack of the 1-mm space in bone led the restoration to end on the raw-cut dentine, with the long-term adverse consequence of marginal caries (arrowed).

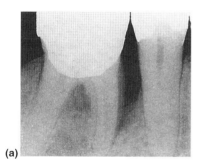

(a)

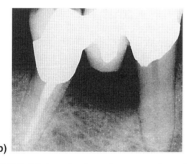

(b)

**Figure 12.24** (a) Angular bone loss extending close to the apex of the mesial root of the mandibular first molar. The widely displayed roots made hemisection suitable. (b) The mesial root has been removed, and the distal root after root canal treatment and surgery has been used as a bridge abutment.

## Bicuspidization

Bicupidization, when indicated, is the separation of the roots of a multirooted tooth. This procedure is primarily used in mandibular molars (Fig. 12.25). Adequate length and width of the root and clinical crown are primary considerations in case selection. The cut should be vertically directed to the middle of the furcation. It is necessary to expose the margin of the cut surface to facilitate later crown preparation. When there is close root proximity, it is necessary to separate the roots by orthodontic techniques (Fig. 12.26). Both roots are then restored as single units to simulate two premolars.

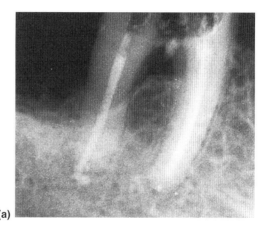

(a)

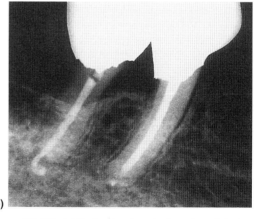

(b)

**Figure 12.25** (a) Perforation into the furcation of the lower molar necessitated bicuspidization. (b) Recall examination after six years; the enlarged furcation space permitted effective oral hygiene.

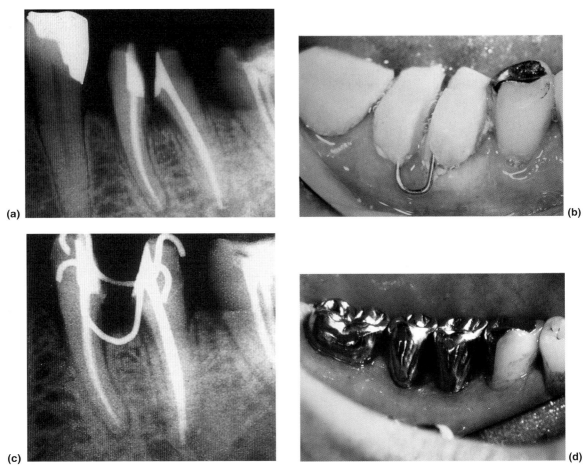

**Figure 12.26** (a) Bicuspidization could only be achieved by root separation; radiograph immediately after sectioning. (b) The roots were separated orthodontically. (c) Radiograph after separation. (d) After cementation of the separate crowns.

## REFERENCES

1. Abbott P (1998) Endodontic management of combined endodontic-periodontal lesions. *Journal of the New Zealand Society of Periodontology* **83**, 15–28.
2. Adriaens PA, Deboever JA, Loesche WJ (1988) Bacterial invasion in root cementum and radicular dentin of periodontally diseased teeth in humans. A reservoir of periodontopathic bacteria. *Journal of Periodontology* **59**, 222–230.
3. Adriaens PA, Edwards CA, Deboever JA, Loesche WJ (1988) Ultrastructural observations on bacterial invasion in cementum and radicular dentin of periodontally diseased human teeth. *Journal of Periodontology* **59**, 493–503.
4. Baumgartner JC, Falkler WA (1991) Bacteria in the apical 5 mm of infected root canals. *Journal of Endodontics* **17**, 380–383.
5. Belk CE, Gutmann JL (1990) Perspectives, controversies and directives on pulpal–periodontal relationships. *Journal of the Canadian Dental Association* **56**, 1013–1017.
6. Bender IB, Seltzer S (1972) The effect of periodontal disease on the pulp. *Oral Surgery, Oral Medicine, Oral Pathology* **33**, 458–474.
7. Bergenholtz G, Lindhe J (1978) Effect of experimentally induced marginal periodontitis and periodontal scaling on the dental pulp. *Journal of Clinical Periodontology* **5**, 59–73.
8. Blomlof L, Lengheden A, Lindskog S (1992) Endodontic infection and calcium hydroxide–treatment. Effects on periodontal healing in mature and immature replanted monkey teeth. *Journal of Clinical Periodontology* **19**, 652–658.
9. Buhler H (1988) Evaluation of root-resected teeth. Results after 10 years. *Journal of Periodontology* **59**, 805–810.
10. Burch JG, Hulen S (1974) A study of the presence of accessory foramina and the topography of molar furcations. *Oral Surgery, Oral Medicine, Oral Pathology* **38**, 451–455.

11. Czarnecki RT, Schilder H (1979) A histological evaluation of the human pulp in teeth with varying degrees of periodontal disease. *Journal of Endodontics* **5**, 242–253.

12. Dahle UR, Tronstad L, Olsen I (1996) Characterization of new periodontal and endodontic isolates of spirochetes. *European Journal of Oral Sciences* **104**, 41–47.

13. De Deus QD (1975) Frequency, location and direction of the lateral, secondary and accessory canals. *Journal of Endodontics* **1**, 361–366.

14. Dongari A, Lambrianidis T (1988) Periodontally derived pulpal lesions. *Endodontics and Dental Traumatology* **4**, 49–54.

15. Gold SI, Moskow BS (1987) Periodontal repair of periapical lesions: the borderland between pulpal and periodontal disease. *Journal of Clinical Periodontology* **14**, 251–256.

16. Gutmann JL (1978) Prevalence, location, and patency of accessory canals in the furcation region of permanent molars. *Journal of Periodontology* **49**, 21–26.

17. Haapasalo M, Ranta H, Ranta K, Shah H (1986) Black-pigmented Bacteroides spp. in human apical periodontitis. *Infection and Immunity* **53**, 149–153.

18. Jansson L, Ehnevid H (1998) The influence of endodontic infection on periodontal status in mandibular molars. *Journal of Periodontology* **69**, 1392–1396.

19. Jansson L, Ehnevid H, Blomlof L, Weintraub A, Lindskog S (1995) Endodontic pathogens in periodontal disease augmentation. *Journal of Clinical Periodontology* **22**, 598–602.

20. Jansson L, Ehnevid H, Lindskog S, Blomlof L (1995) The influence of endodontic infection on progression of marginal bone loss in periodontitis. *Journal of Clinical Periodontology* **22**, 729–734.

21. Jansson LE, Ehnevid H, Lindskog SF, Blomlof LB (1993) Radiographic attachment in periodontitis-prone teeth with endodontic infection. *Journal of Periodontology* **64**, 947–953.

22. Kipioti A, Nakou M, Legakis N, Mitsis F (1984) Microbiological findings of infected root canals and adjacent periodontal pockets in teeth with advanced periodontitis. *Oral Surgery, Oral Medicine, Oral Pathology* **58**, 213–220.

23. Kirkham DB (1975) The location and incidence of accessory pulpal canals in periodontal pockets. *Journal of the American Dental Association* **91**, 353–356.

24. Langeland K, Rodrigues H, Dowden W (1994) Periodontal disease, bacteria, and pulpal histopathology. *Oral Surgery, Oral Medicine, Oral Pathology* **37**, 257–270.

25. Langer B Stein SD, Wagenberg B (1981) An evaluation of root resections: a ten-year study. *Journal of Periodontology* **52**, 719–722.

26. Lowman JV, Burke RS, Pelleu GB (1973) Patent accessory canals: incidence in molar furcation region. *Oral Surgery, Oral Medicine, Oral Pathology* **36**, 580–584.

27. Mazur B, Massler M (1964) Influence of periodontal disease on the dental pulp. *Oral Surgery, Oral Medicine,*

*Oral Pathology* **17**, 592–603.

28. Paul BF, Hutter JW (1997) The endodontic-periodontal continuum revisited: new insights into etiology, diagnosis and treatment. *Journal of the American Dental Association* **128**, 1541–1548.

29. Pitt Ford TR, Torabinejad M, McKendry D, Hong CU, Kariyawasam SP (1995) Use of mineral trioxide aggregate for repair of furcal perforations. *Oral Surgery, Oral Medicine, Oral Pathology, Oral Radiology, Endodontics* **79**, 756–763.

30. Ross IF, Thompson RH (1978) A long term study of root retention in the treatment of maxillary molars with furcation involvement. *Journal of Periodontology* **49**, 238–244.

31. Rubach WC, Mitchell DF (1965) Periodontal disease, accessory canals and pulp pathosis. *Journal of Periodontology* **36**, 34–38.

32. Rupf S, Kannengiesser S, Merte K, Pfister W, Sigusch B, Eschrich K (2000) Comparison of profiles of key periodontal pathogens in periodontium and endodontium. *Endodontics and Dental Traumatology* **16**, 269–275.

33. Seltzer S, Bender IB, Nazimov H, Sinai I (1967) Pulpitis-induced interradicular periodontal changes in experimental animals. *Journal of Periodontology* **38**, 124–129.

34. Seltzer S, Bender IB, Ziontz M (1963) The inter-relationship of pulp and periodontal disease. *Oral Surgery, Oral Medicine, Oral Pathology* **16**, 1474–1490.

35. Simon JH, Glick DH, Frank AL (1972) The relationship of endodontic-periodontic lesions. *Journal of Periodontology* **43**, 202–208.

36. Simon JHS, Dogan H, Ceresa LM, Silver GK (2000) The radicular groove: its potential clinical significance. *Journal of Endodontics* **26**, 295–298.

37. Solomon C, Chalfin H, Kellert M, Weseley P (1995) The endodontic-periodontal lesion: a rational approach to treatment. *Journal of the American Dental Association* **126**, 473–479.

38. Sundqvist G (1992) Associations between microbial species in dental root canal infections. *Oral Microbiology and Immunology* **7**, 257–262.

39. Sundqvist G, Johansson E, Sjogren U (1989) Prevalence of black-pigmented Bacteroides species in root canal infections. *Journal of Endodontics* **15**, 13–19.

40. Thilo BE, Baehni P, Holz J (1986) Dark-field observation of the bacterial distribution in root canals following pulp necrosis. *Journal of Endodontics* **12**, 202–205.

41. Torabinejad M, Kiger RD (1985) A histologic evaluation of dental pulp tissue of a patient with periodontal disease. *Oral Surgery, Oral Medicine, Oral Pathology* **59**, 178–200.

42. Trope M, Tronstad L, Rosenberg ES, Listgarten M (1988) Darkfield microscopy as a diagnostic aid in differentiating exudates from endodontic and periodontal abscesses. *Journal of Endodontics* **14**, 35–38.

43. Wong R, Hirsch RS, Clarke NG (1989) Endodontic effects of root planing in humans. *Endodontics and Dental Traumatology* **5**, 193–196.

# Problems in endodontic treatment

## T. R. Pitt Ford and P. J. C. Mitchell

**Emergency treatment**  237
   Acute pulpitis  237
   Acute apical periodontitis  238
   Acute periradicular abscess  238
   Acute flare-up  239

**Failure of anaesthesia in acute inflammation**  239
   Alternative anaesthetic techniques  239

**Problems with preparation of the root canal system**  241
   Access cavity preparation  241
   Problems with primary preparation of the root canal system  241
   Problems with preparation of the previously treated root canal (root canal retreatment)  243

**Problems with filling of the root canal system**  247
   Non-iatrogenic problems with root canal filling  247
   Iatrogenic problems with root canal filling  249

**References**  249

## EMERGENCY TREATMENT

It is important that a patient who is in pain is rendered comfortable as soon as possible. The practice of treating the patient with antibiotics and analgesics without attempting to make a correct diagnosis and treat effectively the cause of the pain is bad practice.

Even in the emergency situation, where the cause of the problem appears to be obvious, an accurate diagnosis must be established before any treatment is provided. This can only be achieved by taking a careful history and conducting a thorough clinical examination, followed by appropriate radiographic examination and special tests. If the clinician has no idea precisely what is the cause of the pain at the end of the initial examination, active treatment should be delayed, as it might be incorrect and may cause the patient harm [18]. This should be explained to the patient, and analgesics prescribed until symptoms change and the diagnosis becomes clearer.

Although the following three conditions, acute pulpitis, acute apical periodontitis and acute periradicular abscess, cause patients to present as an emergency, it must be remembered that other non-endodontic conditions can cause pain, e.g. food packing, sinusitis and temporomandibular joint syndrome.

Where the diagnosis is clear, the emergency treatment consists of applying one or more of the basic surgical principles, which are:

- remove the cause of pain;
- provide drainage if fluid exudate is present;
- prescribe analgesics if required;
- adjust the occlusion if indicated.

### Acute pulpitis

The causes of pulp injury, its prevention and treatment have been discussed in Chapter 4. The question is often asked: at what stage should palliative treatment cease and be replaced by pulp extirpation? Ideally the treatment should be related to the state of the pulp, but this can only be determined indirectly. The clinician thus relies on the history given by the patient and a thorough examination. As a rule of thumb, if the pulp of a mature permanent tooth causes severe and prolonged pain after exciting factors such as thermal stimuli or the patient is woken at night, then it is likely that the pulp has been irreversibly injured and pulp extirpation is indicated. Emergency pulpotomy can usually achieve relief of pain, if the clinician does not have time to extirpate the entire pulp [21]. It may be difficult to anaesthetize an acutely inflamed pulp and this problem is covered later in this chapter.

## Acute apical periodontitis

This may be defined as acute inflammation of the periodontium. It is often a direct result of irritation through infection of the root canal [20], and may be associated with acute pulpitis.

A purulent exudate is not present periapically, and treatment consists of removing any pulp remnants from the root canals, irrigation of the canal system with sodium hypochlorite, drying the canals, sealing in an antibacterial dressing, and closure of the access cavity. The importance of cleaning the canal system thoroughly cannot be overemphasized, and the use of ultrasonic instruments that have an internal irrigating facility helps considerably. This approach to treatment has been widely adopted by practising endodontists [11,12].

Care must be taken not to irritate the periapical tissues by extruding infected intracanal material through the apical constriction. Likewise, over-medicating the canal with an irritant drug may cause it to diffuse periapically and cause inflammation. Indeed, the necessity of using a potent medicament within the canal has long been questioned if the irrigating solution used to clean the canal is antiseptic, e.g. sodium hypochlorite (see Chapter 7). When a medicament is used, there is little evidence to show that the choice of medicament has any influence on postoperative periapical pain [45,50].

The tooth may be slightly extruded and the occlusion can be relieved by grinding either the tooth itself or, in exceptional circumstances, the opposing tooth. The guiding principle on occlusal reduction should be to do no permanent harm. Clinically, heavily worn or heavily restored teeth that require root canal treatment should be protected against fracture by placement of an orthodontic band; in these cases the occlusion should be adjusted. The importance of preventing a tooth from fracturing by placing a band cannot be overemphasized.

## Acute periradicular abscess

This condition may develop as a sequel to acute apical periodontitis or present as an acute phase of chronic apical periodontitis. Diagnosis may sometimes be difficult. It is common for adjacent teeth to be tender to pressure. It is essential to pulp test adjacent teeth so that the correct tooth is treated. Radiography may not be helpful as acute lesions do not become radiologically visible until bone, including the cortical plates, has been resorbed.

Where a soft tissue swelling exists, the diagnosis is generally easier, but it is important to verify to which tooth the swelling relates. Relief of pain can be obtained speedily by obtaining drainage and adjusting slightly the occlusion of the causative tooth. The practice of prescribing antibiotics without obtaining drainage is incorrect, and unnecessarily prolongs the patient's misery. Opening into the pulp chamber may cause considerable discomfort because of vibration, but this can be minimized by stabilizing the tooth with fingers, and obtaining access with a small round bur in the turbine handpiece.

Ideally, the tooth should be allowed to drain until the discharge stops and then the canals irrigated gently with sodium hypochlorite, cleaned of debris and prepared fully, dressed and sealed as normal. Such a regime rarely leads to complications [4]. However, this is not always possible either because of lack of time or because the tooth is exceedingly tender and there is copious discharge of exudate. In this case it is permissible to leave the tooth on open drainage for no longer than 24 h. At the end of this period the patient should be seen again and, if comfortable, the canals cleaned of debris, irrigated with sodium hypochlorite and shaped with files prior to closure [52]. It is important that the root canal is cleaned and sealed as soon as possible so that food does not pack into the canal and invading microorganisms cause a further acute flare-up. The practice of leaving the canal open for weeks, if not months, has nothing to commend it [5] and usually leads to periodic 'flare-ups' due to reinfection from the oral cavity by microorganisms that may be more difficult to eliminate. Leaving the access cavity open for a long period may lead to caries in the pulp chamber and may make subsequent restoration of the tooth very difficult if not impossible.

If a tooth is symptom-free while on open drainage but flares up as soon as it is sealed, then the thoroughness of debridement must be questioned. This is probably the commonest cause of postoperative flare-up, for no tooth will settle until the canal is thoroughly cleaned. The coronal seal must be effective so if the clinical crown contains caries or inadequate restorations, these must be removed. It is also remotely possible that a tooth adjacent to the one being treated has a periradicular abscess, which communicates with that on the first tooth.

Sometimes because of anatomical difficulties or because there is an immovable obstruction in the root canal it may not be possible to obtain drainage through the canal. In such instances emergency treatment will depend on the presence or absence of swelling. If the swelling is fluctuant, incision and drainage, or aspiration through a large bore needle into a syringe, are advisable and generally relieve acute pain. If there is no swelling, supportive antibiotic therapy may be appropriate, followed by root canal retreatment or surgical treatment when the acute symptoms have subsided (see Chapter 9).

### Acute flare-up

Following instrumentation of a symptomless tooth, in the majority of cases, the patient can expect little pain. If the patient has severe pain or a periapical lesion prior to treatment, the likelihood of severe postoperative pain is higher [16,45]. The intensity of pain will reduce with time and is substantially helped by prescribing analgesics such that pain is of a low order after 24 h. Patients who present with pain and swelling during a flare-up are best managed by prescribing analgesics and antibiotics [45]. Flare-ups are more likely to occur in teeth with necrotic pulps [30,50,51], and in those patients who suffer from allergies [48]. The incidence of flare-ups has been reported to be as low as 2.5% of teeth undergoing root canal treatment [50]. This is a reflection of a high standard of treatment. A much higher incidence of pain could be expected where treatment is inadequate, or infected debris is extruded through the apical foramen. The incidence of extrusion of debris through the apical foramen is lower when the root canal is prepared by a crowndown approach and with a balance force technique, than with a filing technique and a stepback approach [2].

## FAILURE OF ANAESTHESIA IN ACUTE INFLAMMATION

Profound analgesia is essential for pulpotomy or vital pulp extirpation, yet there are occasions where, in spite of normally sufficient dosage and technique, adequate analgesia is not obtained. Such occasions are distressing to the patient and embarrassing to the dentist. The main reasons for failure are given below, but the subject has been reviewed [54].

The term 'hot tooth' has been used to describe such a situation. The tooth may be excessively stimulated by heat or cold, and may be tender to bite on; it may be difficult, if not impossible, to achieve analgesia of sufficient depth despite repeated injections. The reasons for this failure are not entirely clear although various explanations have been proposed:

- Pulpal inflammation in the affected tooth produces chemical mediators which cause hyperexcitability of the nerve fibres, particularly C fibres. The local anaesthetic solution is therefore unable to block the conduction of all these impulses [1].
- There is usually increased vascularity of the tissues in the region of the inflamed tooth and hence the local anaesthetic may be more rapidly removed by the bloodstream, shortening its period of duration [29].
- It has been shown that there is a tendency for inflammation to increase sensory nerve transmission so countering the effects of anaesthetics [36].
- There is a possible spread of inflammatory mediators along the myelin sheaths of nerves, which restrict the absorption of the local anaesthetic; this is likely to contribute only a small part [22].
- The pH of inflammatory products in the region of the tooth may be more acidic, thus making the local anaesthetic solution potentially less effective; however, this is considered unlikely [29].

### Alternative anaesthetic techniques

In endodontic practice, the failure to obtain analgesia ultimately is an infrequent occurrence, and when it does occur is likely to be in a mandibular molar tooth [9]. It must be noted that an acutely inflamed pulp can remain very painful in spite of what appears to be an otherwise satisfactory mandibular block injection. In such infrequent instances several alternative techniques are available:

- application of a sedative dressing to the pulp;
- intrapulpal anaesthesia;
- intraosseous anaesthesia;
- sedation.

### Application of a sedative dressing to the pulp

The kindest management of the patient is to accept failure of local anaesthesia, dress the tooth to reduce pulpal inflammation and attempt pulpal extirpation on a subsequent occasion. The pulp may be sedated with a zinc oxide–eugenol dressing [24], or with a corticosteroid antibiotic dressing [13,39].

If the pulp has been exposed and is inflamed, it bleeds copiously and should be allowed to do so for 2–3 min to wash out inflammatory mediators. The exposure is then covered with a pledget of cotton wool damped by a medicament such as Ledermix (Lederle Laboratories, Gosport, UK). The cotton wool is covered by a fortified zinc oxide–eugenol cement. On the subsequent visit a local anaesthetic should again be given, and when it appears effective the pulp should be extirpated. It is usually possible to achieve effective anaesthesia, when it had not been on the previous occasion.

### Intrapulpal anaesthesia

This may be used to supplement existing inadequate anaesthesia. The technique consists of injecting local anaesthetic solution into the pulp. The needle is advanced into the pulp chamber and the solution injected under pressure; initial pain may be reduced by placing topical anaesthetic gel on the exposed pulp prior to injection. Most topical anaesthetic gels contain either benzocaine or lidocaine (lignocaine) at concentrations of 20–30%. Intracanal use of a topical anaesthetic is also useful when 'hot' vital pulp tissue is encountered apically.

### Intraosseous anaesthesia

Intraosseous injections of anaesthetic may be delivered either via the periodontal ligament or through the cortical plate. They may be used to supplement existing inadequate anaesthesia [9]. In the case of periodontal ligament injections, special syringes allow small preset increments of anaesthetic solution to be injected intraosseously through the periodontal ligament. The anaesthetic capsule is inserted into an autoclavable protective sleeve to guard against breakage and a 30-gauge ultrashort needle used to inject the solution into the ligament. Prior to injection, the gingival sulcus must be disinfected and the soft tissues anaesthetized to reduce discomfort during injection. The primary injection is given on the distal aspect of the tooth, and the needle with the bevel towards the root face is slid into the periodontal ligament space until it is stopped by alveolar bone. The lever is squeezed extremely slowly and 0.2 ml of anaesthetic deposited. The procedure may be repeated on the mesial aspect of the tooth, and in the case of molars on other surfaces.

Intraosseous anaesthetic techniques such as the Stabident system (Fairfax Dental, FL, USA) use a small disposable 'perforator' to create a hole in the cortical plate of bone through the attached gingiva. The soft tissues must be adequately anaesthetized first. Anaesthetic is then delivered into the cancellous bone, within the mandible or maxilla, with a matching needle.

Both periodontal ligament injection and injection through the cortical plate produce effective and rapid intraosseous anaesthesia.

These techniques have some disadvantages:

- Infection can be introduced into the tissues unless the soft tissues have been disinfected.
- The injections are painful unless surface anaesthetic and /or conventional anaesthetic has been used.
- Adrenaline (epinephrine) injected intraosseously is rapidly absorbed intravenously. This may result in a noticeable tachycardia. It may therefore be wise to use non adrenaline (epinephrine)-containing anaesthetics for these injections in patients with cardiac conditions.
- Periodontal ligament injections alter the occlusion of the tooth very slightly by raising it out of its socket, and a careful check of the occlusion of the temporary restoration must be made.
- The anaesthetic is usually only effective for periods of up to 30 min.

## Sedation

There are rare and exceptional cases where the use of relative analgesia or intravenous sedation is the only way that a vital pulp can be extirpated, or an abscess drained. Generally the reasons are not related to the effectiveness of local anaesthesia but to the attitude of the patient. In such instances, before embarking on such a course, the clinician must be satisfied that the patient is fit enough, the tooth is of sufficient importance to the patient's well-being, and that the patient will accept subsequent treatment without recourse to further intravenous sedation. For further information on sedation the reader is referred elsewhere [34,35,40,43].

## PROBLEMS WITH PREPARATION OF THE ROOT CANAL SYSTEM

### Access cavity preparation

The preoperative radiograph must be examined carefully prior to beginning root canal treatment in order to detect the position of the coronal pulp chamber, the position of the canals and the presence of any obstructions that might prevent instrumentation. Access cavity position may vary in teeth that have been 'occlusally realigned' with cast restorations. It is essential to prepare a sufficiently large access cavity so that visual and physical access are not restricted; the entire roof of the pulp chamber should be removed. If the tooth has been restored with a satisfactory crown, it may be left in place during endodontic treatment. Removal of the crown with a crown and bridge remover (see below) may improve access but hinder rubber dam placement. Use of magnification and axial light will eliminate most access problems when working through a crown. If the crown is technically deficient or secondary caries is present, the crown should be removed, along with any caries, prior to endodontic treatment.

### Problems with primary preparation of the root canal

During primary (non-retreatment) preparation of the root canal, the clinician may encounter various natural problems, which may hinder biomechanical debridement of the entire root canal system. These include intracanal hard tissue formation and acute canal curvature.

### Intracanal hard tissue formation

*Pulp stones.* Pulp stones are not uncommon and may be identified from the preoperative radiograph; they normally present little difficulty in removal when ultrasonic instrumentation is utilized. The instrument should be worked around the edge of the stone until it becomes loose. It is more difficult however, to remove a stone from a root canal, particularly if it is attached to the wall. In such an instance, if a file can be passed alongside the stone, it may be removed by careful filing.

*Irritation dentine.* Irritation dentine is formed as a sequel to microbiological or physical trauma. Careful examination of the pulp space on the preoperative radiograph will show its size and to what extent it has been filled with irritation dentine. The depth of the floor of the pulp chamber from the occlusal surface of the tooth should be assessed from the preoperative radiograph. This should help prevent damage to the floor of the pulp chamber. Irritation dentine in the original pulp space should be removed carefully with an ultrasonic instrument or a long-shanked bur in the slow-speed handpiece. Diamond-coated CPR ultrasonic tips (EIE Analytic Technology, CA, USA) or PS periodontal scaling tips (EMS, Forestgate, TX, USA) are particularly well suited to removing irritation dentine. They are designed for use in a piezoelectric scaling unit and should be used with a copious water supply; inadequate cooling may cause burning of the dentine.

Good lighting and magnification is helpful as this dentine is normally very different in colour and texture to primary dentine; it may vary from being porous and yellow in colour to hard, dark and dense. Use of an endodontic probe (DG16) is highly recommended to feel for the canal orifices. Periodically, the operator should stop and assess whether the cavity is in the correct position. Where the pulp chamber is only partially obliterated, the patent canal orifices are useful landmarks for orientation. If a canal orifice remains elusive, a radiograph should be taken to check that the cavity is not deviating off course in a mesiodistal direction. Once the probe

241

will stick in the canal orifice it is usually possible to negotiate the canal with a fine file (ISO size 06).

Canals that are completely calcified from the pulp chamber to the apical foramen are very rare. Calcification normally begins in the pulp chamber and continues in an apical direction as a result of mild pulpal inflammation. Sometimes canals that look completely calcified on a radiograph can be instrumented because a very fine pathway remains within the calcified material. This may not be visible on the radiograph because of inadequate contrast or large film-grain size. For this reason, where endodontic treatment is indicated, an attempt should always be made to negotiate this fine canal using a fine file (ISO size 06), rather than opting for surgery (Fig. 13.1). The irritation dentine which occludes the canal should be removed with an ultrasonic instrument or a long-shanked bur in a slow-speed handpiece. Intracanal irritation dentine is usually much darker than primary dentine, and so magnification and illumination are once again, of great help. Once the canal is patent, preparation is

relatively simple. A lubricant with chelating properties such as File-Eze (Ultradent products, South Jordan, UT, USA) will help to reduce the resistance of a file in a fine canal.

It should be made quite clear that a symptomless tooth with a calcified canal but no periradicular radiolucency does not require root canal treatment [25].

### Acute canal curvature

Canals with acute curvature are more demanding to prepare both for the clinician, and on the instruments used. As well as the degree of curvature, the more coronal the position, the harder preparation is. Some preparation techniques and the inherent inflexibility of some endodontic instruments tend to straighten the root canal causing procedural errors such as stripping, ledging, zipping and blockages. Canal transportation is less likely when a crowndown preparation technique is used [31]. If possible, the coronal third of the canal should be

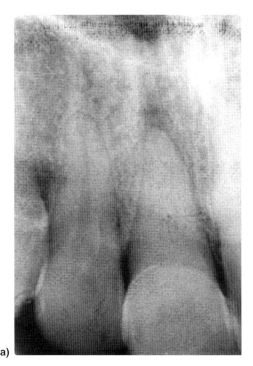

(a)

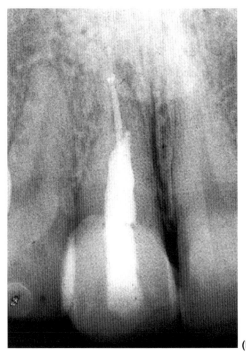

(b)

**Figure 13.1** A non-vital central incisor with a sclerosed root canal. **(a)** Preoperative radiograph. **(b)** Removal of irritation dentine coronally enabled access to the root canal, which has been filled.

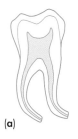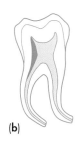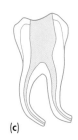

**Figure 13.2** (**a**) Root canals with acute curvature can be difficult to negotiate. (**b**) Removal the shaded area during preparation of the access cavity and coronal part of the root canal leads to straight line access to the middle third of the canal (**c**). This reduces stress on the instrument and the likelihood of canal transportation during preparation of the apical canal.

opened sufficiently in order to allow straight line access to the middle third of the canal (Fig. 13.2). This should not be done at the expense of perforating the canal wall. If the canal is to be prepared with hand instruments, better results are achieved with a reciprocal technique, such as the balanced force technique, rather than with a filing action [41]. The cross-sectional design and material of manufacture of the instrument is of importance in order to ensure maximum flexibility. In general, stainless steel files with a triangular cross-sectional design (e.g. Flexofiles) and nickel-titanium files are most effective [3,14]. Instruments should have a non-cutting tip to reduce the likelihood of ledge formation [37]; they should be discarded regularly as cyclical fatigue has been shown to be associated with instrument failure [19]. Recapitulation is essential in order to prevent debris build up in the apical portion of the canal and subsequent blockage. Lubricants such as File-Eze help to increase cutting ability and reduce instrument damage [55].

## Problems with preparation of the previously treated root canal (root canal retreatment)

Iatrogenic obstructions in root canal retreatment include extracoronal prostheses, posts, ledges and blocked canals, root filling materials and broken root canal instruments.

### Extracoronal prostheses

The decision to remove a satisfactory crown prior to root canal treatment may be made to improve access or prevent damage to the crown during access cavity preparation. Improved access is required for locating additional canals and removing broken root canal instruments. There are various devices currently available which may help remove a crown intact. Most rely on the application of a sharp axial force on the crown margin. The force may be provided by a sliding weight (e.g. Morrell crown remover, Henry Schein, Gillingham, UK), a spring-loaded system (e.g. Schuler crown and bridge remover, Henry Schein, Gillingham, UK) or by compressed air (e.g. Kavo crown and bridge remover, Kavo, Germany). In general, alloy crowns are easier and more predictable to remove than metal-ceramic crowns, which may fracture.

### Posts

If a post is present and it obstructs root canal retreatment, it should normally be removed. The method of removal will depend on the type of post present.

*Metal posts.* Parallel- or tapered-sided, passively retained posts may be removed with ultrasonic vibration, a post puller, or a Masserann trepan (Micro-Mega, Besançon, France). Ultrasonic energy may be imparted to the post or its cement lute, via an ultrasonic scaler, in order to remove it (Fig. 13.3). In general, Piezoelectric driven units are more efficient than magnetostrictive units at doing this; they should be operated at high power with water-spray cooling. If cement remains after post removal in the bottom of the hole, it may be removed with an ultrasonic scaler tip.

243

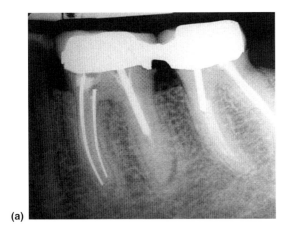

(a)

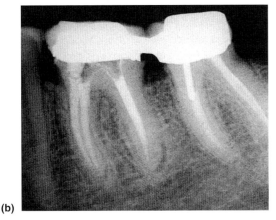

(b)

**Figure 13.3** A first molar with both silver points and a post requiring root canal retreatment. (**a**) Preoperative radiograph. (**b**) The cylindrical post in the oval distal canal was easy to remove with ultrasonic instrumentation. The canals were prepared by a stepdown technique and filled with vertical compaction of gutta-percha.

Post pullers such as the Thomas Gonon post remover (Panadent, Orpington, UK) and the Ruddle post remover (EIE Analytic Technology, CA, USA) work by tapping onto the head of the post and extracting it axially using special forceps; the root face is used as an anchorage point. They are efficient at removing both posts that extend above the canal and posts that have fractured within the canal. It is inappropriate to try to remove screw posts with axial loading.

The Masserann trepan, which is available in different diameters, fits over the post and aims to cut

away the cement lute; it works best on parallel-sided posts, and least satisfactorily on oval and tapered cast posts. The Masserann trepan has the potential disadvantage of being destructive as circumferential dentine may be removed with the cement lute.

If a screw post is present, the cement around the head of the post should initially be removed with an ultrasonic instrument. If possible, the type of post should be ascertained and the relevant spanner which was used for placement can be used for removal. Alternatively, the post can be rotated using fine forceps. The tap component of the Ruddle post removal system is designed to screw on to the post end in an anticlockwise direction. This can be utilized with a torque bar, to give a greater moment, to unscrew the post.

*Posts made from other materials.* Modern post materials such as glass fibre and carbon fibre are designed to be cemented with bonded luting agents. This method of luting, allied with the fact that these materials are less rigid than metal alloys means that they are unsuitable for removal with ultrasonic instruments or post pullers. Carbon fibre posts can be split vertically by drilling through with a small Gates-Glidden bur. The resin within the root canal may still cause problems in removal. A tooth restored with a resin cemented glass fibre post may be better managed by surgery than by root canal retreatment. It is helpful to try and find out what luting agent was used prior to starting treatment.

### Ledges and blocked canals

Ledges and blockages within canals often occur simultaneously. Inadequate use of irrigant and lack of attention to preparation of a glide path or recapitulation lead to a build up of debris within the canal. The file, having lost its natural passage to the working length will then create a ledge within the wall of the root canal. Once created, ledges are very difficult to bypass. If patency to full working length is to be re-established, the canal should first be filled with a lubricant such as File-Eze. A small curve should be placed in the last 3 mm of a size 10 file and it should be moved circumferentially around the canal in a watch-winding motion. The file should be of a design with a non-cutting tip, such as a Flexofile. Eventually, the file should encounter 'tight resistance'; the file is now no longer loose in the canal and is engaging the canal beyond the ledge. The file should be worked up and down in a watch-winding action until loose. The next file should easily pass the ledge, and root canal treatment can proceed as normal.

### Root filling materials

*Gutta-percha*. Gutta-percha may be removed mechanically, thermomechanically or chemically. If the existing gutta-percha points have been poorly condensed, it is often possible to negotiate a file alongside and withdraw them after engaging the gutta-percha with a quarter-turn clockwise action. Well-condensed gutta-percha should be removed from the coronal portion of the root canal with Gates-Glidden burs or Profile orifice shapers (Dentsply Maillefer, Ballaigues, Switzerland). The remaining gutta-percha can be removed efficiently using rotary nickel-titanium instruments such as Profiles in the presence of chloroform [15]. Increasing the speed of the instrument to 300–600 rpm may facilitate quicker removal of gutta-percha. Care should be taken to use an instrument with a small tip size, however, so that it does not engage dentine; cutting of dentine at such high speeds is likely to cause instrument separation.

Alternatively, the remaining gutta-percha may be removed with hand files in conjunction with softening agents such as chloroform, methyl chloroform or xylol [53]. Care should be taken not to allow the chloroform to contact the rubber dam as it will be damaged. A file will then pass easily into the mass of gutta-percha, which clings to the file as it is withdrawn. This should be cleaned off before the file is reinserted.

The use of rotary nickel-titanium files in conjunction with chloroform works particularly well for removing Thermafil. The gutta-percha around the carrier should be removed allowing the carrier to be removed in the same way as a silver point (see below).

With the canal full of chloroform, the last traces of gutta-percha may be removed with a paper point; this is known as 'wicking'. After all the gutta-percha has been removed, canal preparation proceeds as for initial treatment.

*Silver points*. Silver points are rarely used as a root filling material today as they do not fill the canal well and corrode easily [7]. They are often easy to remove, particularly if the head of the point protrudes into the coronal pulp chamber. Great care should therefore be taken not to damage the points when removing the core; an ultrasonic scaler should be used to remove the last remnants of the core. Once the access cavity is clean, the points may be gripped with either a pair of Steiglitz forceps (Henry Schein, Gillingham, UK) or a Masserann extractor and removed. Gentle and even pressure should be applied as the silver is very soft and may otherwise break.

If the silver point is entirely within the root canal, removal is more difficult; one or two Hedstrom files may be passed around the point in order to engage it, facilitating removal. Occasionally, silver points may have been cemented with resin-based sealers such as AH26. These may prove very difficult to remove and require long periods of ultrasonic vibration. Unfortunately, because of the softness of the metal, this often causes disintegration of the silver point within the canal. For further information on silver point removal, the reader is referred to a review [23].

*Cement root fillings*. Soft pastes such as Endomethasone rarely prove difficult to remove (Fig. 13.4); endodontic instruments tend to pass straight through them. Hard setting materials, e.g. AH 26 and SPAD, are very difficult to remove; in a straight canal it may be possible to remove such a material with an ultrasonically energized file. Occasionally, one may find a void in the material through which a small file will pass. Once the canal is patent, root canal retreatment is relatively straightforward. If a hard-setting paste proves impossible to bypass, a surgical approach to retreatment may be indicated.

### Broken root canal instruments

The use of rotary nickel-titanium canal preparation systems is now commonplace; research has shown that instrument separation is a small problem and most commonly occurs in the hands of inexperienced practitioners [28]. Management of separated instruments may be considered according to where in the canal the instrument has separated. In essence, the likelihood of removal of the separated instrument

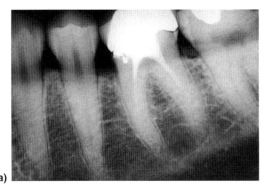 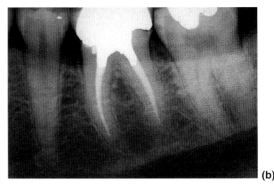

(a) (b)

**Figure 13.4** Endomethasone root fillings are soft and do not normally create problems for retreatment. (**a**) Preoperative radiograph of a mandibular molar, the canals of which were filled with Endomethasone. (**b**) Postoperative radiograph showing completed root canal retreatment using gutta-percha and placement of an amalgam core in the access cavity.

depends on whether it can be seen; with good illumination and magnification this is dependent on whether the instrument has separated in the straight part of the canal or beyond the curve.

*Within the straight part of the canal.* If an instrument is present in the pulp chamber, it may be possible, provided access is sufficiently large, to grip it with Steiglitz forceps or a Masserann extractor (Fig. 13.5) and withdraw it.

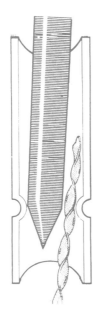

**Figure 13.5** Diagram of a Masserann extractor, which consists of a tube with a constriction; into this a stylet is inserted to trap the broken instrument against the constriction.

If the instrument is entirely within the canal, removal is more difficult; these cases are best treated by specialists. The most conservative and efficient way of retrieving these instruments is by using ultrasonic instrumentation [32]. The access should be enlarged and the instrument vibrated using slender ultrasonic tips, e.g. ProUltra titanium tips (Dentsply Maillefer, Baillaigues, Switzerland). As most separated endodontic files have flutes which are wound in a clockwise direction, the ultrasonic tip should be worked in an anticlockwise direction around the instrument until it works loose (Fig. 13.6). In the case of spiral fillers, however, the reverse is true. Care should be taken not to work in a completely dry field as ultrasonic energy can create significant heat build up, which may potentially damage the tooth and periodontium.

Sometimes, if removal is impossible, an instrument may be bypassed, in which case preparation should then proceed as normal. There is no evidence that such an action adversely affects the prognosis [10].

*Beyond the curve.* If an instrument is not visible because it has separated within the curved part of a canal, removal is unpredictable, but sometimes possible with ultrasonic instrumentation; great care should be taken, however, as significant damage to the root may occur. If it is not possible to remove the instrument, attempts should be made to bypass it and incorporate it into the root canal filling. In some cases it may only be possible to clean, shape and fill the canal to the fractured end of the instrument [18];

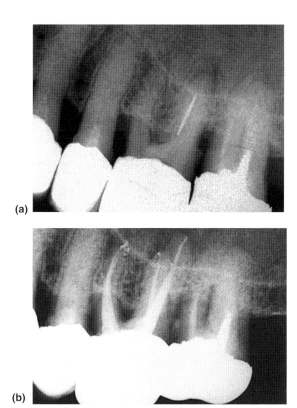

(a)

(b)

**Figure 13.6** Separated instruments within the middle third of the canal are best removed with ultrasonic instruments. **(a)** Preoperative radiograph showing a Gates-Glidden bur in the palatal canal of a first molar. **(b)** Postoperative radiograph. Note the widening of the canal in the mid root area; this was caused by ultrasonic instrumentation around the separated instrument to facilitate its removal.

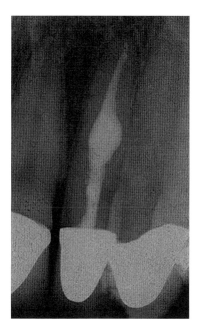

**Figure 13.7** Intracanal irregularities are best filled with thermoplastic gutta-percha techniques. Note the internal resorption in this lateral incisor, which has just been filled.

in teeth without periradicular radiolucencies this does not adversely affect the prognosis [10,17].

Should the patient continue to experience pain, swelling, or a discharging sinus tract after root canal retreatment, then assessment for endodontic surgery is needed. It is worth pointing out that the instrument is very likely to be made from a non-corrodible alloy (e.g. stainless steel or nickel-titanium), therefore it is not the instrument that causes any continued inflammation, but the associated infection.

*Prevention of instrument fracture*

Rotary nickel-titanium instruments appear to break because of cyclical fatigue, i.e. they have been used too many times [19]. It has been recommended that they should be used a maximum of five times [8]. Some clinicians have decided to use these files on a single tooth only. Likewise, fine hand files (ISO size 06–20) should preferably be used for only one tooth and then discarded. Larger sizes may be cleaned, autoclaved and used again provided that they have been examined carefully and discarded if the blades show any irregularity; this being an indication of overuse. If the tip of a fine file becomes bent at a sharp angle during use, it should not be straightened but discarded. The breaking of an instrument in a root canal is distressing to the operator and may alarm the patient; its retrieval is very time-consuming. For these reasons, the use of damaged instruments is a false economy.

## PROBLEMS WITH FILLING OF THE ROOT CANAL SYSTEM

Complications during treatment and retreatment can create particular problems in filling the root canal system. Non-iatrogenic problems as a result

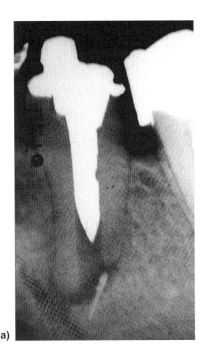

(a)

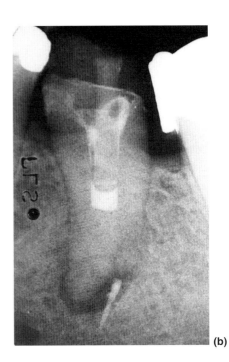

(b)

**Figure 13.8** Mandibular premolar with a wide apex and evidence of apical disease. (**a**) Preoperative radiograph. (**b**) The post has been removed, the canal cleaned and filled apically with mineral trioxide aggregate (at the time of treatment, the available material was radiolucent; the commercially available material is radiopaque). On the coronal surface of the MTA is a layer of IRM (which is radiopaque). (**c**) One year postoperatively, there is almost complete radiological healing and no clinical symptoms. An extruded piece of gutta-percha remains; this does not appear to be affecting the healing process.

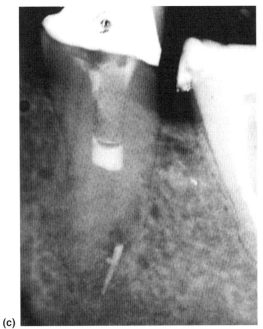

(c)

of inflammatory processes or the death of the pulp in an immature tooth may also pose a challenge.

## Non-iatrogenic problems with root canal filling

Chronic inflammatory processes within the pulp may lead to internal hard tissue resorption (internal resorption). This process ceases following pulpectomy. The root canal shape following preparation, however, is irregular and difficult to fill without a plastic root filling material. Warm gutta-percha filling techniques lend themselves to this type of problem (Fig. 13.7).

Resorption of dental hard tissue is common in the presence of chronic apical periodontitis [27]; this is known as external inflammatory resorption. In severe cases of external inflammatory resorption, the apical constriction may be lost. This leads to difficulty in creating a tapered preparation. Overfilling and a poor apical seal are likely to occur. This problem may be overcome by employing a root-end closure technique such as is used in immature teeth (see Chapter 10). Alternatively, a material such as mineral trioxide aggregate (MTA) may be used to fill the canal apically (Fig. 13.8). Mineral trioxide aggregate is biocompatible [46,47], creates a good seal [49] and stimulates hard tissue formation [42].

## Iatrogenic problems with root canal filling

During root canal retreatment, irregularities within the root canal, such as ledges and elbows are often encountered. According to Schilder [38], an evenly tapered root canal is easiest to fill. The use of a warm gutta-percha technique enables three-dimensional filling of irregular canals where cold lateral condensation would not be effective. Dealing with perforations within the root canal system can create a challenge for the operator. Traditionally, materials such as amalgam and gutta-percha have been used to repair these defects; these materials have been associated with high rates of failure [6], probably due to microleakage. Modern perforation repair materials such as MTA appear to give good results in the absence of infection [26,33,44].

In general, coronally placed perforations should be cleaned well with sodium hypochlorite to dis-

infect the dentine and sealed as early as possible; this prevents extrusion of infected material through the defect during preparation of the root canal and will reduce interappointment microleakage. Deeper perforations may have been created by stripping the inner wall of a curved canal (strip perforations) or injudicious post placement. These are often extremely difficult to manage and should be referred to a specialist. Magnification and good illumination are essential in deep perforation repair.

## REFERENCES

1. Ahlberg KF (1978) Influence of local noxious heat stimulation on sensory nerve activity in the feline dental pulp. *Acta Physiologica Scandinavica* **103**, 71–80.
2. al-Omari MA, Dummer PM (1995) Canal blockage and debris extrusion with eight preparation techniques. *Journal of Endodontics* **21**, 154–158.
3. al-Omari MA, Dummer PM, Newcombe RG, Doller R (1992) Comparison of six files to prepare simulated root canals. 2. *International Endodontic Journal* **25**, 67–81.
4. August DS (1977) Managing the abscessed tooth: instrument or close? *Journal of Endodontics* **3**, 316–318.
5. Bence R, Meyers RD, Knoff RV (1980) Evaluation of 5000 endodontic treatments: incidence of the opened tooth. *Oral Surgery, Oral Pathology, Oral Medicine* **49**, 82–84.
6. Benenati FW, Roane JB, Biggs JT, Simon JH (1986) Recall evaluation of iatrogenic root perforations repaired with amalgam and gutta-percha. *Journal of Endodontics* **12**, 161–166.
7. Brady JM, del Rio CE (1975) Corrosion of endodontic silver cones in humans: a scanning electron microscope and X-ray microprobe study. *Journal of Endodontics* **1**, 205–210.
8. Buchanan LS (2001) The standardized-taper root canal preparation – Part 2; GT file selection and safe handpiece-driven file use. *International Endodontic Journal* **34**, 63–71.
9. Cohen HP, Cha BY, Spangberg LSW (1993) Endodontic anesthesia in mandibular molars: a clinical study. *Journal of Endodontics* **19**, 370–373.
10. Crump MC, Natkin E (1970) Relationship of broken root canal instruments to endodontic case prognosis: a clinical investigation. *Journal of the American Dental Association* **80**, 1341–1347.
11. Dorn SO, Moodnik RM, Feldman MJ, Borden BG (1977) Treatment of the endodontic emergency: a report based on a questionnaire – part I. *Journal of Endodontics* **3**, 94–100.
12. Dorn SO, Moodnik RM, Feldman MJ, Borden BG (1977) Treatment of the endodontic emergency: a report based

on a questionnaire – part II. *Journal of Endodontics* **3**, 153–156.

13. Ehrmann EH (1965) The effect of triamcinolone with tetracycline on the dental pulp and apical periodontium. *Journal of Prosthetic Dentistry* **15**, 144–152.

14. Esposito PT, Cunningham CJ (1995) A comparison of canal preparation with nickel-titanium and stainless steel instruments. *Journal of Endodontics* **21**, 173–176.

15. Ferreira JJ, Rhodes JS, Pitt Ford TR (2001) The efficacy of gutta-percha removal using ProFiles. *International Endodontic Journal* **34**, 267–274.

16. Genet JM, Wesselink PR, Thoden van Velzen SK (1986) The incidence of preoperative and postoperative pain in endodontic therapy. *International Endodontic Journal* **19**, 221–229.

17. Grossman LI (1968) Fate of endodontically treated teeth with fractured root canal instruments. *Journal of the British Endodontic Society* **2**, 35–37.

18. Gutmann JL, Dumsha TC, Lovdahl PE (1992) *Problem Solving in Endodontics; Prevention, Identification, and Management.* St Louis, MO, USA: Mosby-Year Book.

19. Haikel Y, Serfaty R, Bateman G, Senger B, Allemann C (1999) Dynamic and cyclic fatigue of engine-driven rotary nickel-titanium endodontic instruments. *Journal of Endodontics* **25**, 434–440.

20. Hashioka K, Yamasaki M, Nakane A, Horiba N, Nakamura H (1992) The relationship between clinical symptoms and anaerobic bacteria from infected root canals. *Journal of Endodontics* **18**, 558–561.

21. Hasselgren G, Reit C (1989) Emergency pulpotomy: pain relieving effect with and without the use of sedative dressings. *Journal of Endodontics* **15**, 254–256.

22. Hudson N (1960) Inflammatory conditions. In: *Digest Report.* London, UK: Society for the Advancement of Anaesthesia in Dentistry.

23. Hülsmann M (1990) The retrieval of silver cones using different techniques. *International Endodontic Journal* **23**, 298–303.

24. Hume WR (1988) In vitro studies on the local pharmacodynamics, pharmacology and toxicology of eugenol and zinc oxide–eugenol. *International Endodontic Journal* **21**, 130–134.

25. Jacobsen I, Kerekes K (1977) Long-term prognosis of traumatized permanent anterior teeth showing calcifying processes in the pulp cavity. *Scandinavian Journal of Dental Research* **85**, 588–598.

26. Lee SJ, Monsef M, Torabinejad M (1993) Sealing ability of a mineral trioxide aggregate for repair of lateral root perforations. *Journal of Endodontics* **19**, 541–544.

27. Lomcali G, Sen BH, Cankaya H (1996) Scanning electron microscopic observations of apical root surfaces of teeth with apical periodontitis. *Endodontics and Dental Traumatology* **12**, 70–76.

28. Mandel E, Adib-Yazdi M, Benhamou LM, Lachkar T, Mesgouez C, Sobel M (1999) Rotary Ni-Ti Profile systems for preparing curved canals in resin blocks: influence of operator on instrument breakage. *International Endodontic Journal* **32**, 436–443.

29. Meechan, JG, Robb, ND, Seymour RA (1998) *Pain and Anxiety Control for the Conscious Dental Patient.* Oxford, UK: Oxford University Press.

30. Mor C, Rotstein I, Friedman S (1992) Incidence of interappointment emergency associated with endodontic therapy. *Journal of Endodontics* **18**, 509–511.

31. Morgan LF, Montgomery S (1984) An evaluation of the crown-down pressureless technique. *Journal of Endodontics* **10**, 491–498.

32. Nagai O, Tagi N, Kayaba Y, Kodama S, Osada T (1986) Ultrasonic removal of broken instruments in root canals. *International Endodontic Journal* **19**, 298–304.

33. Pitt Ford TR, Torabinejad M, McKendry DJ, Hong CU, Kariyawasam SP (1995) Use of mineral trioxide aggregate for repair of furcal perforations. *Oral Surgery, Oral Medicine, Oral Pathology, Oral Radiology, Endodontics* **79**, 756–762.

34. Roberts GJ (1990) Inhalation sedation (relative analgesia) with oxygen/nitrous oxide gas mixtures: 1. Principles. *Dental Update* **17**, 139–146.

35. Roberts GJ (1990) Inhalation sedation (relative analgesia) with oxygen/nitrous oxide gas mixtures: 2. Practical techniques. *Dental Update* **17**, 190–196.

36. Rood JP, Pateromichelakis S (1982) Local anaesthetic failures due to an increase in sensory nerve impulses from inflammatory sensitisation. *Journal of Dentistry* **10**, 201–206.

37. Sabala CL, Roane JB, Southard LZ (1988) Instrumentation of curved canals using a modified tipped instrument: a comparison study. *Journal of Endodontics* **14**, 59–64.

38. Schilder H (1974) Cleaning and shaping the root canal. *Dental Clinics of North America* **18**, 269–296.

39. Schroeder A (1962) Cortisone in dental surgery. *International Dental Journal* **12**, 356–373.

40. Scully C, Cawson RA (1993) *Medical Problems in Dentistry.* 3rd edn. Oxford, UK: Butterworth-Heinemann.

41. Sepic AO, Pantera EA, Neaverth EJ, Anderson RW (1989) A comparison of Flex-R files and K-type files for enlargement of severely curved molar root canals. *Journal of Endodontics* **15**, 240–245.

42. Shabahang S, Torabinejad M, Boyne PP, Abedi H, McMillan P (1999) A comparative study of root-end induction using osteogenic protein-1, calcium hydroxide and mineral trioxide aggregate in dogs. *Journal of Endodontics* **25**, 1–5.

43. Skelly AM (1992) Sedation in dental practice. *Dental Update* **19**, 61–67.

44. Torabinejad M, Chivian N (1999) Clinical applications of mineral trioxide aggregate. *Journal of Endodontics* **25,** 197–205.

45. Torabinejad M, Cymerman JJ, Frankson M, Lemon RR, Maggio JD, Schilder H (1994) Effectiveness of various medications on postoperative pain following complete instrumentation. *Journal of Endodontics* **20**, 345–354.

46. Torabinejad M, Hong CU, Pitt Ford TR, Kariyawasam SP (1995) Tissue reaction to implanted super-EBA and mineral trioxide aggregate in the mandible of guinea

pigs: a preliminary report. *Journal of Endodontics* **21**, 569–571.

47. Torabinejad M, Hong CU, Pitt Ford TR, Kettering JD (1995) Cytotoxicity of four root end filling materials. *Journal of Endodontics* **21**, 489–492.

48. Torabinejad M, Kettering JD, McGraw JC, Cummings RR, Dwyer TG, Tobias TS (1988) Factors associated with endodontic interappointment emergencies of teeth with necrotic pulps. *Journal of Endodontics* **14**, 261–266.

49. Torabinejad M, Watson TF, Pitt Ford TR (1993) Sealing ability of a mineral trioxide aggregate when used as a root end filling material. *Journal of Endodontics* **19**, 591–595.

50. Trope M (1990) Relationship of intracanal medicaments to endodontic flare-ups. *Endodontics and Dental Traumatology* **6**, 226–229.

51. Trope M (1991) Flare-up rate of single-visit endodontics. *International Endodontic Journal* **24**, 24–27.

52. Walker RT (1984) Emergency treatment – a review. *International Endodontic Journal* **17**, 29–35.

53. Wennberg A, Ørstavik D (1989) Evaluation of alternatives to chloroform in endodontic practice. *Endodontics and Dental Traumatology* **5**, 234–237.

54. Wong MK, Jacobsen PL (1992) Reasons for local anesthesia failures. *Journal of the American Dental Association* **123**, (1) 69–73.

55. Yguel-Henry S, Vannesson H, von Stebut J (1990) High precision, simulated cutting efficiency measurement of endodontic root canal instruments: influence of file configuration and lubrication. *Journal of Endodontics* **16**, 418–422.

# 14

# Restoration of endodontically treated teeth

R. J. Ibbetson

Introduction  253

Effects of endodontic treatment on the tooth  253

Timing the restorative procedure  254

Anterior teeth  254
   Conservative restoration of anterior teeth  254
   Tooth reinforcement  255
   Anterior crowns without posts  257
   Previously crowned anterior teeth  257

Posterior teeth  257
   Conservative restoration of posterior teeth  257
   Adhesive restorations for posterior root-filled
     teeth  258
   Indirect tooth-coloured adhesive restorations  260
   Cast restorations for extensively damaged
     teeth  260
   Cores for cast restorations  261
   Position of the preparation margin  265

Posts  265
   Selecting a post  265
   How long should the post be?  266
   Preservation of the apical seal  266
   Form of the post  266

Metal posts with cast cores  268
   Tooth preparation  268
   Construction of the post and core  271
   Try-in and cementation  273
   Cast cores and posts for multirooted teeth  274

Endodontically treated teeth as abutments  275

Elective devitalization  275

Conclusions  275

References  276

## INTRODUCTION

Modern root canal treatment has a high rate of success: teeth with vital pulps have a successful outcome >90% [41]; the same study showed that if there was an inadequate root canal filling already present at the beginning of treatment and a periapical radiolucency, the success rate was approximately 60%. Such information is important in timing when to restore the root-treated tooth. It is unfortunate that there is little information about how successful restorative procedures are for root-treated teeth when compared with their vital counterparts. There are many methods of restoring root-treated teeth; some of these are traditional, but the availability of modern adhesive techniques has expanded options for treatment.

## EFFECTS OF ENDODONTIC TREATMENT ON THE TOOTH

The failure rate of restored root-treated teeth is higher than that for vital teeth [38]. There has always been the belief that pulp removal from a tooth changes the physical properties of the tooth structure. Terms such as brittle are used to describe root-treated teeth and this is often given as the major reason why fractures are common. There is a reduction in moisture content in dentine following loss of the pulp. However, apart from perhaps a very small increase in the modulus of elasticity [22], which could be interpreted to be consistent with making the tooth more brittle, most other research has failed to show any change in the physical properties of dentine [40]. This does not necessarily mean that there is none; it may be a reflection of the difficulties in carrying out tests on small samples of tooth structure. Alternatively, it is known that teeth undergo rapid post-mortem changes after extraction and it may be that by the time tests of extracted teeth take place, significant changes in the physical properties of the teeth have already occurred.

Teeth with vital pulps are brittle; the dental hard tissues have generally high compressive but low tensile strength, which characterize them as brittle. It is possible that fractures of endodontically treated teeth are due to major loss of tooth structure combined with fatigue fracture of remaining enamel and dentine.

In practical terms, whether the tooth structure has undergone some fundamental alteration or not is probably of little consequence. The major effect of root canal treatment is the removal of tooth structure. Many teeth that undergo root canal treatment have previously been extensively restored. Modern root canal treatment requires access cavities that are not only correctly positioned but are large enough to allow straight-line access into the root canal system. Stresses generated in restorative and endodontic procedures may also contribute to failure by promoting cracks and fractures. Endodontic procedures such as the condensation of gutta-percha may produce stress, the consequences of which cannot be determined but are certainly undesirable [32]. The previous treatment procedures therefore have a cumulative weakening effect on the tooth and, in the absence of any firm data on the effects of removing the pulp, the most helpful concept to bear in mind is one of restoring an extensively damaged tooth. In such cases, there is a need to:

- preserve and protect useful remaining tooth structure;
- minimize stress within both tooth and restoration.

## TIMING THE RESTORATIVE PROCEDURE

It is essential that endodontic treatment is part of an overall strategy for treatment of the patient. It would be better to consider extraction and construction of a fixed prosthesis supported by a tooth or implant if the condition of the tooth to be root-canal-treated made it unrestorable. When the costs of the endodontic treatment and restoration are compared with those of a prosthesis and reviewed in the light of the prognosis for the tooth, extraction and replacement may be preferable to preservation. However, once the decision to root treat and restore has been taken, a further decision will need to be made as to how long to wait after root canal treatment before placing the final restoration. There is no set answer and the following factors need to be considered:

- The pre-existing endodontic status.
- The quality of the root canal filling.
- The site of the tooth in the mouth.
- The type of restoration to be placed.

Given a satisfactory technical result on the final radiograph of the root-filled tooth and an absence of symptoms, it would be reasonable to proceed immediately to placement of the final restoration where the pulp had previously been vital. In contrast, if there had been acute apical periodontitis prior to treatment associated with an unsatisfactory root canal filling, root canal retreatment would not give the same chance of success. In cases where the prognosis is in doubt, it would be sensible to delay final restoration until there is clinical evidence of healing, and in some cases radiological evidence. However, where the decision is taken to wait for evidence of healing, little will be seen radiologically before 12 months. During this time, the remaining tooth structure must be protected by an adequate interim restoration, which also prevents coronal leakage [19,35].

## ANTERIOR TEETH

### Conservative restoration of anterior teeth

On many occasions, the restorative procedure required following endodontic treatment is simple and under such circumstances there is nothing to be gained by delay. Should further endodontic treatment become necessary, the restoration can easily be removed to allow access to the root canal filling.

This is true for many anterior teeth where there has been little previous restoration. Such teeth may be restored using a combination of composite resin placed over a base of glass ionomer cement. Composite resin is the most appropriate material for restoring the access cavity, given its physical properties and a high quality surface finish, together with a good seal achieved by bonding procedures. Care must be taken to ensure that the root canal filling is removed from the crown of the tooth if potential discoloration of the dentine due to endodontic sealers containing eugenol is to be prevented.

## Tooth reinforcement

There is no indication for the placement of a metal post within the root canal of a relatively intact anterior tooth. The idea that such a post can reinforce a tooth and therefore protect against fracture has been shown to be untrue [23]. A clinical study has shown that posts have no reinforcing effect [44]. In an in vitro study of extracted teeth where those that were root treated were compared with those that had additionally received a post, the results showed no difference in their resistance to fracture whilst, in the group with posts, the fractures occurred further apically near the end of the post [15]. Translating this into clinical practice indicates that the presence of the post not only confers no advantage but in the event of fracture may make the tooth more difficult to restore. The data relating to the use of carbon fibre and quartz fibre posts is more difficult to evaluate. Their use with an adhesive resin cement may have some potential with regard to protecting the remaining tooth structure but evidence of their efficacy has only been demonstrated in relatively short follow-up periods [13,14]. With the increased range of adhesive techniques available for restoring anterior teeth, together with the lack of benefit of placing posts, there is every indication for a conservative approach to the restoration of even extensively damaged root-canal-treated anterior teeth. Figure 14.1 shows a root-treated anterior tooth that has discoloured some time following treatment; this was successfully treated by internal bleaching.

An alternative method of bleaching the root-treated tooth is to use carbamine peroxide and a vacuum-formed matrix. This is a modification of

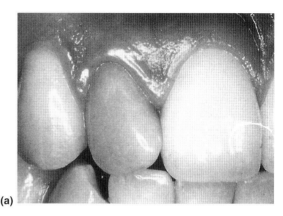
(a)

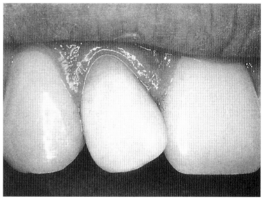
(b)

**Figure 14.1** (a) Maxillary lateral incisor discoloured following root canal treatment. (b) Maxillary lateral incisor following internal bleaching.

the technique used for vital bleaching. The vacuum-formed matrix is produced from a study cast where the stone surface of the tooth to be bleached has been coated with spacer to allow the carbamine peroxide gel to be held round the tooth. After completion of the root filling, the base of the access cavity is covered with a resin-modified glass iomer cement. The access cavity is left open and the patient shown how to syringe a small amount of the peroxide gel into the access cavity and into the matrix where it covers the tooth to be bleached. This can then be used by the patient on a daily basis until the desired colour is produced. The technique is effective, although there is an increased likelihood of coronal leakage and a risk of fracture of unsupported coronal tooth structure.

Sometimes a tooth is relatively immature with a wide root canal (Fig. 14.2); post placement not only has little to offer under such circumstances but

255

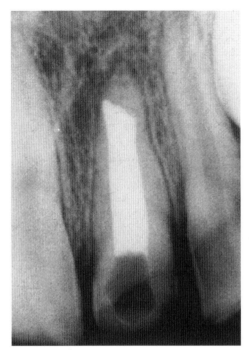

**Figure 14.2** Periapical radiograph of a tooth with an immature root for which a post crown is contraindicated.

would be clearly damaging. If bleaching of such a discoloured tooth were unsuccessful, it could be restored using a combination of composite resin in the access cavity together with a labial porcelain veneer.

If posts do not strengthen teeth, there are good reasons to avoid post placement in anterior teeth, particularly in younger patients where wide root canals mean that there is little radicular dentine. Figure 14.3 shows tetracycline-discoloured incisors of a 16-year-old whose maxillary left central incisor had received a vital pulpotomy at the age of ten years. The dimensions of the root canal made post placement inadvisable and there was furthermore no indication for root canal treatment as the pulp was vital. This tooth was restored with a directly placed composite resin; and seven years later this was in turn replaced with a porcelain veneer. The restoration continued to perform well and the pulp of the tooth remained vital 20 years after the initial pulpotomy. It could be argued that had a post been placed when the patient was ten-years-old, the tooth might by this time have been lost. The worst outcome for any of the conservative restorative

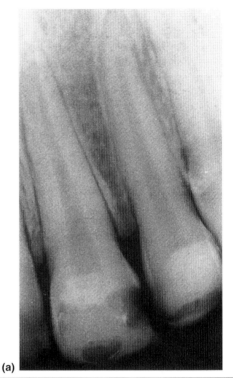

(a)

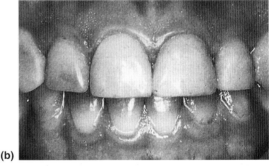

(b)

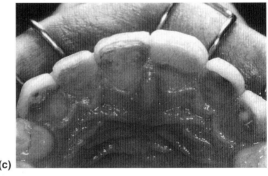

(c)

**Figure 14.3** Anterior teeth discoloured due to tetracycline. (a) Radiograph showing maxillary central incisor that had a coronal pulpotomy six years previously. (b) Labial view of completed direct composite resin restorations. (c) Palatal view of completed restorations.

procedures that were undertaken would have been fracture of the remnants of the coronal tooth tissues with loss of the restoration. This would have still left the opportunity for placement of a post-retained crown.

## Anterior crowns without posts

There are occasions when a crown is required for a root canal-treated anterior tooth but the tooth may not necessarily require placement of a post. Where anterior teeth are in normal occlusion, it is the palatal wall of dentine in maxillary anteriors and the labial wall for mandibular anteriors that are particularly important in providing retention and resistance form, and, in the root-filled tooth, resistance to fracture of the remaining coronal tooth structure.

The labiolingual dimension of mandibular incisors is small at the junction between the crown and the root. The combination of the loss of tooth structure produced by the endodontic access cavity and the crown preparation generally removes such a large percentage of the coronal tissue that very often a post will be necessary to support a crown. Maxillary central incisors are larger at the amelo-cemental junction, and when the endodontic access cavity is sited carefully, there is often sufficient coronal tissue remaining after crown preparation to allow the dentine core to support the crown with-out the need to place a post. The further incisally that the endodontic access cavity is placed, the more palatal dentine will remain. By making access to the pulp chamber through the incisal edge, or just palatal to it, dentine is preserved in this critical area. If the tooth being root canal treated is also to be crowned, the access cavity should be cut on the labial side of the incisal edge. This is even more conservative of palatal dentine whilst still allowing straight-line access into the root canal (Fig. 14.4).

## Previously crowned anterior teeth

The pulp in a crowned maxillary anterior tooth may become non-vital. A common error in making access through the crown and preserving the porcelain incisal edge of the tooth is to place the cavity too far palatally. After root canal preparation has been completed, the result is that little palatal wall dentine

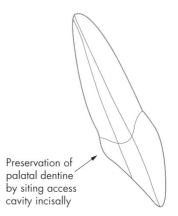

Preservation of palatal dentine by siting access cavity incisally

**Figure 14.4** Diagram to show that incisally placed access cavity preserves palatal dentine.

remains, and it is therefore not surprising that later fracture of the dentine core occurs with loss of the crown.

There is considerable benefit in removing the existing crown particularly if it is defective prior to root canal treatment after discussing the reasons with the patient (Fig. 14.5). This allows the access cavity to be sited incisally or incisolabially, thus preserving as much palatal dentine as possible (Fig. 14.5a). It is important that the palatal finishing line of the new crown is sited to allow coverage of a reasonable length of the axial wall (Fig. 14.5b). Such an approach works well for single crowns but should be used with greater caution where the tooth is to be a bridge abutment where torsional and shear forces are increased.

## POSTERIOR TEETH

## Conservative restoration of posterior teeth

The wider the isthmus of an occlusoapproximal cavity, the lower the resistance to fracture of the tooth [51]. The endodontically treated posterior tooth has lost the roof of its pulp chamber and both coronal and radicular dentine. Added to this is the loss of dentine associated with previous restorations. These teeth, even if previously lightly restored, can be considered to have been much weakened. Posterior teeth that have been endodontically treated require restorations that will:

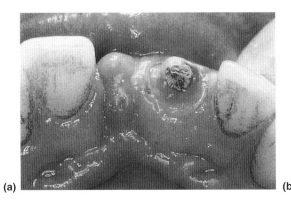

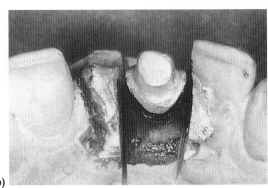

(a)

(b)

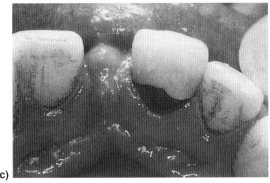

(c)

**Figure 14.5** (a) The existing porcelain jacket crown on a maxillary central incisor was removed so that the access cavity could be made through the incisal edge; a cermet fills the access cavity. (b) The die of the new crown preparation. (c) Palatal view of the new metal-ceramic crown.

- preserve and/or protect remaining tooth structure;
- maintain occlusal stability.

The reasons for protecting the remaining tooth structure are obvious, whilst stability in the occlusion is necessary to control the loads. Where contacts between opposing teeth alter, there is risk of unwanted changes in the position of the restored tooth or its antagonists. Such changes in position may create interferences on mandibular movement, which, particularly in the case of those on the non-working side, are associated with increased loads that may damage the teeth or restorations.

## Adhesive restorations for posterior root-filled teeth

The endodontic access cavity in a posterior tooth not only removes the roof of the pulp chamber but also creates a wide occlusal isthmus. Consequently, even if both marginal ridges remain intact, the tooth must be considered at some risk from fracture. Composite resin placed using an adhesive tech-

nique increases the resistance to fracture of root-filled teeth compared with non-adhesive restorations [11].

An endodontically treated maxillary first premolar restored with a disto-occlusal composite restoration is shown in Figure 14.6. The reasons for this restoration being chosen are easy to understand, as given the nature of the occlusal contacts the only aesthetic alternative would be a metal-ceramic crown. Furthermore, the preparation for this type of crown would have removed much axial tooth tissue and, coupled with the dentine loss in preparing the access cavity, would have necessitated the use of a post and core to support the crown. In addition, there is recession of the buccal gingival tissues that would have made aesthetic margin placement and its maintenance unpredictable. Whilst the reasons for this treatment decision are clear, the question remains as to whether it represents the best option, particularly in terms of protecting the remaining tooth structure and maintaining stability in the occlusion. It can be argued that composite resin represents the best option when restoring small cavities in the occlusal surfaces of posterior teeth. The operative field can generally be

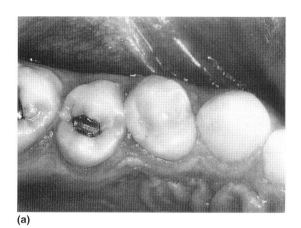

(a)

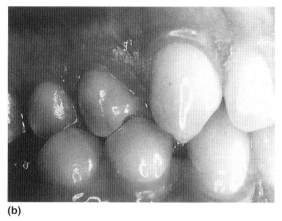

(b)

**Figure 14.6** (**a**) Occlusal view of a disto-occlusal composite resin restoration in a root-filled maxillary first premolar. (**b**) Buccal view with the teeth in intercuspal position.

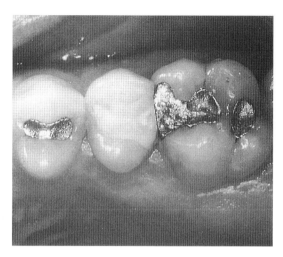

**Figure 14.7** Maxillary second premolar containing five-year-old composite resin restoration.

well controlled, the margins of the cavity are all in enamel and a small restoration is not often required to replace a large number of occlusal contacts. However, all dentists are aware of the operative difficulties raised by using composite resin in larger cavities in posterior teeth, especially those involving approximal surfaces. In particular, isolation and control of approximal form are often difficult. From an occlusal standpoint, large composite resin restorations present problems because the ultimate shaping and finishing of the occlusal surface must be carried out with rotary instruments. Precise occlusal functional form is unlikely to be produced by such means. Further factors affecting stability in the occlusion will be the resistance of the composite resin to wear and also its effect on the wear of opposing teeth. There is evidence to suggest that

the further posterior the restoration in the mouth, the more it is likely to wear [28]. Figure 14.7 shows a moderately sized disto-occlusal composite resin restoration in a maxillary premolar. This restoration was only five-years-old but already displayed wear both occlusally and approximally.

It is generally agreed that modern posterior composite resins are not as abrasive on opposing natural tooth structure as their predecessors. Any strengthening effect of composite restorations will only be possible if the material is durably and effectively bonded to the enamel and dentine. The polymerization shrinkage of composite resin induces stresses within the adjacent tooth structure. In teeth already severely weakened by root canal treatment, additional stress would seem to be best avoided.

Retrospective data covering a 20-year period of restoring root-treated posterior teeth with silver amalgam or composite resin have been reported [17,18]. At the five- and ten-year points, there were fewer tooth fractures in the composite resin group than in the amalgam group. However, at the 20-year interval there was no difference between the two materials. Both showed that, without cuspal coverage, fracture of the teeth at the ten-year period was 16% for amalgam and 13% for composite resin. However, at the 20-year period the incidence of fracture was over 25% for both groups. It was concluded that the incidence of tooth fracture was so high that posterior endodontically treated teeth should be restored with cuspal coverage. This data comes from a relatively old study; unfortunately no more up-to-date studies are available.

The production of extensive amalgam restorations combining cuspal coverage with good occlusal form is difficult. Where cusps are onlayed with amalgam, at least 2 mm of coverage must be used. It is difficult to create the appropriate occlusal form together with good axial contours. Such restorations are adequate to protect the remaining tooth structure and may also be considered as interim restorations when time is required to evaluate the success of root canal treatment or when financial considerations prevent placement of a crown. The principle of protecting the remaining tooth structure in a root-treated tooth using a restoration with an onlay component is fundamental. The fracture resistance in vitro of intact premolar teeth has been compared with those endodontically treated, those endodontically treated and restored with composite resin, and those endodontically treated and restored with onlays [53]. The teeth restored with traditional MOD onlay restorations in cast gold were the most resistant to fracture.

## Indirect tooth-coloured adhesive restorations

The introduction of indirect posterior composite restorations addressed many of these problems. They provide an opportunity to improve physical properties by up to 30% through a greater degree of polymerization. The effects of polymerization shrinkage on the tooth structure are virtually eliminated by employing an indirect technique, and restorations can be made with accurate occlusal contacts. However, they are expensive and, compared with conventional techniques for gold and porcelain restorations, the precision of fit is disappointing. Any strengthening effect from these restorations will be reliant on the stability of the composite luting agent. Ceramic inlays represent a further alternative (Fig. 14.8). There appears to be growing agreement that, particularly where the isthmus is large, onlay, rather than inlay, construction is preferred for both composite resin and ceramic restorations. The tooth preparation for a tooth-coloured onlay appears radical requiring 2 mm of occlusal reduction. It should have generally rounded form to minimize

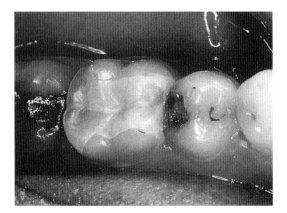

**Figure 14.8** Cast ceramic inlay in a root-canal-treated mandibular first molar.

stresses and facilitate the laboratory procedure. The finish line is best made as a wide chamfer in the area of the supporting cusp which blends smoothly into the proximal boxes. The non-supporting cusp is finished as a butt joint.

This review leads to two main conclusions regarding predictability in the restoration of endodontically treated posterior teeth:

- Cuspal coverage is necessary to minimize the possibility of fracture.
- Onlay restorations in cast metal are more likely to produce long-term occlusal stability than those made from composite resin or ceramic.

## Cast restorations for extensively damaged teeth

A cast onlay provides a conservative method for restoring and protecting the root-treated posterior tooth. It is important not to regard a full ceramic-coverage metal–ceramic restoration in the same way, because heavy tooth reduction to create the necessary room is likely to remove the majority of remaining coronal dentine.

The use of partial and full-coverage restorations in yellow gold remains an appropriate method for the restoration of endodontically treated posterior teeth where there is a reasonable quantity of coronal dentine remaining. The beneficial effect of crowns in preventing fracture of root-treated posterior teeth has been emphasized in a study where the incidence of posterior tooth fracture was nearly 60% when crowns were not used [43].

## Cores for cast restorations

The loss of coronal tissue by previous restorations and root canal treatment is frequently so great as to require a core to support the final crown. There is a need to provide adequate retention for the core. The general principles of core retention apply in the same way as for vital teeth, such as maximal use being made of the remaining tooth structure by providing boxes, rails and other retentive features within the bulk of dentine. However, there are virtually no indications for the use of self-threading pins in endodontically treated teeth. There is usually an inadequate bulk of dentine at the line angles of the teeth where pins would normally be placed as the access cavity will very often have reduced or undermined the dentine remaining in these areas. Furthermore, self-threading pins create stresses in both the tooth structure and the core [10,46]. The effect of these stresses within the reduced bulk of tooth structure is to enhance crack propagation, bringing with it the increased likelihood of tooth fracture or loss of core retention. Only if access cannot be gained to the root canals should pins be considered. If their use is absolutely necessary, they should be retained by a cement lute to avoid creating stresses in the tooth. However, they need to extend 4 mm into dentine to provide adequate retention, and this depth can make them difficult to place safely.

In contrast, the pulp chamber and root canals provide areas where retention and resistance for cores may be obtained relatively easily and with minimal generation of stress. As with anterior teeth, even if there has been considerable loss of coronal tooth structure it is not always necessary or advisable to place a post in order to retain a core. It may be said that the placement of a post is generally the last thing that is done to a tooth before it is finally extracted. Whilst this is not always true, it underlies an approach that places emphasis on the unpredictable nature of post crowns.

If root canal treatment fails and the root contains a long post, it is probable that the tooth will be lost unless the post can be removed or the site is accessible for surgery. It is sensible to avoid a post where possible as such an approach allows access for root canal retreatment. Figure 14.9 shows a periapical radiograph of two molar teeth; the first molar is the abutment for a fixed bridge; it has a failed root canal

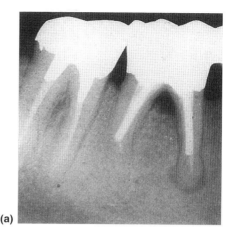

**(a)**

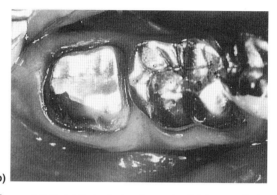

**(b)**

**Figure 14.9** (**a**) Periapical radiograph of right mandibular first and second molars showing posts in the first molar and an amalgam dowel core in the second molar. (**b**) Crown preparation of mandibular second molar containing amalgam dowel core (mirror view).

treatment, signs of a possible perforation on the distal aspect of the mesial root and two posts present. The chances of successful post removal and root canal retreatment are low. In contrast, the second molar is also root-canal treated but contains an amalgam core that extends 2 mm down each of the root canals. If this root canal treatment were to fail, there would be a reasonable chance of removing the core to allow access for root canal retreatment. The completed amalgam core is shown in Figure 14.9b; it reveals the remaining buccal wall and the amalgam core. This is an *amalgam dowel core* [31].

### Amalgam dowel core

This technique works well in posterior teeth where a minimum of one cusp with a good dentine base remains and will still be present following crown preparation [31]. If no cuspal dentine remains there is a danger that the amalgam core could fracture at the level of the roof of the pulp chamber. The clinical technique is shown in Figure 14.10, where an amalgam dowel core was placed in a maxillary first molar. The following points should be noted:

- All the root canal filling material must be removed from the pulp chamber.
- Gutta-percha is removed from the coronal 2 mm of the root canals using a Gates-Glidden drill, the dimensions of which are the same size or slightly larger than the coronal aspect of the root canal. The Gates-Glidden drill should be

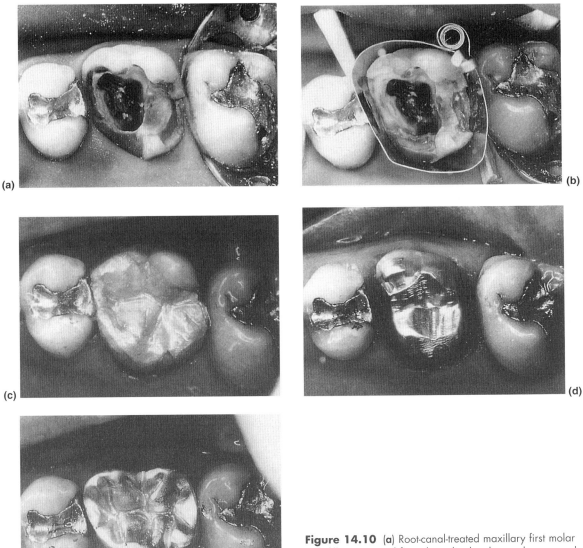

(a)

(b)

(c)

(d)

(e)

**Figure 14.10** (a) Root-canal-treated maxillary first molar with filling removed from the pulp chamber and gutta-percha from the coronal 2–3 mm of root canals. (b) Matrix band in place; note the groove and distal box providing additional resistance form. (c) Completed amalgam dowel core. (d) Tooth prepared to receive 7/8 gold veneer crown. (e) Completed gold veneer crown.

run at low speed and high torque to melt the gutta-percha ahead of the blunt tip.

- Extension of the amalgam more than the recommended 2 mm will not improve the retention of the core but will make later removal of the amalgam much more difficult should root canal retreatment be required.
- Optimal use should be made of the pulp chamber to make sure that it provides retention from opposing walls.
- Figure 14.10b shows that retention and resistance form have been improved by the use of further auxiliary retentive features in the coronal aspect of the tooth. A groove has been placed in the dentine palatal to the access cavity and the features of the distal box have been sharpened.
- Condensation of the amalgam alloy into the coronal aspects of the root canals requires appropriately sized amalgam condensers.
- Figure 14.10d shows the amount of coronal dentine which remains and the final preparation for a 7/8 gold veneer. The technique will not work consistently in the absence of coronal dentine.

Where there is a significant amount of remaining coronal dentine and a definitive pulp chamber, there is no requirement to extend the core into the root canals. Once again, such an approach improves the possibility for root canal retreatment if this should prove necessary.

### Use of plastic core materials with prefabricated posts

The core takes on an increasingly structural role as the amount of coronal dentine decreases. Where there is considerable bulk of dentine, the mechanical demands placed on the core are of a generally low order and hence the choice of material is not critical. This is not the case where little dentine remains, as both the possibility of core failure and dentine fracture become more likely.

It is important that the clinician imagines the appearance of the crown preparation prior to preparation. The appropriate time to consider the final form of the preparation is when the core is placed. Figure 14.11 shows a root-canal-treated maxillary

second molar; the decision was made to place a cemented, serrated stainless-steel post in the palatal root canal and to place two amalgam dowels in the coronal 2–3 mm of the buccal root canals (Fig. 14.11b). The reasons for this become clearer when the preparation for a metal–ceramic restoration is examined (Fig. 14.11c,d). The only bulk of coronal dentine remaining is in the area of the palatal cusp. The tooth was to serve as an abutment for a fixed bridge to replace the maxillary first molar and would therefore receive greater loading. The cemented post was placed to increase the resistance of the tooth to torsional and shear forces. Prior to cementation, the length of the post was adjusted to ensure that it was long enough to extend coronal to the pulp chamber but not so long as to be exposed by the subsequent crown preparation. Exposure of a pin or post during crown preparation weakens the core material. After the cement had set, all the excess was cleared from the pulp chamber so that the amalgam core was supported on a dentine base and could be well-condensed around the post and also into the coronal aspects of the two buccal root canals.

### Choice of core material

The demands on the core vary depending on its size and also the loads it will receive. Where a large bulk of coronal dentine remains, the choice of core material is not critical, but it becomes increasingly so as the amount of remaining dentine decreases. The critical point is empirical but when less than one wall of a posterior tooth remains, the core can be assumed to have a considerable structural role. Under such circumstances, composite resins, resin-modified glass ionomer cements and cermets are risky choices.

*Composite resin* has always performed well in tests in vitro of core materials [4,24], but concerns have been expressed about its dimensional and hydrolytic stability [33]. This lack of stability may explain the clinical impression of large composite resin cores tending to become loose beneath cast restorations.

*Resin modified glass ionomer cements* are marketed as being suitable as core materials. They provide significantly improved physical properties compared with conventional glass ionomer cements, but they are inferior to composite resins. As such, they are likely to be suitable for cores when a significant

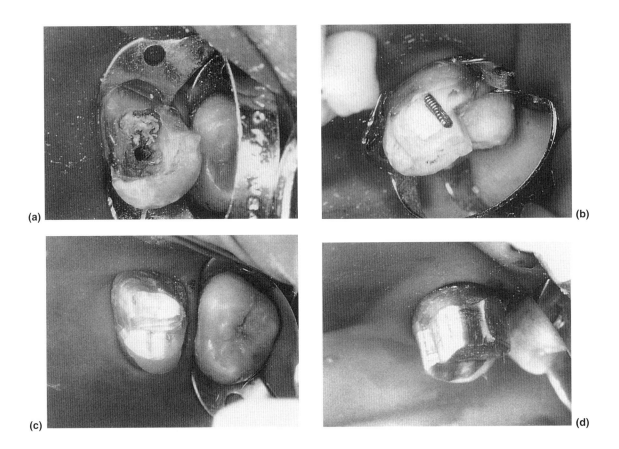

**Figure 14.11** (a) Occlusal view of right maxillary second molar after removal of gutta-percha from palatal root canal. (b) Stainless-steel post cemented within palatal canal. (c) Completed preparation. (d) Buccal view of crown preparation to show position of margin extending well onto sound tooth.

amount of coronal dentine remains but are contra-indicated when little tooth structure remains.

*Cermets*, being glass ionomer cement derivatives, possess adhesive properties and these provide good resistance to microleakage. However, fracture strength values are low, being approximately 20% of those obtained using composite resin [5]. Furthermore, whilst these may be very useful materials for small cores, they should be used with caution when the core is large.

*Silver amalgam* as a core material remains popular because of its physical properties. Data are lacking regarding the clinical performance of core materials. However, in an in vitro study, endurance testing of extracted root-treated premolar teeth restored with posts, cores of composite resin, cermet or amalgam, and then crowns showed failure of 60% in the composite resin group, 90% in the cermet group and 30% in the amalgam group [26]. It is often stated that amalgam is not a practical core material as it cannot be prepared at the same visit as it is placed. However, if a fast-setting alloy is used, the bulk of the initial preparation can be made with an amalgam carver and completed using a turbine with light pressure under waterspray. There is evidence that this does not adversely affect the properties of the set amalgam. Silver amalgam remains the plastic material of choice for large cores in posterior teeth.

### Adhesion for cores

The continuing developments in dentinal adhesion indicate that this should be employed when placing core materials. Cermets adhere readily to clean dentine and enamel surfaces, whilst resin-modified glass ionomer cements and silver amalgam require the use of specific adhesives. The literature has indicated that these are as effective as dentine pins or cavity design features in providing retention, but may be more effective when used in combination with mechanical retention. Reliance should not be placed on adhesion alone, firstly because the strongest bond is to enamel and much remaining enamel is removed during crown preparation, and secondly because long-term data on the performance of dentinal adhesives remains incomplete.

## Position of the preparation margin

Whatever core material is used, the position of the axial margins of the crown is important as it is a site of stress concentration [7]. This is also likely to be true for the margin of a core. One aim of the crown preparation must be to position the margin so that stresses received by the crown are transferred to the root of the tooth; this helps to minimise the loads on the core. When different cores on extracted root-treated teeth were tested without final crowns covering them, there were quite marked differences in their resistance to failure [21]. However, when the tests were repeated with final crowns in place, and their margins were extended 2 mm onto sound tooth structure, there was little difference between groups. It is an important principle that to distribute loads and hence minimise stress concentration, the margins of the final preparation should extend well onto sound tooth structure (Fig. 14.11d). This may sometimes require that a surgical crown-lengthening procedure is carried out prior to crown preparation to provide visible tooth structure apical to the margins of the core.

## POSTS

### Selecting a post

It is clear that when the amount of coronal dentine is very much reduced, a large core may be required which needs a post placed within one of the root canals to retain it. The choice of post is important but there are few indicators as to what the best post

may be. There is an enormous range of makes and types of post that are available. This indicates that there is not one post that is superior in all situations to any other. It is difficult to make an informed choice based on clinical data because such reports are limited [20].

The main information comes from in-vitro studies, and because a whole range of different tests have been used comparison is difficult. A brief review is helpful in choosing a post. Classical studies [6] of retention of posts have shown that:

- the longer the post, the greater the retention;
- parallel-sided posts have greater retention than tapered posts;
- roughening the post increases its retention;
- threaded posts are more retentive than posts with other surface finishes.

Many studies have examined the performance of posts and cores under angled compression as this has been regarded as more representative of the clinical situation [1]. Variations in post design have been associated with different levels of resistance to failure; however, failure occurred in the tooth structure rather than in the post [1,25]. Recent evidence indicates that teeth with quartz-fibre posts fail at higher loads, and in a way that permits repair compared with other posts [1]. The limiting factor in the performance of post systems is the amount of tooth structure remaining rather than the post itself [42]. The preservation of even small amounts of tooth structure is helpful [12], as is the ferrule effect [2]. Further information has been derived from stress analysis studies using either photo-elastic or computer-generated finite element tests. The information from these can be summarized:

- increased post length leads to decreased stress;
- tapered posts produce greater stresses than parallel-sided posts;
- parallel-sided posts produce higher apical stresses [47];
- posts that are both tapered and threaded are associated with high levels of stress, particularly on insertion [9];
- posts have a role not only in retention but also in stress distribution [36].

Reasonable conclusions about the desirable characteristics of a post are that:

- it should be of adequate length;
- it should, if possible, be parallel-sided [49,50];
- its surface should be roughened or serrated.

Furthermore, posts that rely on the elasticity of dentine for their retention, namely self-threading posts, should be avoided.

## How long should the post be?

A frequently asked question is what is the appropriate length for a post? There are many recommendations:

- as long as the crown;
- two-thirds the length of the root;
- one-half the root length surrounded by bone;
- as long as possible.

To establish which of these is correct, further thought must be given to the functions of the post. These are:

- retention for the core;
- stress distribution.

Considerable research into posts has looked at their ability to distribute stress. The post distributes stresses not only into the dentine of the root but also into the surrounding alveolar bone via the periodontal ligament [36]. The most appropriate recommendation for the length of a post appears to be one that relates length to the level of alveolar bone surrounding the root.

## Preservation of the apical seal

Post length cannot be considered without reviewing the length of the root canal filling that must remain if the apical seal is to be preserved [8]. The minimum acceptable length of gutta-percha is 5 mm [29], but it is based on the use of traditional root canal sealers and luting cements for posts. A maxillary central incisor may be 22 mm long with a crown length of 7 mm. If the root canal filling is 1 mm short of the anatomical apex, this leaves 14 mm of root, 5 mm of which needs to be occupied by root canal filling material. This will allow 9 mm for the post, which is adequate, but the situation can radically change if:

- the root canal filling is short of ideal length;
- periodontal bone levels are reduced;
- the root is short.

It was assumed until comparatively recently that if slightly less than the optimal length of root canal filling remained, this would probably not be of great consequence if a post were subsequently cemented into the canal. However, if the length of root canal filling falls below 3 mm, the incidence of periapical radiolucency increases significantly [27]; this may reflect on the method of gutta-percha removal [16]. This does present a restorative dilemma – whether to compromise the length of root canal filling or the length of the post. At present there does not appear to be a satisfactory answer to this question, particularly when there is insufficient information.

## Form of the post

### Tapered versus parallel-sided

There is laboratory evidence that parallel-sided posts are better retained and distribute stresses more easily than those that are tapered [44]. However, this conclusion is simplistic. It is reasonable to suggest that if all other factors are equal the use of a parallel-sided post represents the better option. However, much will depend on the anatomy of the filled root canal. It is clearly unwise to widen a root canal that is already broad in its apical region in order to make it parallel-sided. To do so can often risk weakening the apical part of the root. Stresses are concentrated at the apical end of the post and there would an increased risk of an apical root fracture. A clinical study reported superiority of parallel-sided over tapered posts [43]. However, teeth that were unsuitable for parallel-sided posts were provided with tapered posts. Such teeth would have tended to be those with relatively wide-tapering root canals; teeth of this type possess less dentine and would be more prone to root fracture. There is no doubt from a clinical point of view that tapered posts can function very well when there is adequate radicular dentine [52]; the same is also true of parallel-sided posts. However, to choose to use a tapered post when both types are appropriate seems illogical.

### Threaded posts

*Self-threading designs.* Earlier mention was made of self-threading posts, which rely on dentinal elasticity for their retention, exerting high stresses on the root of the tooth [9]. Posts of this design are generally very retentive; however, they may also lead the user to believe that retention is the only important requirement. Some of these types of post display the characteristics of being short, markedly tapered and relatively coarsely threaded. Such posts screwed into somewhat undersized root canals will produce high stresses. The form of the threads may also serve to concentrate stresses, whilst the short post length makes them of limited benefit in terms of stress distribution throughout the root and alveolar bone.

A number of improved variants of self-threading posts are available. Some resemble the traditional self-threading post but have been refined to reduce their taper and coarseness of thread, whilst also matching them to appropriately sized twist drills (Fig. 14.12). An alternative design consists of a self-threading post with a longitudinal incomplete split (Fig. 14.13). The intraradicular part of the post compresses on insertion, thereby reducing the stress. Additionally, the post is tapered only at its tip, being parallel-sided over the rest of its length. However, concerns have been expressed that it may concentrate stresses coronally because it is not well adapted inside the canal [3]. One further design recognizing the stresses induced by tapered posts uses a matched system of twist drills and parallel-

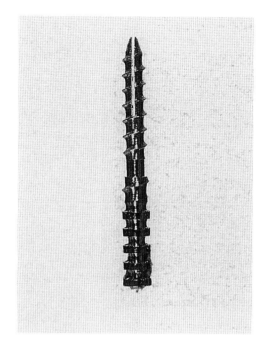

**Figure 14.13** Flexipost.

sided self-threading posts (Fig. 14.14). There are few data on the performance of these posts. However, it is suggested that they should be used with great caution, if at all.

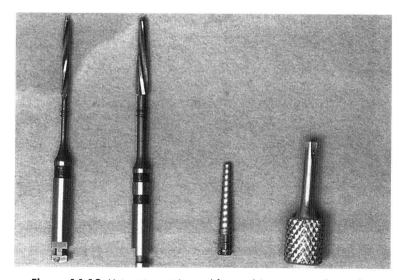

**Figure 14.12** Unimetric post (second from right), reamers and wrench.

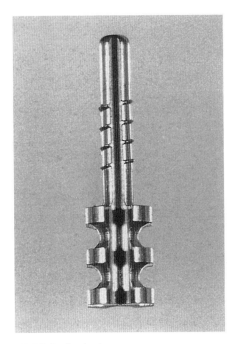

**Figure 14.14** Radix Anchor.

*Threaded posts used with taps.* A number of threaded posts are designed for use in conjunction with a thread previously tapped into dentine. Such posts have been shown to distribute stresses well following placement and to be retentive even over shorter lengths [48]. Care is required in tapping the thread within the root when high stresses can be generated if instructions about regular cleaning of the tap and removal of the swarf are not observed [39]. Threaded posts of this type do carry the advantage of being well-retained, but their resistance to torsional forces that tend to unscrew them is a continued problem, particularly if the design incorporates a prefabricated core. There is a further potential problem: as retention is good, there can sometimes be a tendency to compromise post length. This must be avoided so that the post distributes stress.

## METAL POSTS WITH CAST CORES

Prefabricated posts designed to be used with a core 'build-up' material are unsuitable for the majority of anterior teeth or for posterior teeth where no coronal tissue remains. Therefore, the treatment of choice is the provision of a post and core that are integral with one another – either a cast post and core, or a wrought post with a cast-on core. There are advantages in using one of the commercial systems, which provide a matched system of twist drills, impression posts, pattern posts and, in some instances, temporary posts (Fig. 14.15). The important features of such systems are that they provide a useful range of sizes and are easy to use, while at the same time allowing a correctly designed post and core to be made.

### Tooth preparation

The principles of preparation for a post and core are that:

- all useful tooth structure should be preserved;
- the apical seal is maintained;
- stress is minimized within the tooth and the post and core.

The stages in preparation are:

1. Establishing post length.
2. Primary coronal preparation.
3. Complete post preparation, both length and width.
4. Develop antirotation features.
5. Finishing procedures.

### *Establishing post length*

This should be carried out once the temporary restoration has been removed from the tooth. At this stage, the coronal landmarks remain; these will previously have provided the reference points used for the root canal treatment. The length can only be determined from a clinical examination and reference to a good quality postoperative endodontic radiograph, from which the following can be determined:

- the overall shape of the root, particularly its width in the apical third;
- the apparent width of the root canal;
- the length of the clinical crown;
- the level of alveolar bone surrounding the root;
- the approximate length of the root itself.

The shape of the root and the width of the root canal will determine whether the post can be

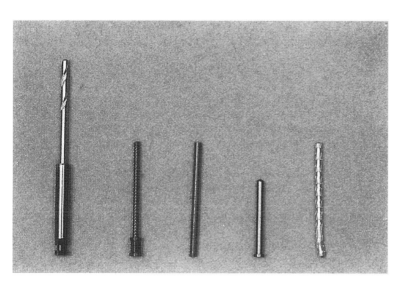

**Figure 14.15** Part of a matched parallel-sided post system: Whaledent's Parapost. Left to right: twist drill, burn out pattern, impression post, temporary post, and wrought post.

parallel-sided or whether a tapered design should be used. The post should occupy no more than one-third of the radiographic width of the root at the apical end of the post. If the width of the root canal apically were such that this proportion would be exceeded, then a tapered post should be used. The other factors will also influence the decision regarding the size of the post.

## Removal of the root canal filling

A root canal filling of gutta-percha can be removed either immediately following placement, or at the time of preparation for the post if this takes place later; this is a matter of convenience for the operator. Some studies show that there is damage to the apical seal by immediate removal, while others show no effect [8]. A number of techniques for removing gutta-percha have been described using heat, solvents or rotary instrumentation. Solvents are best avoided as they have the potential to damage the root canal filling material that remains. Heat is a safe and effective way of removing gutta-percha but it may be slow. Rotary instrumentation is quick, but may have the potential to risk root perforation if carried out incorrectly; a number of instruments are available for this purpose, but the commonest are the Peeso Reamer and the Gates-Glidden drill. The initial diameter of the Gates-Glidden drill should be approximately the diameter of the canal in the mid-root (Fig. 14.16).

## Coronal preparation

This is the second stage. Coronal preparation should never consist of simply cutting off the clinical crown of the tooth; the concept of an elective 'roof-top' preparation is not good practice. The objective of coronal preparation is to create the appropriate amount of space for the final coronal restoration. This requires that full occlusal and axial reduction should be carried out at this stage and not left until cementation of the post and core; this ensures that a full and accurate evaluation of the remaining tooth structure can be made prior to post cementation. Any axial wall of dentine that is taller than it is wide may be considered weak, and should be reduced in height.

Exact rules are inappropriate and clinical judgement is important. The axial tooth structure will require further evaluation and finishing once the intraradicular preparation has been completed. However, axial reduction should be completed as well as the site of the marginal finishing line for the crown; this has a considerable bearing on the axial reduction.

## Completion of post preparation

The length and diameter of the post should have been decided at the beginning of the preparation. The factors affecting its length have already been considered, and broadly it has been suggested that

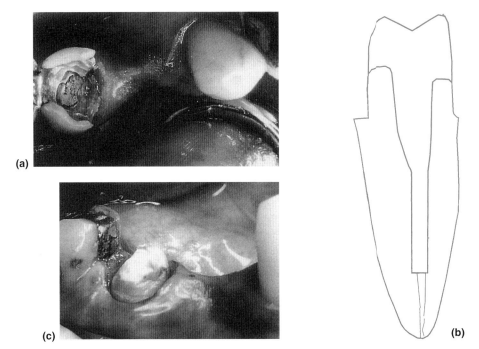

**Figure 14.16** (a) Root-treated mandibular second premolar following removal of the coronal temporary restoration. (b) Diagram to represent ideal preparation of a mandibular second premolar for a cast post and core (Digitized tooth outline – copyright P. Setchell). (c) Occlusal view of completed preparation. (d) Buccal view of the completed preparation.

the apical part of the post should occupy no more than one-third the width of the root. There are limits imposed by tooth anatomy on the dimensions of the post. Correspondingly, there are limitations imposed on the physical properties of the post by its own size. It is generally true that for type III cast-gold alloys, coronal diameters of post <1 mm predispose the post to fracture. It is poor clinical practice to remove excessive amounts of dentine to make a cast post strong enough, particularly where roots are narrow; in such teeth it is more appropriate that a wrought precious-metal post be used and a core cast onto it.

The form of the post preparation is important for dentine to be preserved and stresses to be minimized within the tooth and the post. A tapered post will reflect the essential anatomy of the root canal. It will be wide coronally to increase the bulk of the post, particularly at the point where the post joins the core. The width will reflect the normal anatomy of the root canal and will be greatest buccolingually in the coronal half of the root. This flaring of the canal should not be overemphasized to avoid unnecessary

dentine loss. Such enlargement of the canal may best be achieved by use of an appropriately sized Gates-Glidden drill. These instruments will not produce sharp angles and thus will minimize stress concentration.

Where the post is parallel-sided, the post space should be tapered in its coronal part, reflecting the normal anatomy of the root canal. There is little to commend an intraradicular preparation that has sharp internal form. Rapid changes in bulk of material and consequently sharp line angles will promote stress concentration and will increase the possibility of fracture of either the tooth or post (Fig. 14.16).

The apical part of the post preparation should be completed before the coronal part. If previous preparation has been carried out with Gates-Glidden drills, little extra work is required to complete this part. The final apical preparation is made with a parallel-sided twist drill, which cuts at its tip. It is preferably used by hand to minimize the risk of root perforation and with a safety device to protect the patient; this part of the preparation is quick to complete by hand, and rotary instrumentation is best avoided. When using twist drills, they should be withdrawn from the canal at frequent intervals and cleaned of swarf. Accurate depth markers are required. The original coronal reference point will probably have been removed during extracoronal preparation, therefore establishing the new working length is essential.

The coronal part of the root canal is then finished and blended into the more apical part, such that sharp changes in direction are avoided and stress minimized. For the tapered post, resistance to torsional forces is gained by removing dentine to emphasize the normal anatomy of the root canal. This normally provides all the necessary antirotation and there is no indication for notching the root canal, as this is detrimental in terms of stress concentration. Care should be taken to ensure that the canal is clean of debris following preparation and that the internal walls are smooth. Visual and tactile inspection are required to ensure that no gutta-percha remains on the axial walls of the post preparation. The preparation of the post space will have thinned the walls of remaining coronal dentine, which need to be re-evaluated.

### Finishing procedures

The coronal aspect of the axial walls of the preparation are then bevelled. The aim is to create a ferrule effect around the coronal aspect of the preparation. In order to achieve this, the bevel should be reasonably long. However, such acute angles of metal are only sensible where the thickness of the coronal axial wall dentine is relatively large. In most circumstances, the bevel is necessarily not greater than 45° so as to avoid producing a coronal spike of tooth structure that would be difficult to reproduce on a die and would be prone to fracture (Fig. 14.16).

The other important area for finishing is at the coronal aspect of the root canal in cases where there is little or no coronal dentine remaining. In such circumstances, the junction between the root canal and the root face is a virtual right angle; this should be gently rounded to help both die construction and stress distribution.

A final reassessment is then made of the whole preparation, checks being made for undercut, smoothness of finish and the overall final form.

Particular attention should be given to the positioning and width of the marginal finishing line for the final crown as this should not be significantly altered after the core has been placed.

### Construction of the post and core

After preparation has been completed, a decision is required as to whether the post and core should be made either from a direct pattern or alternatively by an indirect technique on a cast made from an impression. This is only relevant where the construction of the post and core is treated as a separate procedure from the crown. The shape of the core should not be the responsibility of the dental technician. A post and core may not seat as well following cementation as it did at the try-in stage. The difficulties in cement escape from the apical part of the post space make this improbable, and such failure to seat is likely to affect the seating of the final restoration. Furthermore, making a direct pattern gives an opportunity to assess accurately the intraradicular part of the post, and gives control over the final form of the core.

### Direct technique

Self-curing acrylic resin, which does not leave a residue, is the material of choice. It is easy to use, trimmable with rotary instruments, sufficiently sturdy, and dimensionally stable to withstand being transported to a dental laboratory for investing and casting. It may be used with a proprietary pattern post or wrought precious post from the system chosen.

The post should be tried-in to check whether it seats to the full depth of the preparation. If not, the most likely cause is debris, which should be removed. Lubricant is provided with the self-curing acrylic resin and can be applied to the walls of the post space with a paper point.

The resin may be carried to the preparation using a paintbrush and a standard Nealon technique. With the post fully seated, resin is applied to the intraradicular part of the post: the resin should not be too dry and the plastic pattern post may be bent gently to one side to allow the tip of the brush to reach the base of the antirotation feature. Once this is filled, further resin is added to ensure that it is well anchored to the post. However, no attempt should be made to build up the coronal aspect of the core; the resin should be allowed to polymerize (Fig. 14.17). The resin exposed directly to air will cure more rapidly than that in the depths of the preparation. Once hardened, the post is withdrawn and the intraradicular part of the pattern checked for completeness. Gross deficiencies demand a remake; very minor deficiencies can be rectified by adding a small amount of wax after the coronal part of the pattern has been completed. If the post resists withdrawal from the tooth or fails to reseat, it is a sign that there may be an undercut intra-radicularly. Careful checks on alignment and path of withdrawal will usually demonstrate where this is.

The coronal part is formed by further additions of resin once the post has been reseated. The paint-brush is again used to carry the resin and to help form it in the desired shape. Once cured, the pattern may be trimmed in situ; generous waterspray must

be used to avoid overheating of the pattern. The final form of the coronal preparation is created and the occlusal clearance checked before removing the pattern, and inspecting for completeness (Fig. 14.17). Once satisfied with the pattern, it should be placed in a small plastic box or similar container and sent to the laboratory to be cast in a hard precious alloy.

### Indirect technique

This is indicated when the margins of the core are not easily visible, because they are subgingival or when the design of the post and core is complicated such that a direct technique would be time-consuming or even impossbile. Figure 14.18 shows a maxillary canine that has fractured subgingivally: the post and core are better made using an indirect technique as verification of the margins is possible.

The stages in the preparation are identical to those for direct techniques. However, in commercial

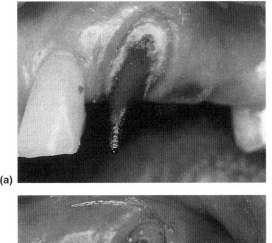

(a)

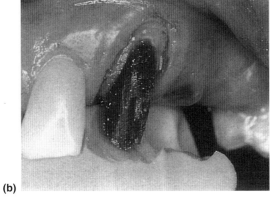

(b)

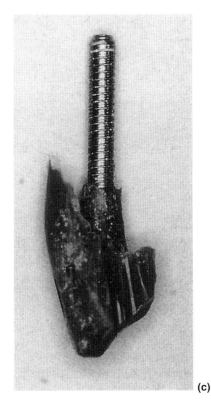

(c)

**Figure 14.17** (a) Root-canal-treated maxillary canine with wrought precious metal post and Duralay intraradicularly. (b) Completed pattern (with contour matrix in position). (c) Completed pattern on removal from the tooth.

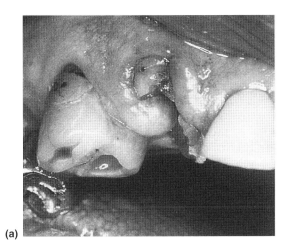

(a)

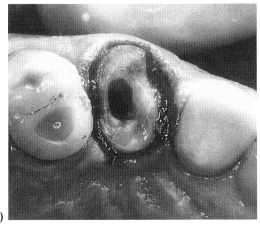

(b)

**Figure 14.18** (a) Fractured crown of root-canal-treated maxillary canine with gingival proliferation. (b) Following electrosurgery to expose the margins and preparation for a post and core.

systems an impression post is often substituted for the pattern post, as it is generally slightly wider to facilitate the laboratory procedures. Dentists who favour all-cast tapered posts sometimes make impressions of the root canal without the use of an impression post matched to the size of the prepared canal. This may appear to have the benefit of being quick and simple, and indeed it is for the clinical technique; however, it may make difficulties for the technician as the impression will record the full detail of the inside of the root canal. The resultant die will reflect this and with possible undercut, complicating removal of the pattern. The cast post may then only seat in its die by abrasion of the stone; as

such abrasion will not happen inside the root canal, difficulties in seating may be encountered clinically. Systems which use standardized impression and pattern posts, minimize such potential difficulties.

The impression post generally requires modification. It should not protrude beyond the level of the adjacent teeth, otherwise it may contact the impression tray, leading to possible distortion; it should also have a retentive head. Both objectives may be accomplished by using a heated wax knife to create a retentive button coronally, whilst at the same time shortening the post. Additionally, the top of the post should be coated with impression tray adhesive prior to use, with adequate time being allowed for it to dry.

Most operators place the post in the preparation before the impression material is syringed around it. It appears logical to seat the post fully before placing impression material, as it avoids the risk of a small amount of impression material being trapped beyond the end of the post. This small plug of material may be lost before the die is made in the laboratory. It is more sensible to seat the post fully before syringing the impression material into the preparation. If the post is pushed gently to one side, impression material can be injected into the remaining post space; good detail will result. On removal of the impression, detail should be checked. Marginal detail is important, because the technician must have sufficiently well-defined margins to be able to visualize the form of the final restoration if errors in contour are to be avoided. On occasions voids may be found on the intraradicular part of the impression corresponding to the antirotation features within the preparation. If these are small, it is reasonable to block these with wax, or to ask the technician to do so. If the void is larger the impression should be remade. Indirect techniques require that the technician has sufficient occlusal information to create an accurate core; normally, full-arch impressions will be necessary.

## Try-in and cementation

If a casting has been made from a direct pattern, it should need minimal finishing. The fitting surface should be inspected under magnification for spherical excesses, and if present these should be removed using a small round bur under magnification.

The temporary post crown should be removed and the preparation cleaned of temporary cement. This usually requires the use of the final twist drill used to prepare the root canal to ensure that no cement remains apically. The preparation must also be thoroughly washed and dried before being inspected to ensure that no debris remains. The fitting surface of the post should have been lightly sand-blasted to provide a matt surface, so that if it binds on seating a burnished area will result that can be seen more easily, thereby facilitating adjustment. The post should be seated using only light finger pressure, as heavy seating forces may cause root fracture. If the post does not seat, the root canal should be inspected for debris. The core should not require adjustment; minor finishing may be carried out after cementation. The tooth itself and the core should need no further preparation.

### Cements and cementation

There is a choice between using the more traditional acid-base cements such as zinc phosphate, poly-carboxylate or glass ionomer, and a resin cement. Higher retentive values can be obtained with resin cements, particularly when there is some form of dentinal adhesion [30]. However, tests in vitro may not replicate the conditions found within the root canal intraorally, particularly in relation to contami-nation with materials used in root canal treatment or biofilms. Furthermore, too great an emphasis placed on retentive values is unhelpful. Small gains in retention where posts are of reasonable dimen-sions have no particular clinical benefit, whereas if post length is lacking, improvements in reten-tion do not improve stress distribution, which is probably the most important function of the post. The case for resin cements for luting posts has not been clearly established; they make future post removal extremely difficult.

The aim of post cementation is to ensure com-plete seating with minimal stress being applied to the root. The post is unlikely to seat completely because of the difficulties of venting the cement over the entire length of the post. Heavy seating pressures should be avoided to reduce the risk of root fracture. Complete seating is aided by the post having a longitudinal vent; some posts have these as a design feature, but this may be negated when

an antirotation feature has been added to the post. It is good practice to provide a vent by making a longitudinal groove in the post using a fine cut disc or bur.

Complete seating will also be enhanced by correct mixing of the cement to provide maximal working time. Cements with longer working times are to be preferred: zinc phosphate cement is still commended. A cold slab and incremental mixing provide good working time. It is important to take active steps to fill the canal with cement if voids in the film are not to result. The post preparation should be clean and dry; once the cement is mixed, the post is coated with cement and placed on the cold slab. Cement is then carried to the post space and the internal walls coated using a long probe or an endodontic plugger. This must be carried out quickly and the post placed using only light finger pressure. The pressure must be maintained until the cement begins to set, otherwise the post may rebound out of the preparation. The cement should be left until fully set before excess is removed.

## Cast cores and posts for multirooted teeth

On occasions there may be such a lack of coronal dentine in a posterior tooth that the demands placed on a plastic core material become unrealistic. It is not possible to be dogmatic about this decision, as it depends on:

- the amount of remaining coronal tooth structure;
- the quality of dentine;
- the loads that will be placed on the restoration and tooth.

As a broad guide, when the amount of dentine is less than one cusp, there is a strong indication for a cast core.

### Number of posts

The availability of more than one root canal has traditionally often meant that more than one post is placed. Many of the techniques described reflect more the ingenuity of the dentist and technician, rather than necessarily being of benefit to patients [34]. Additional posts may help to distribute stresses to the roots in which they are placed, but this needs to be balanced against a reduction in dentine and posts not providing reinforcement. Where a post is required, it should be placed in the largest root available and the post should be of appropriate length.

### Antirotation features

Resistance to rotation is generally more easily achieved in multirooted than single-rooted teeth as the shape of the pulp chamber naturally provides this feature. Where this needs to be enhanced internally, it should be carried out where the bulk of dentine is present. Such enhancement of the resistance form should not undermine useful remaining coronal dentine, nor should the floor of the pulp chamber be modified.

### Indications for multiple posts

Two situations arise when more than one post may be required:

- the root selected for the post is short or the anatomy of the root prevents it being used to the required length.
- there is little in the way of pulp chamber to provide antirotation.

However, these situations are uncommon.

## ENDODONTICALLY TREATED TEETH AS ABUTMENTS

The root-treated tooth may be required to act as the abutment for a fixed or removable prosthesis. Abutments show an increased level of failure compared with other endodontically treated teeth [45], whilst post-retained crowns used as bridge retainers have a higher failure rate than partial or full-veneer retainers on teeth with vital pulps [38]. The higher rate of failure is probably due to the increased loads acting on teeth where the amount of dentine is reduced. This information on prognosis should influence the use of such teeth as abutments and also the prognosis that the patient is given for the lifespan of the prosthesis. The use of implants

may be a better option than attempting to use an extensively damaged root-filled tooth as an abutment.

## ELECTIVE DEVITALIZATION

This procedure is sometimes incorrectly employed as a technique for improving retention of the final restoration. Its use is a symptom of a lack of crown height, and the solution is to increase the height available and use axial grooves, rather than employ the root canal for retention.

Its use has been recommended in teeth where the existing intracoronal restoration is deep and the tooth is to act as an abutment for a fixed prosthesis [37]. The suggestion was made because a small number of teeth suffered loss of pulp vitality subsequent to bridges being placed. These teeth were generally those that had previously had a history of pulpal inflammation or had had deep cavities. When root canal treatment was carried out through the retainer, this was followed by fracture of the remaining coronal dentine in a number of instances. These fractures were considered to be due to the endodontic access cavity removing much of the core dentine. It was therefore suggested that where long-term pulp vitality was in doubt and the tooth was to be used as a bridge abutment, elective devitalization should be carried out. Such a suggestion needs to be seen against the success of endodontically treated teeth as abutments.

## CONCLUSIONS

There have been advances in the methods available for restoring endodontically treated teeth. Many of these are adhesive in nature; however, there is an improved understanding of the behaviour of endodontically treated teeth in response to continued loading within the mouth. Two major conclusions can be drawn:

- Stress within the tooth and restoration must be kept to a minimum.
- The preservation of useful tooth structure should be seen as a prime objective, both during endodontic procedures and the subsequent restoration.

## REFERENCES

1. Akkayan B, Gulmez T (2002) Resistance to fracture of endodontically treated teeth restored with different post systems. *Journal of Prosthetic Dentistry* **87**, 431–437.
2. Barkhordar RA, Radke R, Abbasi J (1989) Effect of metal collars on resistance of endodontically treated teeth to root fracture. *Journal of Prosthetic Dentistry* **61**, 676–678.
3. Burns DA, Krause WR, Douglas HB, Burns DR (1990) Stress distribution surrounding endodontic posts. *Journal of Prosthetic Dentistry* **64**, 412–418.
4. Cohen BI, Condos S, Deutsch AS, Musikant BL (1994) Fracture strength of three different core materials in combination with three different endodontic posts. *International Journal of Prosthodontics* **7**, 178–182.
5. Cohen BI, Pagnillo MK, Condos S, Deutsch AS (1996) Four different core materials measured for fracture strength in combination with five different designs of endodontic posts. *Journal of Prosthetic Dentistry* **76**, 487–495.
6. Colley IT, Hampson EL, Lehman ML (1968) Retention of post crowns. An assessment of the relative efficiency of posts of different shapes and sizes. *British Dental Journal* **124**, 63–69.
7. Craig RG, Farah JW (1977) Stress analysis and design of single restorations and fixed bridges. *Oral Sciences Reviews* **10**, 45–74.
8. DeCleen MJ (1993) The relationship between the root canal filling and post space preparation. *International Endodontic Journal* **26**, 53–58.
9. Deutsch AS, Cavallari J, Musikant BL, Silverstein L, Lepley J, Petroni G (1985) Root fracture and the design of prefabricated posts. *Journal of Prosthetic Dentistry* **53**, 637–640.
10. Dhuru VB, McLachan K, Kasloff Z (1979) A photoelastic study of stress concentrations produced by retention pins in amalgam restorations. *Journal of Dental Research* **58**, 1060–1064.
11. Eakle WS (1986) Fracture resistance of teeth restored with Class II bonded composite resin. *Journal of Dental Research* **65**, 149–153.
12. Fernandes AS, Dessai GS (2001) Factors affecting the fracture resistance of post-core reconstructed teeth: a review. *International Journal of Prosthodontics* **14**, 355–363.
13. Ferrari M, Vichi A, Mannocci F, Mason PN (2000) Retrospective study of the clinical performance of fiber posts. *American Journal of Dentistry* **13**, (special issue), 9B–13B.
14. Fredriksson M, Astback J, Pamenius M, Arvidson K (1998) A retrospective study of 236 patients with teeth restored by carbon fiber-reinforced epoxy resin posts. *Journal of Prosthetic Dentistry* **80**, 151–157.
15. Guzy GE, Nicholls JI (1979) In vitro comparison of intact endodontically treated teeth with and without endo-post reinforcement. *Journal of Prosthetic Dentistry* **42**, 39–44.
16. Haddix JE, Mattison GD, Shulman CA, Pink FE (1990) Post preparation techniques and their effect on the apical seal. *Journal of Prosthetic Dentistry* **64**, 515–519.
17. Hansen EK, Asmussen E (1990) In vivo fractures of endodontically treated posterior teeth restored with enamel-bonded resin. *Endodontics and Dental Traumatology* **6**, 218–225.
18. Hansen EK, Asmussen E, Christiansen NC (1990) In vivo fractures of endodontically treated posterior teeth restored with amalgam. *Endodontics and Dental Traumatology* **6**, 49–55.
19. Heling I, Gorfil C, Slutzky H, Kopolovic K, Zalkind M, Slutzky-Goldberg I (2002) Endodontic failure caused by inadequate restorative procedures: review and treatment recommendations. *Journal of Prosthetic Dentistry* **87**, 674–678.
20. Heydecke G, Peters MC (2002) The restoration of endodontically treated, single-rooted teeth with cast or direct posts and cores: a systematic review. *Journal of Prosthetic Dentistry* **87**, 380–386.
21. Hoag EP, Dwyer TG (1982) A comparative evaluation of three post and core techniques. *Journal of Prosthetic Dentistry* **47**, 177–181.
22. Huang TJG, Schilder H, Nathanson D (1991) Effects of moisture content and endodontic treatment on some mechanical properties of human dentin. *Journal of Endodontics* **18**, 209–215.
23. Johnson ME, Stewart GP, Nielsen CJ, Hatton JF (2000) Evaluation of root reinforcement of endodontically treated teeth. *Oral Surgery, Oral Medicine, Oral Pathology, Oral Radiology, Endodontics* **90**, 360–364.
24. Kantor ME, Pines MS (1977) A comparative study of restorative techniques for pulpless teeth. *Journal of Prosthetic Dentistry* **38**, 405–412.
25. King PA, Setchell DJ (1990) An in vitro evaluation of a prototype CRFC prefabricated post developed for the restoration of pulpless teeth. *Journal of Oral Rehabilitation* **17**, 599–609.
26. Kovarik RE, Breeding LC, Caughman WF (1992) Fatigue life of three core materials under simulated chewing conditions. *Journal of Prosthetic Dentistry* **68**, 584–590.
27. Kvist T, Rydin E, Reit C (1989) The relative frequency of periapical lesions in teeth with root canal-retained posts. *Journal of Endodontics* **15**, 578–580.
28. Leinfelder KF, Wilder AD, Teixeira LC (1986) Wear rates of posterior composite resins. *Journal of the American Dental Association* **112**, 829–833.
29. Mattison GD, Delivanis PD, Thacker RW, Hassell KJ (1984) Effect of post preparation on the apical seal. *Journal of Prosthetic Dentistry* **51**, 785–789.
30. Mendoza DB, Eakle WS (1994) Retention of posts cemented with various dentinal bonding cements. *Journal of Prosthetic Dentistry* **72,** 591–594.
31. Nayyar A, Walton RE, Leonard LA (1980) An amalgam coronal-radicular dowel and core technique for endodontically treated posterior teeth. *Journal of Prosthetic Dentistry* **43**, 511–515.
32. Obermayr G, Walton RE, Leary JM, Krell KV (1991) Vertical root fracture and relative deformation during

obturation and post cementation. *Journal of Prosthetic Dentistry* **66**, 181–187.

33. Oliva RA, Lowe JA (1986) Dimensional stability of composite used as a core material. *Journal of Prosthetic Dentistry* **56**, 554–561.

34. Pameijer JHN (1985) *Periodontal and Occlusal Factors in Crown and Bridge Procedures.* Amsterdam: Dental Center for Postgraduate Courses, p. 217.

35. Ray HA, Trope M (1995) Periapical status of endodontically treated teeth in relation to the technical quality of the root filling and the coronal restoration. *International Endodontic Journal* **28**, 12–18.

36. Reinhardt RA, Krejci RF, Pao YC, Stannard JG (1983) Dentin stresses in post-reconstructed teeth with diminishing bone support. *Journal of Dental Research* **62**, 1002–1008.

37. Reuter JE, Brose MO (1984) Failure in full crown retained dental bridges. *British Dental Journal* **157**, 61–63.

38. Roberts DH (1970) The failure of retainers in bridge prostheses. An analysis of 2,000 retainers. *British Dental Journal* **128**, 117–124.

39. Ross RS, Nicholls JI, Harrington GW (1991) A comparison of strains generated during placement of five endodontic posts. *Journal of Endodontics* **17**, 450–456.

40. Sedgley CM, Messer HH (1992) Are endodontically treated teeth more brittle? *Journal of Endodontics* **18**, 332–335.

41. Sjogren U, Hagglund B, Sundqvist G, Wing K (1990) Factors affecting the long-term results of endodontic treatment. *Journal of Endodontics* **16**, 498–504.

42. Sorensen JA, Engelman MJ (1990) Ferrule design and fracture resistance of endodontically treated teeth. *Journal of Prosthetic Dentistry* **63**, 529–536.

43. Sorensen JA, Martinoff JT (1984) Intracoronal reinforcement and coronal coverage: a study of endodontically treated teeth. *Journal of Prosthetic Dentistry* **51**, 780–784.

44. Sorensen JA, Martinoff JT (1984) Clinically significant factors in dowel design. *Journal of Prosthetic Dentistry* **52**, 28–35.

45. Sorensen JA, Martinoff JT (1985) Endodontically treated teeth as abutments. *Journal of Prosthetic Dentistry* **53**, 631–636.

46. Standlee JP, Caputo AA, Collard EW (1971) Retentive pins installation stresses. *Dental Practitioner and Dental Record* **21**, 417–422.

47. Standlee JP, Caputo AA, Collard EW, Pollack MH (1972) Analysis of stress distribution by endodontic posts. *Oral Surgery, Oral Medicine, Oral Pathology* **33**, 952–960.

48. Standlee JP, Caputo AA, Hanson EC (1978) Retention of endodontic dowels: effects of cement, dowel length, diameter and design. *Journal of Prosthetic Dentistry* **39**, 400–405.

49. Stockton LW (1999) Factors affecting retention of post systems: a literature review. *Journal of Prosthetic Dentistry* **81**, 380–385.

50. Torbjorner A, Karlsson S, Odman PA (1995) Survival rate and failure characteristics for two post designs. *Journal of Prosthetic Dentistry* **73**, 439–444.

51. Vale WA (1956) Cavity Preparation. *Irish Dental Review* **2**, 33–41.

52. Weine FS, Wax AH, Wenckus CS (1991) Retrospective study of tapered, smooth post systems in place for 10 years or more. *Journal of Endodontics* **17**, 293–297.

53. Wendt SL, Harris BM, Hunt TE (1987) Resistance to cusp fracture in endodontically treated teeth. *Dental Materials* **3**, 232–235.

# Index

Abscess, 3
    acute periradicular, 238–9
Access cavity preparation, 81–3
    instruments, 56
    problems of, 241
    *see also* Root canal preparation
Accessory canal, 19–20
*Actinobacillus actinomycetemcomitans*, 216
*Actinomyces* spp., 97
Acute periodontitis, 238
Acute periradicular abscess, 238–9
Acute pulpitis, 237–8
Adhesive restorations, 258–60
Age, and pulp size, 18
Aldehydes, 99
Alpha-Seal system, 130
Amalgam dowel cores, 261–3
Amoxycillin, 11, 12, 14
Anaerobic culture, 3
Anaesthesia, 146–7
    alternative techniques, 239–41
    intraosseous, 240, 249
    intrapulpal, 240
    sedation, 241
    sedative dressings, 240
Anaesthesia, failure of, 239–41
Analgesia, 14–15, 97
Anatomical redesigning, 228–34
    bicuspidization, 233–4
    contraindications, 228–9
    indications, 228
    root amputation, 229–31
    tooth resection, 231–3
Ancient Greece, endodontic treatment in, 1
Ancient Rome, endodontic treatment in, 1
Antibacterial dressing, 101–2
Antibiotics, 14, 98–9
Antisepsis, 96
Anxiety, control of, 14–15
Apex
    barrier formation coronal to, 210
    electronic locators, 63–5, 85
    *see also* Apical
Apical closure, 33
Apical constriction, 18
Apical dentine plug, 132
Apical foramina, 18, 20–1

Apical periodontitis, 4, 95, 101
    acute, 238
Apical seal, 2
    preservation of, 266
*Arachnia* spp., 41, 97
Asepsis, 96
Aspirin, 14, 15
Augmentin, 14
Auto-transplantation, 207–8
Avulsion, 205–6

Bacteria
    leakage, 42–3
    mechanical reduction, 106–7
    and periodontitis, 95
    pulpal, 97–8
    resistance, 100–1
    *see also individual types*
*Bacteroides* spp., 3
*Bacteroides forsythicus*, 216
Barbed broaches, 57
Bicuspidization, 228, 233–4
Bleeding, 97, 104
Bone morphogenic proteins, 187
Burs, 56

Calcium hydroxide, 96, 99, 100
    with antimicrobial additives, 100
    application on dressings, 107
    pulpotomy, 187
    toxicity, 106
Calcium hydroxide sealers, 116
Cancellier extractor, 66
Canines
    mandibular, 28
    maxillary, 23
    primary, 32
Caries
    management, 43–4
    as pulpal irritant, 40–1
Cast onlays, 260
Cavi-Endo unit, 60
Cavity preparation
    as pulpal irritant, 41–2
    without anaesthesia, 40
Cement
    glass ionomer, 163, 263–4

root fillings, 245
    silicate, 42
    zinc oxide-eugenol, 43, 44
Cermets, 264
Cervical root fracture, avoidance of, 210–11
Children, 183–93
    direct pulp capping, 184–5
    indirect pulp capping, 184
    pulpectomy, 187–8
    pulpotomy
        bone morphogenic proteins, 187
        calcium hydroxide, 187
        ferric sulphate, 187
        formocresol, 185–6
        glutaraldehyde, 186
        mineral trioxide aggregate, 187
    treatment of immature permanent teeth,
        188–91
        non-vital teeth, 189–91
        surgery, 191
        vital teeth, 188–9
    treatment of primary teeth, 183–4
    vital pulpotomy, 185
Chinese, worm theory, 1
Chlorhexidine, 99, 100
Chlorine, 99
Chloroform, 131
Clamp forceps, 53, 54
Clamps, 53, 54
Clindamycin, 12, 14, 99
Clinical tests, 39–40
    application of cold, 39
    application of heat, 39
    assessment of blood flow, 40
    cavity preparation without anaesthesia,
        40
    electric current application, 39
    radiographs, 39–40
Cocaine, 1
Cold application, 39
Composite resin
    cores, 263
    irritant properties, 42
Concussion, 202
Cores for cast restorations, 261–5
    adhesion for cores, 264–5
    amalgam dowel cores, 261–3

Cores for cast restorations (*contd*)
  choice of material, 263–4
  plastic core materials with prefabricated
    posts, 263
Corticosteroids, 135
Critical crestal zone, 170
Crown fractures, 197, 198
Crown preparation, 80–1
Crown-root fracture, 200
Crowndown technique, 87–8
Crowns without posts, 257
Curative endodontics, 95
Cusps, cracked, 45
Cytokines, 4

Dens evaginatus, 21
Dens invaginatus, 21
*Dental Practitioners' Formulary*, 15
Dentine
  drug penetration, 105
  exposure of, 43
  fracture, 198–9
  fracture with pulp exposure, 199–200
  intratubular, 18
  irritation, 18, 21, 241–2
  secondary, 18
Dentine bonding agents, irritant properties,
    42
Dentine-bonded composite resin, 163
Depression, 11
Devitalization, 275
Diagnosis of pulp disease, 5, 38–40
Diaket, 163
Dihydrocodeine, 14, 15
Discoloration, 210
  primary teeth, 198
Disinfectants, 99–100
Disinfection, 96–7, 101–3
  antibacterial dressing, 101–2
  antibacterial effects of irrigation, 101
  controlled, 102
  follow-up studies, 102
  instrumentation, 71–2, 101
  predictable, 102
  single-visit endodontics, 102
  treatment of non-infected teeth, 102–3
Distobuccal canal, 26
Dressings
  antibacterial, 101–2
  calcium hydroxide, 107
  disinfectant, 107
  sedative, 240
Drug resistance, 100–1

*Eikenella corrodens*, 216
Elective devitalization, 275
Electric pulp testing, 39
Electronic apex locators, 63–5, 85
Emergency treatment, 237–9
  acute apical periodontitis, 238
  acute flare-up, 239
  acute periradicular abscess, 238–9
  acute pulpitis, 237–8
Enamel
  fracture, 198–9

fracture with pulp exposure, 199–200
  infractions, 198
Endodontic triad, 78
Endoring II system, 71
*Eubacterium* spp., 41
European Society of Endodontology, 4
Extracoronal prostheses, 243
Extrusive luxation, 203
Exudation, 97, 104

Ferric sulphate pulpotomy, 187
Fibre-optic lights, 73
Files, 58–60
  Flexofile, 58
  GT hand files, 59
  Hedstrom file, 58–9
  K-file, 58
  K-flex file, 58
  nickel-titanium, 59
  Series 29, 59–60
Flexipost, 267
Flexofile, 59
Fluticasone, 13
Forceps, 66–7
Formocresol, 99
  pulpotomy, 185–6
Fractures
  permanent teeth, 198–202
    crown-root fracture, 200
    enamel and dentine, 198–9
    infractions and fracture of enamel, 198
    intra-alveolar root fracture, 200–2
    pulp exposure, 199–200
  primary teeth, 197–8
    crown fractures, 197, 198
    intra-alveolar root fracture, 197
Frames, 54, 55
Friction grip burs, 56
*Fusobacterium* spp., 97, 98
*Fusobacterium nucleatum*, 216

Gates-Glidden burs, 56, 57
Glass bead (salt) heater, 73
Glass ionomer cement, 163
  cores, 263–4
Glass ionomer sealers, 117
Glutaraldehyde pulpotomy, 187
GORE-TEX, 173
GT hand files, 60
Guided-tissue regeneration, 173
Gutta-percha, 118–32, 245
  canal filling, 118
  carrier devices, 70–1
  cold techniques, 118–25
    lateral condensation, 119–25
  heat-softened techniques, 125–30
    continuous wave of condensation,
      125–7
    extracanal, 127–30
    intracanal, 125–7
    operator-coated carrier-condenser,
      129–30
    precoated carriers, 127–9
    rotating condenser, 127
    thermoplastic delivery systems, 129

warm vertical condensation, 127
  solvent-softened, 130–2
  thermomechanical compaction, 69
  thermoplasticized injectable, 69–70
Gutta-percha points, 68, 120
  master point, 121

Haemostasis, 146–7
Halogens, 99–100
Hand instruments, 57–60
  barbed broaches, 57
  files, 58–60
  reamers, 57–8
Hard tissue barrier, 97, 103
Heat application, 39
Hedstrom file, 59–60
History of pulp treatment, 1–2
Hollow tube theory, 2
Hot tooth, 239
Human immunodeficiency virus, 9
Hunter, William, 2

Ibuprofen, 14
Idiopathic orofacial pain, 10–11
Incisors
  mandibular, 27–8
  maxillary, 22–3
  primary, 32
Infection, 4
  *see also* Bacteria; and individual infections
Infective endocarditis, 12–13
Inflammatory mediators, 4
Instrument fracture, 245–7
  prevention of, 247
Instruments, 51–76
  access cavity preparation, 56
  basic instrument pack, 51
  burs, 56
  disinfection, 71–2, 101
  fibre-optic lights, 72–3
  irrigant delivery devices, 66
  loupes, 72–3
  nickel-titanium, 60, 90
  operating microscopes, 72–3
  retrieval of broken instruments and posts,
    66–8
  root canal filling, 68–71
  root canal preparation, 57–63
    hand instruments, 57–60
    power-assisted instruments, 60–3
  rubber dam, 51–5
  storage and sterilization, 71–2
  surgery, 145–6
  working length determination, 63–6
Intermediate restorative material, 162–3
International Normalized Ratio, 13
International Organization for
    Standardization (ISO), 57
Intra-alveolar root fracture, 197
  permanent teeth, 200–2
Intra-alveolar surgery, pulp response to, 46
Intracoronal hard tissue formation, 241–2
Intraosseous anaesthesia, 240
Intrapulpal anaesthesia, 240
Intratubular dentine, 18

Intrusive luxation, 204–5
Iodine, 99, 100
Irrigant delivery devices, 65, 66
Irrigation, 85–6
  antibacterial effect, 101
  drug application by, 107
Irritants, 40–3
  bacterial leakage, 42–3
  cavity preparation, 41–2
  dental caries, 40–1
  dental materials, 42
  exposure of dentine, 43
  pulp response to, 37–8
Irritation dentine, 18, 241–2
  effect on pulp space, 21–2

K-file, 59
K-flex file, 59
Kerr M4 Safety handpiece, 60
Kloroperka, 132

Lactobacillus spp., 41
Laser Doppler flowmetry, 5, 40
Lateral canal, 19–20
Lateral condensation, 68, 119–25
Lateral luxation, 203–4
Ledermix, 104, 105, 240
Ledges, 244
Leukotrienes, 4
Lidocaine, 15
Loupes, 73
Luebke-Ochsenbein flap, 150
Luxation injuries
  permanent teeth, 202–6
    avulsion, 205–6
    concussion, 202
    extrusive luxation, 203
    intrusive luxation, 204–5
    lateral luxation, 203–4
    subluxation, 202
  primary teeth, 198

Mandibular canine, 28
  surgery, 169
Mandibular incisors, 27–8
  surgery, 169
Mandibular molars, 30–2
  access cavities, 32
  surgery, 169
Mandibular premolars, 29–30
  access cavities, 30
  surgery, 169
Masserann trepan, 67, 244, 246
Maxillary canine, 23
  surgery, 168
Maxillary incisors, 22–3
  access cavities, 23
  surgery, 168
Maxillary molars, 27
  access cavities, 27
  surgery, 168–9
Maxillary premolars, 23–7
  access cavities, 25
  surgery, 168
Maxillary sinus, 11

Medication, 95–112
  antimicrobial agents, 98–100
    antibiotics, 98–9
    disinfectants, 99–100
  application of, 107
  asepsis, antisepsis and disinfection, 96–7
  diffusion and solubility, 105
  history, 96
  penetration of dentine, 105
  resistance to, 100–1
  smear layer, 105
  tissue distribution, 105
  tissue toxicity, 106
Mesiobuccal canal, 26
Metronidazole, 14, 98
Microorganisms, 3–4
Microscopes, operating, 72
MicroSeal system, 130
Midazolam, 15
Mineral trioxide aggregate, 5, 44, 132, 164
  pulp capping and apexification, 190
  pulpotomy, 187
Molars
  mandibular, 30–2
  maxillary, 27
  primary, 33
Mucoperiosteal tissue flap
  full, 148–50
  limited, 150

Nickel-titanium alloys, 5
Nickel-titanium instruments, 90
  files, 60
Nitrous oxide, 15
Nomenclature, 18–19

Obtura II system, 70, 129
Oil of eucalyptus, 131
Operating microscopes, 73
Oraseal caulking agent, 52
Orthodontic treatment, 211
Osteomyelitis, 4

Pain
  differential diagnosis, 9–11
  endodontic, 103–4
  examination, 10
  history, 10
  idiopathic orofacial, 10–11
  pulpitis, 38
Pain control see Analgesia
Palatal canal, 26
Paracetamol, 14, 15
Paraformaldehyde, 99, 135
Partsch incision, 147
Paste fillers, 134–5
Penicillin, 98
Peptostreptococcus spp., 97
Periodontal disease, pulp response to, 45–6
Periodontitis, 215–35
  acute, 238
  anatomical redesigning, 228–34
    bicuspidization, 233–4
    contraindications, 228–9
    indications, 228

    root amputation, 229–31
    tooth resection, 231–3
  anatomy, 215
  apical, 4, 95, 101, 238
  classification, 217–27
    retrospective, 226
  combined lesions, 226
  complications, 227–8
    diagnosis, 227–8
    treatment, 228
  effect on pulp, 216
  primary endodontic lesion, 217
    with secondary periodontal
      involvement, 217–21
  primary periodontal lesion, 221–2
    with secondary endodontic
      involvement, 2225
  prognosis, 226–7
Periodontium, effect of necrotic pulp,
    215–16
Periradicular abscess, 238–9
Periradicular curettage, 152
Periradicular surgery see Surgery
Permanent teeth
  fractures, 198–202
    crown-root fracture, 200
    enamel and dentine, 198–9
    infractions and fracture of enamel, 198
    intra-alveolar root fracture, 200–2
    pulp exposure, 199–200
  immature, 188–91
  luxation injuries, 202–6
    avulsion, 205–6
    concussion, 202
    extrusive luxation, 203
    intrusive luxation, 204–5
    lateral luxation, 203–4
    subluxation, 202
  pulp space, 22–32
  trauma, 198–206
Pethidine, 14, 15
Phenols, 99, 100
Phenoxymethyl penicillin, 14
Piezon-Master 400 unit, 60
Polymerase chain reaction, 3
Porphyromonas spp., 97, 98
Porphyromonas gingivalis, 216
Post removal devices, 67
Posts, 243–4, 265–8
  length of, 266
  metal, 243–4
  metal with cast cores, 268–75
    completion of post preparation, 269–71
    construction of post and core, 271–3
    coronal preparation, 269
    finishing procedures, 271
    multirooted teeth, 274–5
    post length, 268–9
    removal of root canal filling, 269
    tooth preparation, 268–71
    try-in and cementation, 273–4
  preservation of apical seal, 266
  selection of, 265–6
  tapered versus parallel-sided, 266
  threaded, 266–8

Potassium oxalate, 43
Power-assisted instruments, 60–3
    reciprocating handpieces, 60
    rotary handpiece and motor, 63
    rotary instruments, 60–3
    ultrasonic Instruments, 61
Precoated carriers, 127–9
Premolars
    mandibular, 29–30
    maxillary, 23–7
Preventive endodontics, 95
*Prevotella* spp., 3, 97, 98
*Prevotella intermedia*, 216
*Prevotella oralis*, 4
Primary teeth
    canines, 32
    discoloration, 198
    endodontic treatment, 183–4
    fractures, 197–8
        crown fractures, 197, 198
        intra-alveolar root fracture, 197
    incisors, 32
    luxation injuries, 198
    molars, 33
    pulp space, 32–3
    pulpotomy, 185–7
*Propionibacterium* spp., 41
Prostaglandins, 4
Prosthetic hip joints, 13
Pulp, 37–49
    clinical tests, 39–40
        application of cold, 39
        application of heat, 39
        assessment of blood flow, 40
        cavity preparation without anaesthesia,
            40
        electric current application, 39
        radiographs, 39–40
    diagnosis of damage, 38–40
    exposure, 44–5, 199–200
    irritants, 40–3
        bacterial leakage, 42–3
        cavity preparation, 41–2
        dental caries, 40–1
        dental materials, 42
        exposure of dentine, 43
    microbes, 97–8
    responses to
        intra-alveolar surgery, 46
        irritants, 37–8
        periodontal disease, 45–6
    trauma, 45
Pulp canal, 18
Pulp capping, 44
    direct, 184–5
    indirect, 184
Pulp chamber, 18
Pulp disease, 5
Pulp horns, 18
Pulp necrosis, 202
    effect on periodontium, 215–16
Pulp space, 18
    access cavities, 22–32
    alteration with age, 18
    anatomy, 21

effects of irritation dentine on, 21
    permanent teeth, 22–32
    primary teeth, 32–3
Pulp stones, 241
Pulpectomy, 187–8
Pulpitis, 38
    acute, 237–8
Pulpotomy, 44–5
    bone morphogenic protein, 187
    calcium hydroxide, 187
    children, 185–7
    ferric sulphate, 187
    formocresol, 185–6
    glutaraldehyde, 186
    immature permanent teeth, 188–9
    mineral trioxide aggregate, 187
    primary teeth, 185–7
    vital, 185
Punches, 52–3

Quality assurance, 4–5

Radial lands, 63
Radicular anomalies, 227–8
    diagnosis, 227–8
    treatment, 228
Radiography, 39–40
    root canal length, 63, 64
Radix Anchor, 268
Reamers, 57–8
Reciprocating handpieces, 60
Regenerative procedures, 172–3
Replantation, 171–2
Resin sealers, 116–17
Restorations, 253–77
    anterior teeth, 254–7
        anterior crowns without posts, 257
        conservative restoration, 254–5
        previously crowned teeth, 257
        tooth reinforcement, 255–7
    effects of endodontic treatment on teeth,
        253–4
    elective devitalization, 275
    endodontically treated teeth as
        abutments, 275
    metal posts with cast cores, 268–75
        cast cores and posts for multirooted
            teeth, 274–5
        construction of post and core, 271–3
        tooth preparation, 268–71
        try-in and cementation, 273–4
    posterior teeth, 257–65
        adhesive restorations, 258–60
        cast restorations for extensively
            damaged teeth, 260
        conservative restoration, 257–8
        cores for cast restorations, 261–5
        indirect tooth-coloured adhesive, 260
        position of preparation margin, 265
    posts, 265–8
        form of, 266–8
        length of, 266
        preservation of apical seal, 266
        selection of, 265–6
    timing of restorative procedure, 254

Retreatment, 174–5, 210
    problems of, 243–7
        broken instruments, 245–7
        extracoronal prostheses, 243
        ledges and blocked canals, 244
        posts, 243–4
        root filling materials, 245
Reye's syndrome, 15
Root amputation, 228, 229–31
Root canal, 18
    bleeding, 97, 104
    blockage, 244
    calcification, 89
    configuration, 19
    curvature, 242–3
    disinfectants, 99–100
    exudation, 97, 104
    infection, 4
    medication, 95–112
    orifice, 83–4
Root canal filling, 68–71, 113–42
    access and canal preparation, 114
    anatomy, 114
    apical dentine plug, 132
    criteria for, 114–15
    criteria of success, 135
    follow-up, 135
    gutta-percha, 118–32
        carrier devices, 70
        cold techniques, 118–25
        heat-softened, 125–30
        solvent-softened, 130–2
    iatrogenic problems, 249
    lateral condensation method, 68
    materials, 115
    mineral trioxide aggregate, 132
    non-instrumentation methods, 132–3
    paste fillers, 134–5
    problems of, 247–9
        iatrogenic, 248–9
        non-iatrogenic, 247–8
    restoration of root filled tooth, 135
    sealers, 115–17
        calcium hydroxide, 116
        functions of, 115–16
        glass ionomer, 117
        resin, 116–17
        zinc oxide-eugenol, 116
    silver points, 133–4
    smear layer, 117–18
    thermomechanical compaction, 69
    thermoplasticized injectable gutta-percha,
        70
    vertical condensation method, 68–9
Root canal preparation, 77–94
    access cavity *see* Access cavity
        preparation
    apical patency filing, 91
    cleaning and shaping, 90–1
    hand instruments, 57–60
        barbed broaches, 57
        files, 58–9
        reamers, 57–8
    instrumentation techniques, 86–9
        calcified canals, 89

Root canal preparation (*contd*)
    crowndown technique, 87–8
    stepback technique, 88–9
irrigation, 85–6
nickel-titanium instruments, 90
number of visits, 91
power-assisted instruments, 60–3
    reciprocating handpieces, 60
    rotary handpiece and motor, 63
    rotary instruments, 61–2
    ultrasonic instrumentation, 60
preoperative assessment, 78–80
preparation of clinical crown, 80–1
problems of, 241–7
    acute canal curvature, 242–3
    intracanal hard tissue formation, 241–2
root canal orifices, 83–4
working length determination, 63–6, 84–5
    electronic apex locators, 64–5
    measuring devices, 65
    radiography, 63, 64
Root canal therapy, 1
Root filling materials
    irritant properties, 42
    *see also individual materials*
Root resorption, 97, 104–5
    cervical external, 208–9
    external inflammatory, 208
    external replacement, 209–10
Root-end cavity filling, 159–62
    materials, 162–4
        dentine-bonded composite resin, 163
        Diaket, 163
        glass ionomer cement, 163
        intermediate restorative material, 162–3
        mineral trioxide aggregate, 164
        Super-EBA, 162
Root-end cavity preparation, 157–9
Root-end resection, 153–7
Rotary handpiece, 63
Rotary instruments, 60–3
    core diameter/flute depth, 62
    flute design, 62
    helical flute angle, 62
    non-cutting tip, 63
    radial lands, 63
    rake angle, 62
    variable taper, 60
Rotating condenser, 127
Round burs, 56
Rubber dam, 51–5
    application of, 54–5
    clamp, 53
    clamp forceps, 54
    frame, 54
    punch, 52–3
    split-dam technique, 81

Safe-ended burs, 56
Scope of endodontics, 3
Sealers, 115–17
    calcium hydroxide, 116
    functions of, 115–16
    glass ionomer, 117
    resin, 116–17

zinc oxide-eugenol, 116
Secondary dentine, 18
Sedation, 240
Sedative dressings, 240
Series 29 files, 60–1
Silicate cement, irritant properties, 42
Silver amalgam, 264
Silver points, 133–4, 245
Single-visit endodontics, 102
Sinus, maxillary, 11
Sinusitis, 11
Smear layer, 117–18
Sodium hypochlorite, 99
    application by irrigation, 107
Split-dam technique, 81
Spreaders, 122–3
Stabident, 240
Stepdown technique, 88–9
Sterilization of instruments,
Steroids, 13–14
Storage of instruments, 71
*Streptococcus* spp., 41
Stropko irrigator, 160
Subluxation, 202
Sulpha drugs, 98
Super-EBA, 162
Surgery, 143–81
    anatomy, 169–70
    closure of surgical site, 164–7
    evaluation of success and failure, 173–4
    immature permanent teeth, 191
    indications for, 143–4
    instrumentation, 145–6
    intra-alveolar, 46
    mandibular anterior teeth, 169
    mandibular molars, 169
    mandibular premolars, 169
    maxillary anterior teeth, 168
    maxillary molars, 168–9
    maxillary premolars, 168
    osseous entry and root identification,
        151–2
    periradicular curettage, 152
    postoperative
        examination and review, 168
        patient instructions, 167–8
        radiological assessment, 167
    preoperative assessment, 144–5
    regenerative procedures, 172–3
    repair of perforation, 170–1
    replantation/transplantation, 171–2
    retreatment, 174–5
    root-end cavity filling, 159–62
    root-end cavity preparation, 157–9
    root-end materials, 162–4
        dentine-bonded composite resin, 163
        Diaket, 163
        glass ionomer cement, 163
        intermediate restorative material, 162–3
        mineral trioxide aggregate, 164
        Super-EBA, 162
    root-end resection, 153–7
    soft tissue incision and reflection, 147–50
        full mucoperiosteal tissue flap, 148–50
        limited mucoperiosteal tissue flap, 150

tissue anaesthesia and haemostasis, 146–7
treatment of root face, 164
Suture knots, 167
Suture materials, 166
Systemic disease, 11–14
    infective endocarditis, 12–13
    prosthetic hip joints, 13
    warfarin and steroids, 13–14

Temporary filling, 107–8
Tetracycline, 98–9
Thermomechanical compaction, 69
Thermoplastic delivery systems, 129
Tissue anaesthesia, 146–7
Tissue response to root canal infection, 4
Tooth reinforcement, 255–7
Tooth resection, 228, 231–3
Transplantation, 171–2
Trauma, 45, 195–213
    auto-transplantation of immature
        premolars, 207–8
    complications
        avoidance of cervical root fracture,
            210–11
        barrier formation coronal to apex, 210
        cervical external inflammatory root
            resorption, 208–9
        discoloration, 210
        external inflammatory root resorption,
            208
        external replacement root resorption,
            209–10
        orthodontic treatment, 211
        previous injury, 210
        root canal treatment, 210
    effect on dental tissues, 197
    examination, 195–7
    history, 195–7
    immature teeth, 206–7
    immediate management, 195–7
    permanent teeth, 198–206
        fractures, 198–202
        luxation injuries, 202–6
    primary teeth, 197–8
        discoloration, 198
        fractures, 197–8
        luxation injuries, 198
    types of injury, 197
*Treponema denticola*, 216

Ultrasonic instrumentation, 60

*Veillonella* spp., 97
Vertical condensation, 68–9

Warfarin, 13–14
Warm vertical condensation, 127
Wicking, 166
Working length determination *see* Root
        canal preparation
Working Party of the British Society for
        Antimicrobial Chemotherapy, 12

Zinc oxide-eugenol cement, 43, 44
Zinc oxide-eugenol sealers, 116